Gastrointestinal Pathology: Classification, Diagnosis, Emerging Entities

Editor

JASON L. HORNICK

SURGICAL PATHOLOGY CLINICS

surgpath.theclinics.com

Consulting Editor
JOHN R. GOLDBLUM

September 2013 • Volume 6 • Number 3

ELSEVIER

1600 John F. Kennedy Boulevard • Suite 1800 • Philadelphia, Pennsylvania, 19103-2899

http://www.theclinics.com

SURGICAL PATHOLOGY CLINICS Volume 6, Number 3
September 2013 ISSN 1875-9181, ISBN-13: 978-0-323-18874-6

Editor: Joanne Husovski

Surgical Pathology Clinics (ISSN 1875-9181) is published quarterly by Elsevier Inc., 360 Park Avenue South, New York, NY 10010. Months of issue are March, June, September, and December. Business and Editorial Office: Elsevier Inc., 1600 John F. Kennedy Blvd., Ste. 1800, Philadelphia, PA 19103-2899. Accounting and Circulation Offices: Elsevier Inc., 3251 Riverport Lane, Maryland Heights, MO 63043. Periodicals postage paid at New York, NY and at additional mailing offices. Subscription prices are $191.00 per year (US individuals), $220.00 per year (US institutions), $94.00 per year (US students/residents), $239.00 per year (Canadian individuals), $249.00 per year (Canadian Institutions), $239.00 per year (foreign individuals), $249.00 per year (foreign institutions), and $116.00 per year (international & Canadian students/residents). Foreign air speed delivery is included in all *Clinics'* subscription prices. All prices are subject to change without notice. **POSTMASTER:** Send address changes to *Surgical Pathology Clinics*, Elsevier, 3251 Riverport Lane, Maryland Heights, MO 63043. Customer Service: 1-800-654-2452 (US). From outside the United States, call 1-314-447-8871. Fax: 1-314-447-8029. E-mail: JournalsCustomerServiceusa@elsevier.com (for print support) and JournalsOnlineSupport-usa@elsevier.com (for online support).

Reprints. For copies of 100 or more, of articles in this publication, please contact the Commercial Reprints Department, Elsevier Inc., 360 Park Avenue South, New York, NY 10010-1710. Tel. 212-633-3874; Fax: 212-633-3820; E-mail: reprints@elsevier.com.

Printed in the United States of America.

Contributors

CONSULTING EDITOR

JOHN R. GOLDBLUM, MD
Chairman, Professor of Pathology, Department
of Anatomic Pathology, Cleveland Clinics
Lerner College of Medicine, Cleveland Clinic,
Cleveland, Ohio

EDITOR

JASON L. HORNICK, MD, PhD
Director of Surgical Pathology, Director,
Immunohistochemistry Laboratory,
Department of Pathology, Brigham and
Women's Hospital, Associate Professor of
Pathology, Harvard Medical School, Boston,
Massachusetts

AUTHORS

ANDREW M. BELLIZZI, MD
Clinical Assistant Professor, Department of
Pathology, University of Iowa Hospitals and
Clinics, University of Iowa Carver College of
Medicine, Iowa City, Iowa

JON M. DAVISON, MD
Department of Pathology, University of
Pittsburgh Medical Center, Pittsburgh,
Pennsylvania

VIKRAM DESHPANDE, MD
Associate Professor of Pathology, Harvard
Medical School; Associate Pathologist,
Department of Pathology, Massachusetts
General Hospital, Boston, Massachusetts

LEONA A. DOYLE, MD
Department of Pathology, Brigham and
Women's Hospital, Harvard Medical School,
Boston, Massachusetts

JEFFREY D. GOLDSMITH, MD
Assistant Professor of Pathology, Harvard
Medical School; Director of Surgical Pathology
Laboratory, Department of Pathology, Beth

Israel Deaconess Medical Center; Consultant
in Gastrointestinal Pathology, Children's
Hospital Boston, Boston, Massachusetts

JOEL K. GREENSON, MD
Professor of Pathology, Department of
Pathology, University of Michigan Hospital
and Health Systems, Ann Arbor, Michigan

JASON L. HORNICK, MD, PhD
Director of Surgical Pathology, Director,
Immunohistochemistry Laboratory,
Department of Pathology, Brigham and
Women's Hospital, Associate Professor of
Pathology, Harvard Medical School, Boston,
Massachusetts

ERIC D. HSI, MD
Professor of Pathology, Cleveland Clinic
Lerner College of Medicine, Cleveland Clinic,
Cleveland, Ohio

MADELYN LEW, MD
Clinical Fellow in Pathology, Harvard
Medical School; Department of Pathology,
Massachusetts General Hospital, Boston,
Massachusetts

MIKHAIL LISOVSKY, MD, PhD
Assistant Professor, Department of Pathology,
Dartmouth Hitchcock Medical Center,
Lebanon, New Hampshire

SCOTT R. OWENS, MD
Associate Professor of Pathology, Department
of Pathology, University of Michigan Hospital
and Health Systems, Ann Arbor, Michigan

REETESH K. PAI, MD
Department of Pathology, University of
Pittsburgh Medical Center, Pittsburgh,
Pennsylvania

LAUREN B. SMITH, MD
Assistant Professor, Department of Pathology,
University of Michigan Hospital and Health
System, Ann Arbor, Michigan

AMITABH SRIVASTAVA, MD
Assistant Professor, Department of Pathology,
Brigham and Women's Hospital, Boston,
Massachusetts

ERIC U. YEE, MD
Instructor of Pathology, Harvard Medical
School; Staff Pathologist, Beth Israel
Deaconess Medical Center, Boston,
Massachusetts

Contents

Gastric and gastroesophageal junction adenocarcinomas constitute a major health problem. For localized disease, adjuvant treatment is multidisciplinary and usually includes a combination of surgery, radiation and chemotherapy. Recently, trastuzumab (Herceptin) has been approved for the treatment of metastatic upper gastrointestinal (GI) tract (gastric, esophageal, and gastroesophageal) adenocarcinomas. The purpose of this review is to provide pathologists with practical guidance in HER2 assessment of upper GI tract adenocarcinomas in order to accurately identify patients eligible for trastuzumab therapy.

The gastrointestinal tract is the most common extranodal site of non-Hodgkin lymphoma. Certain lymphomas have a predilection for the gastrointestinal tract, including extranodal marginal zone lymphoma of mucosa-associated lymphoid tissue, mantle cell lymphoma, natural killer/T-cell lymphoma, and enteropathy-associated T-cell lymphoma. Follicular lymphoma may also be primary to the gastrointestinal tract. In addition to diagnosing neoplastic conditions, it is important to differentiate lymphomas from atypical reactive proliferations. Recent research relevant to non-Hodgkin lymphomas involving this location is reviewed with an emphasis on novel and evolving areas of classification.

Mesenchymal tumors involve the gastrointestinal (GI) tract more frequently than other visceral organs. Many such tumors are small, and are benign and increasingly being detected incidentally during colonoscopic screening. Some tumors show distinctive features at this site, such as schwannoma and clear cell sarcoma–like tumor of the GI tract. Without knowledge of these features, recognition of these tumor types can be difficult. This reviews addresses recent developments and diagnostic features of mesenchymal tumors of the GI tract other than gastrointestinal stromal tumor (GIST).

Surgical pathologists need to answer 2 questions when evaluating biopsies from the distal esophagus or gastroesophageal junction in patients with a history of gastroesophageal reflux disease: Are the findings consistent with Barrett esophagus?

and Is there any evidence of dysplasia? Pathologists should be well informed about the controversy around the definition of Barrett esophagus and the common pitfalls that lead to a false-positive diagnosis of Barrett esophagus or Barrett esophagus–associated dysplasia. A concise description of distinct morphologic types of dysplasia in Barrett esophagus and a summary of recent data on the natural history of BE are provided in this review.

IgG4-related disease, a newly established multisystemic disease can affect virtually every organ. Histologically, it is characterized by the presence of a dense lymphoplasmacytic infiltrate, storiform-type fibrosis, and obliterative phlebitis. The disease shows elevated serum and tissue IgG4. The pancreas and hepatobiliary tract are involved far more commonly than the tubular gut. This review summarizes the clinical and pathologic features of the gastrointestinal manifestations of IgG4-related disease and discusses the wide spectrum of diseases that this entity may mimic.

In the clinical context of pediatric diarrheal illness, the interpretation of endoscopic mucosal biopsies varies significantly from that in adults. This review outlines these differences by first describing a host of diarrheal illnesses that are nearly exclusive to the pediatric age group. The final portion of this article describes salient pathologic differences between adult and pediatric idiopathic inflammatory bowel disease. The goal of this review is to provide a brief description of each disease process and focus on practical aspects of diagnosis that are applicable for pathologists working in general practice settings.

This article reviews the major gastrointestinal polyposis syndromes, with an emphasis on the molecular, clinical, and histopathological features of each. Salient features helpful in making or suggesting the diagnosis of these syndromes are discussed, as is the use of ancillary techniques, such as immunohistochemistry and molecular diagnostic studies in diagnosis confirmation and family screening.

Immunohistochemistry (IHC) has broad applications in neoplastic gastrointestinal surgical pathology. Although classically used as a diagnostic tool, IHC increasingly provides prognostic and predictive information. This review highlights 11 key uses of IHC. Emphasis is placed on specific clinical applications and qualitative aspects of interpretation. Common pitfalls are specifically highlighted. The potential application of emerging markers is discussed in relation to several of the 11 topics. In many instances, an immunostain serves as a surrogate for spe-cific molecular genetic events. Survey of relevant articles forms the evidence basis for this review.

SURGICAL PATHOLOGY CLINICS

FORTHCOMING ISSUES

Hematopoietic Neoplasms: Controversies in Diagnosis and Classification
Tracy George and Daniel Arber, *Editors*

Cytopathology
Tarik El Sheikh, *Editor*

Cutaneous Lymphoma
Antonio Subtil, *Editor*

RECENT ISSUES

Liver Pathology
Sanjay Kakar, MD, and Dhanpat Jain, MD, *Editors*

Placental Pathology
Rebecca N. Baergen, MD, *Editor*

Current Concepts in Molecular Oncology
Jennifer Hunt, MD, *Editor*

Breast Pathology: Diagnosis and Insights
Stuart J. Schnitt, MD, and Sandra J. Shin, MD, *Editors*

RELATED INTEREST

Seminars in Oncology, August 2004 (Vol. 31, No. 4)
Pathology of Upper Gastrointestinal Malignancies Original Research Article
Mario Sarbia, Karl Friedrich Becker, Heinz Höfler, *Editors*

DOWNLOAD
Free App!

Review Articles
THE CLINICS

NOW AVAILABLE FOR YOUR iPhone and iPad

Preface

Current Concepts in Gastrointestinal Pathology: Classification, Diagnosis, Emerging Entities

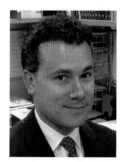

Jason L. Hornick, MD, PhD
Editor

In most departments of anatomic pathology, gastrointestinal pathology represents a high-volume service and a large proportion of all surgical pathology specimens. As such, general surgical pathologists encounter a wide range of gastrointestinal pathology cases on a daily basis. At the same time, the range of diseases that occur in the gastrointestinal tract is as broad as any other organ system, including inflammatory, infectious, hereditary, preneoplastic, and neoplastic conditions. There have been significant advances in our understanding of all of these groups of disorders, which have led to marked improvements in diagnostic pathology practice.

Basic research in immunology, embryology, and molecular biology has provided new tools for the diagnostic pathologist; clinical immunohistochemistry and molecular diagnostic laboratories continually add new tests to our armamentarium. Research relevant to gastrointestinal pathology is published in a wide range of journals, not only pathology and gastroenterology, but also surgery, oncology, immunology, and radiology (among others). It is therefore difficult (at times, seemingly impossible!) to keep up with this rapidly changing field. In terms of oncology, surgical (and gastrointestinal) pathologists play a critical role not only in the traditional areas of diagnosis and prognostication, but also in predictive testing to determine which patients should be treated with specific targeted therapeutic agents.

For this volume of *Surgical Pathology Clinics*, I have invited leaders in gastrointestinal pathology to share some of their particular areas of expertise by providing updates on a broad range of gastrointestinal topics encountered by general surgical pathologists. The possibilities for such topics in this large and diverse field are endless; we have chosen to focus on a group of areas that have evolved especially rapidly in the last few years and therefore would be helpful updates for practicing pathologists. For the most part, these reviews

Surgical Pathology 6 (2013) ix–x
http://dx.doi.org/10.1016/j.path.2013.06.001
1875-9181/13/$ – see front matter © 2013 Elsevier Inc. All rights reserved.

emphasize the role of routine histopathology in the diagnosis and differential diagnosis (the microscope remains our most important tool!), supplemented by ancillary techniques when relevant. I hope you will find these articles useful references for your clinical practices.

I would particularly like to thank the authors of these reviews for their excellent contributions to this volume. I would also like to thank John Goldblum for inviting me to serve as guest editor for this interesting organ system. Finally, I would like to thank Joanne Husovski for her assistance throughout this project.

Jason L. Hornick, MD, PhD
Department of Pathology
Brigham and Women's Hospital
75 Francis Street
Boston, MA 02115, USA

E-mail address:
jhornick@partners.org

HER2 Assessment in Upper Gastrointestinal Tract Adenocarcinoma
A Practical, Algorithmic Approach

Jon M. Davison, MD, Reetesh K. Pai, MD*

KEYWORDS

• HER2 • Trastuzumab • Herceptin • Esophageal adenocarcinoma • Gastric adenocarcinoma

ABSTRACT

Gastric and gastroesophageal junction adenocarcinomas constitute a major health problem. For localized disease, adjuvant treatment is multidisciplinary and usually includes a combination of surgery, radiation, and chemotherapy. For advanced disease, there is no formal consensus or evidence-based rationale regarding the best chemotherapy regimen. Although treatment of patients with unresectable or metastatic disease remains palliative and survival rates low, chemotherapy improves survival and quality of life compared with best supportive care. The purpose of this review is to provide pathologists with practical guidance in HER2 assessment of upper gastrointestinal tract adenocarcinomas to accurately identify patients eligible for trastuzumab therapy.

OVERVIEW OF UPPER GASTROINTESTINAL TRACT ADENOCARCINOMA

Gastric and gastroesophageal junction adenocarcinomas constitute a major health problem. Gastric cancer is the fourth most prevalent malignancy and the second leading cause of cancer death worldwide.[1] In the United States, an estimated 21,000 cases of gastric cancer were diagnosed and 10,570 patients died from this disease in 2010.[2] Carcinoma of the esophagus and gastroesophageal junction is overall less common, but the incidence has risen faster than any other malignancy in the past 25 years in the United States and other Western countries.[3] For localized disease, adjuvant treatment is multidisciplinary and usually includes a combination of surgery, radiation, and chemotherapy. For advanced disease, there is no formal consensus or evidence-based rationale regarding the best chemotherapy regimen. Although treatment of patients with unresectable or metastatic disease remains palliative and survival rates still low, chemotherapy improves survival and quality of life compared with best supportive care.[4] The median time to progression for advanced disease is 4 to 6 months and median overall survival is 7 to 10 months.

Until recently, targeted agents have not shown a significant survival advantage in advanced upper gastrointestinal (GI) tract cancers. Trastuzumab (Herceptin) is a targeted anticancer therapy that functions by binding to the human epidermal growth factor 2 (HER2 and also called HER2/neu) receptor, preventing its constitutive activation, blocking receptor dimerization, and facilitating immune recognition of tumor cells through antibody-dependent cell-mediated cytotoxicity.[5,6] HER2 is a membrane-associated receptor tyrosine kinase that transduces extracellular signals to mitogen-activated protein kinase and phosphatidylinositol 3-kinase intercellular signaling networks, which

Department of Pathology, University of Pittsburgh Medical Center, 200 Lothrop Street, Pittsburgh, PA 15213, USA
* Corresponding author. Department of Pathology, Presbyterian Hospital, University of Pittsburgh, 200 Lothrop Street, Room A-610, Pittsburgh, PA.
E-mail address: pair@upmc.edu

Surgical Pathology 6 (2013) 391–403
http://dx.doi.org/10.1016/j.path.2013.05.001

are major signal transduction pathways stimulating cell growth in many cancer types.[6] HER2 protein may be overexpressed in gastric, gastroesophageal junction, and esophageal adenocarcinomas as well as several other types of tumors, most frequently in breast,[7] and is highly correlated with amplification of the HER2-encoding gene, *ERBB2*, located on chromosome 17 (Chr17).[8] A phase III study investigating trastuzumab was presented by the Trastuzumab for Gastric Cancer (ToGA) investigators first at the 2009 American Society of Clinical Oncology (ASCO) annual meeting and then published.[9] In the ToGA study, 594 patients with HER2-positive, advanced gastric or gastroesophageal junction adenocarcinoma were randomized to standard therapy with a fluoropyrimidine and cisplatin with or without trastuzumab. HER2 positivity was defined by immunohistochemistry (IHC 3+) or amplification by fluorescence in situ hybridization (FISH) (*HER2*:Chr17 ratio >2). Patients receiving trastuzumab had a significantly longer median overall survival (13.8 vs 11.1 months, $P = .0046$), progression-free survival (6.7 vs 5.5 months, $P = .0002$), and response rate (47% vs 35%, $P = .00175$). The ToGA trial also showed evidence of a greater survival benefit for trastuzumab with tumors that expressed higher levels of HER2 protein expression.

Based on the results of the ToGA trial, the US Food and Drug Administration (FDA) has approved the use of trastuzumab for the treatment of metastatic upper GI tract (gastric, esophageal, and gastroesophageal) adenocarcinomas that meet the ToGA inclusion criteria.[10] The European Medicines Agency has approved trastuzumab for IHC 3+ or IHC 2+/FISH-amplified tumors.[11] The optimal protocol for HER2 assessment is rapidly evolving as more information has become available. The purpose of this review is to provide pathologists with practical guidance in HER2 assessment of upper GI tract adenocarcinomas to accurately identify patients eligible for trastuzumab therapy.

SAMPLE COLLECTION AND TISSUE PROCESSING

SPECIMEN TYPE

Because the therapy regimen, including trastuzumab, for upper GI tract adenocarcinoma, is typically reserved for those patients with inoperable locally advanced or metastatic disease in the United States, HER2 assessment is often performed on small endoscopic biopsies. In contrast to breast carcinoma, where there is a high concordance between HER2 assessment in needle core biopsy and subsequent surgical resection,[12,13] HER2 testing can yield discordant results between biopsy and resections in upper GI tract carcinomas. In an analysis by Lee and colleagues,[14] 54 paired biopsy and gastrectomy specimens were analyzed for HER2 and only 87% of cases had concordant results between biopsy and resection specimens. Of the 7 discordant cases, 3 tumors showed 3+ HER2 on the resection specimen but were HER2-negative on the biopsy specimen. The small tissue fragments obtained by endoscopic biopsies of carcinomas allow for only a limited area of each tumor to be analyzed for HER2 expression. Such false-negative HER2 results on biopsy specimen are likely due to the frequent occurrence of heterogeneous HER2 expression in upper GI tract adenocarcinomas. To compensate for heterogeneous HER2 expression, it is recommend that a minimum of 6 to 8 endoscopic biopsy fragments be submitted for HER2 assessment.[15] One potential benefit of assessing HER2 status on endoscopic biopsy specimens is superior antigen preservation in the smaller biopsy fragments due to more complete formalin penetration. In the analysis by Lee and colleagues,[14] 4 of the 7 discordant cases were tumors with negative HER2 results on surgical resection but 3+ HER2 results on preoperative biopsy samples. Whether the advantage of better antigen preservation in biopsy specimens outweighs the disadvantage of sampling error in small biopsy samples from tumors with significant HER2 heterogeneity is a subject of debate in the literature.

Another consideration in HER2 assessment is whether to test the primary carcinoma or sites of metastatic disease.[16–19] Some literature reports have demonstrated discordant HER2 expression between metastatic tumor deposits and the primary tumor. Kim and colleagues[18] tested 250 paired primary and metastatic lesions and demonstrated 6 (2.4%) cases of HER2-positive metastatic disease and HER2-negative primary tumor. Similarly, Perrone and colleagues[16] reported 3/27 (11%) discordance between metastatic tumor deposits and primary tumor. Other literature reports have found a much less frequent (approximately 1.5%) occurrence of discordant results between primary and metastatic tumor with discordant cases. Most discordant results between primary and metastatic tumor reported in the literature are due to positive HER2 conversion in the metastatic tumor. These few data suggest that testing metastatic tumors in addition to the primary tumor may provide a better assessment of HER2 status to identify patients eligible for trastuzumab therapy.

TISSUE PROCESSING

Preanalytic variables, such as cold ischemia and formalin-fixation times, in HER2 assessment have emerged as important factors in the accuracy of HER2 assessment. For breast carcinoma, the ASCO/College of American Pathologists (CAP) guidelines indicate that specimens should be promptly placed into 10% neutral buffered formalin fixative to minimize ischemic time to 1 hour or less, using minimum and maximum fixation times of 6 hours and 48 hours, respectively.[20] Recent data suggest that prolonged fixation time up to 96 hours does not alter HER2 evaluation in breast cancer.[21–23] Because formalin fixation time is an important preanalytic variable, the pathology report should document the total number of hours that samples are fixed in neutral buffered formalin. Although data on preanalytical variables in HER2 assessment in upper GI tract adenocarcinoma are not currently available, it seems reasonable to apply the ASCO/CAP guidelines for breast carcinoma to upper GI tract adenocarcinomas. After appropriate fixation, tissue may be processed in routine fashion for paraffin embedding. It is recommended that fresh 4-μm sections from the paraffin tissue block be cut immediately before HER2 testing and stored no longer than 2 weeks to preserve antigenicity.[15]

HER2 IMMUNOHISTOCHEMISTRY

ANTIBODIES AND KITS FOR HER2 DETECTION

There are 2 FDA-approved and validated kits for HER2 detection in gastric cancer: the HercepTest kit (Dako) and the PATHWAY kit (rabbit monoclonal Ab clone 4B5) (Ventana). The Ventana monoclonal 4B5 antibody and the Dako polyclonal antibody are directed at intracellular domains of the HER2 protein. Other antibodies used to detect HER2 expression in gastroesophageal cancer include the monoclonal antibody clones CB11[24] and SP3.[25] HER2 screening for the ToGA trial used the HercepTest kit and for this reason it can be regarded as a reference. In the authors' experience, the Ventana 4B5 antibody shows excellent concordance with FISH results and sensitivity for detecting amplification.[26] Although published data for upper GI tract cancers are limited, anecdotal experience suggests that the use of a validated kit (eg, HercepTest or PATHWAY) may offer superior results over potentially more cost-effective in-house alternatives when testing upper GI cancers.[15]

SCORING CRITERIA FOR HER2 IHC IN UPPER GI CANCERS

The ToGA trial showed that a combined IHC and FISH protocol could identify HER2-amplified tumors and thereby identify patients who benefit from the addition of trastuzumab to a conventional chemotherapy regimen for the primary treatment of advanced gastric or gastroesophageal junction adenocarcinoma. For this reason and because IHC is considerably less labor intensive than in situ hybridization, most laboratories screen for HER2 amplification by IHC and use an in situ assay for validation of equivocal cases. The criteria for scoring HER2 expression in upper GI tract cancers are outlined in **Table 1**. To correctly score HER2 protein expression, 3 staining variables must be assessed for each sample:

1. Pattern or quality of staining (complete, basolateral, or lateral membranous staining vs luminal, cytoplasmic, or nuclear staining)
2. Intensity of staining (weak, moderate, or strong)
3. Fraction of tumor cells that are positive (a cutoff of 10% is used for resection specimens [discussed later]).

These guidelines were validated in the context of establishing scoring criteria for the ToGA clinical trial with the aim of achieving high concordance between IHC and FISH results.[27]

POSITIVE HER2 STAINING IN UPPER GI CANCER (IHC 3+)

Positive staining requires strong complete, basolateral, or lateral membranous staining in at least 10% of invasive tumor epithelial cells when scoring a surgical specimen (**Fig. 1**). Biopsies are scored positive if at least a single tumor cell cluster shows strong membranous staining (**Fig. 2**). A tumor cell cluster was arbitrarily defined by Ruschoff and colleagues[15] as 5 or more cells.[28] These low cutoffs are intended to minimize false-negative IHC scores. In the authors' experience, HER2 FISH-positive upper GI tract carcinomas have been identified, which exhibit strong, basolateral staining in only 10% to 30% of tumor cells, providing support for the 10% cutpoint for 3+ HER2 in upper GI tract carcinomas (**Fig. 3**).[29] In practice, positive (IHC 3+) expression is readily discerned with a low magnification objective (2× to 4× objective) (**Fig. 4**). The prevalence of IHC 3+ HER2-positive gastric cancer varies widely in the literature from 6.8% to more than 30% (mean 17.6%) (reviewed by Hofmann and colleagues[27]). This variability can most likely be attributed to lack of standardized interpretation criteria and reporting, use of different methods of HER2 detection, and different composition of the cases. More than 3800 cases from multiple countries were evaluated for inclusion in the ToGA trial and 22% were HER2 positive.[30] Their detailed analysis showed that location and histologic type are pathologic factors

Table 1
HER2 scoring criteria in upper gastrointestinal tract adenocarcinoma by specimen type

HER2 IHC Assessment	Scoring Criteria for Surgical Resection[9]	Scoring Criteria for Biopsy Specimen[9]	Magnification Guideline for Staining Intensity Assessment[28]
Negative (0)	• No reactivity or membranous reactivity in <10% of tumor cells	• No reactivity in any tumor cell	Not applicable
Negative (1+)	• Some membranous reactivity in ≥10% of tumor cells; cells may be reactive in only part of their membrane • Faint or barely perceptible intensity	• Some membranous reactivity in ≥1 tumor cell cluster[a] • Faint or barely perceptible intensity	• Membranous staining visible only with high-power (eg, 40×) objective
Equivocal (2+)[b]	• Complete, basolateral, or lateral membranous reactivity in ≥10% of tumor cells • Weak to moderate intensity	• Complete, basolateral, or lateral membranous reactivity in ≥1 tumor cell cluster[a] • Weak to moderate intensity	• Membranous staining visible only with intermediate (eg, 10×–20×) objective
Positive (3+)	• Complete, basolateral, or lateral membranous reactivity in ≥10% of tumor cells • Strong intensity	• Complete, basolateral, or lateral membranous reactivity in ≥1 tumor cell cluster[a] • Strong intensity	• Membranous staining visible with low-power (eg, 2×–4×) objective

[a] Tumor cell cluster is defined as a cluster of 5 or more tumor cells by Ruschoff and colleagues.[28] There is no percentage cutoff in biopsy specimens for upper GI tract HER2 scoring.
[b] Reflex to HER2 in situ testing (see Table 3).

associated with HER2 expression: gastroesophageal junction adenocarcinomas are more frequently HER2 positive in comparison with distal gastric cancers, and gland-forming intestinal type adenocarcinomas are more frequently positive than diffuse-type cancers.[30]

In the authors' experience, more than 90% of IHC 3+ cases are amplified by FISH when both tests are performed.[26] Consequently, when screening for HER2 amplification by IHC, a score of IHC 3+ does not require confirmation by in situ hybridization.

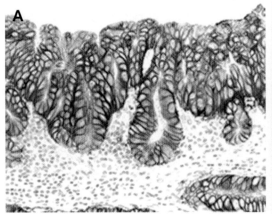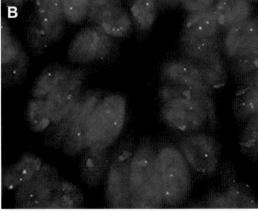

Fig. 1. HER2 staining in upper GI tract adenocarcinoma often exhibits a basolateral or lateral membranous staining pattern ([A] HER2 IHC, 200×). This staining pattern should be interpreted as 3+, because it is always associated with HER2 gene amplification by FISH ([B] HER2 red signal and Chr17 green signal, 1000×).

Fig. 2. In this biopsy specimen of gastric carcinoma, tumor cell clusters demonstrate strong membranous HER2 staining (400×). Strong membranous staining in tumor cell clusters (5 or more cells) should be scored as 3+ (positive). There is no percentage cutoff in biopsy specimens.

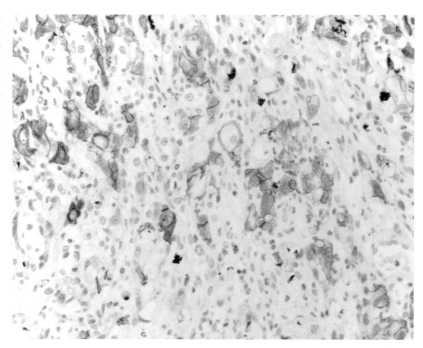

EQUIVOCAL HER2 STAINING IN UPPER GI CANCERS (IHC 2+)

Equivocal staining requires confirmation by in situ hybridization (discussed later) to establish HER2 amplification. In the authors' experience, equivocal HER2 expression (IHC 2+) is amplified by FISH in approximately half of cases. Most equivocal cases are amplified, however, at a low level (HER2:Chr17 centromere ratio 2.2–4.0), whereas HER2-positive cases are usually amplified at a high level (ratio >4.0 [Jon Davison, MD, personal communication 2012]). The circumstances that merit an equivocal (IHC 2+) score include

1. Cases of weak to moderate complete, basolateral, or lateral membranous staining in at least 10% of cells (resection specimens) or in a single tumor cell cluster (biopsy specimens)
2. Cases that, in practice, require an intermediate objective magnification (10×–20×) to confidently discern positive membranous staining should be considered equivocal (see **Fig. 4**).

Other circumstances that could merit additional testing in the form of repeat IHC on the same or a different tumor block[31] and/or confirmatory in situ hybridization are[15]

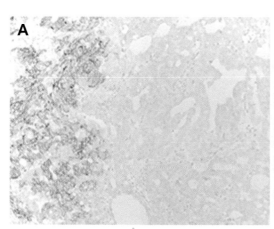
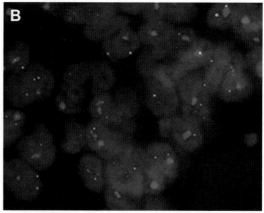

Fig. 3. This HER2-positive tumor only exhibited HER2 protein overexpression in 10% to 30% of tumor cells ([A] 200×) but demonstrated HER2 amplification by FISH ([B]1000×). Patients with this extent of HER2 protein overexpression (10% or greater) are eligible for trastuzumab therapy.

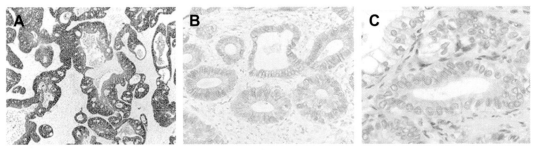

Fig. 4. Assessing the intensity HER2 immunohistochemical staining in upper GI tract carcinoma using magnification guidelines: 3+ HER2 staining is easily identified at 2× (*A*) or 4× objective magnification in this gastric adenocarcinoma. This esophagogastric adenocarcinoma demonstrates moderate (2+) membranous visible with 20× objective magnification. (*B*) This gastric carcinoma demonstrates faint membranous staining (1+) visible only with 40× objective magnification (*C*).

1. Cases of focal areas of strong membranous staining that do not meet the 10% cutoff or tumor cell cluster criteria
2. Difficult cases that are borderline between negative (IHC 1+) and equivocal (IHC 2+) due to staining intensity
3. Cases that are scored IHC 1+ but exhibit extensive weak expression (eg, >50% of tumor cells)
4. Cases of edge effects, nonspecific cytoplasmic staining (**Fig. 5**) or other artifacts, and strong positive staining in normal epithelial cells. Heterogeneity of HER2 expression in gastric cancer can account for equivocal HER2 expression in some of these scenarios.

NEGATIVE HER2 STAINING IN GASTRIC CANCER (IHC 0 OR 1+)

The majority (>70%) of cases stained by IHC are negative. Interpretation of negative staining requires appropriate positive and negative controls with each case. Negative staining is defined as

1. Membranous staining in fewer than 10% of tumor cells in surgical specimens (exceptions discussed previously) or complete absence of staining in biopsy specimens, and
2. Weak, barely visible membranous staining requiring high magnification objectives (40×) to appreciate in greater than 10% of cells in surgical specimens or tumor cell clusters in a

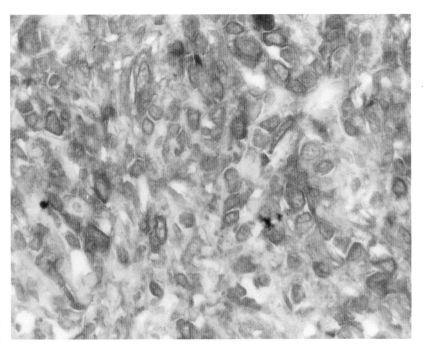

Fig. 5. This diffuse-type gastric adenocarcinoma demonstrated unusual diffuse cytoplasmic HER2 staining with IHC (400×). Given the unusual staining, FISH analysis was performed and demonstrated HER2 gene amplification. This case highlights the importance of having a low threshold for performing confirmatory FISH testing to reduce false-negative HER2 immunohistochemical results.

biopsy sample (scored as IHC 1+; exceptions discussed previously)

Because HER2 IHC is used to select patients for potentially beneficial therapy, it is imperative that false-negative cases be minimized. By in situ hybridization, these cases are rarely positive for HER2 amplification (less than 5%); hence, if a case is deemed negative by IHC, it does not require confirmatory in situ analysis. Cases that are borderline between negative and equivocal, in clinical practice, should be further tested. It is imperative that laboratories monitor concordance between IHC and FISH and aim for greater than 95% concordance between IHC and FISH positive and negative results. In gastric cancer, Hoffman and colleagues[27] showed that a 10% cutpoint for a 3+ HER2 IHC using the HercepTest in gastric adenocarcinoma does not detect rare HER2 FISH-positive cases due to the presence of HER2-amplified tumor subclones.

COMPARING BREAST CANCER AND GASTRIC CANCER HER2 SCORING CRITERIA

There are significant differences in the expression of HER2 protein between upper GI tract and breast cancer that necessitate different IHC interpretation criteria (summarized in **Table 2**). Hofmann and colleagues[27] found that a direct application of breast cancer scoring guidelines[20] would result in unacceptable rates of false-negative scores in gastric cancers due to distinct patterns of HER2 expression in gastric cancer. First, upper GI tract

adenocarcinomas with strong (3+) staining frequently lack complete, circumferential membranous HER2 immunoreactivity and instead exhibit a basolateral or lateral membranous staining pattern that should be scored positive (see **Fig. 1**).[29]

Another major difference with breast cancer concerns the higher frequency of intratumoral heterogeneous HER2 protein expression and HER2 gene amplification in upper GI tract adenocarcinomas (**Fig. 6**). The proportion of upper GI tract carcinomas with intratumoral heterogeneous HER2 expression and amplification varies between 5%[27,29,32] and 50%[14] in the literature, in contrast to the 1% to 2% range for breast carcinoma.[12,27,33–37] In whole tumor sections from upper GI cancer resection specimens, as few as 10% of cells can express HER2 by IHC and still be scored positive. In biopsy specimens from upper GI tract carcinomas, HER2 is scored positive if a single tumor cell cluster demonstrates appropriate HER2 immunoreactivity, regardless of the percentage of positive tumor cells. In contrast, the ASCO/CAP recommendations for HER2 testing in breast cancer set a threshold of 30% of tumor cells for a positive result.[38]

The appropriate thresholds for HER2 amplification by FISH are also different between breast and upper GI tract adenocarcinomas. The ASCO/CAP guideline recommendations for breast carcinoma include a FISH equivocal category for cases of HER2:Chr17 ratios between 1.8 and 2.2. The ToGA investigators did not include the equivocal FISH category and set a cutpoint of 2.0 for positive HER2 amplification by FISH.

Table 2
Comparison of *HER2* scoring in upper gastrointestinal tract adenocarcinoma and breast carcinoma

Feature	Upper GI Tract Adenocarcinoma	Breast Carcinoma
Immunohistochemical Scoring		
Extent of staining	Biopsies: ≥5 cells (cluster) Resection: ≥10% of tumor	≥30% of Tumor
Pattern of staining	Complete membranous, basolateral, or lateral	Complete membranous only
Heterogeneity of staining	Frequently present (~5%)	Infrequent (~1%–2%)
FISH analysis		
Cutpoint for amplification	*HER2*:Chr17 ratio ≥2.0	*HER2*:Chr17 ratio ≥2.2
Heterogeneity of tumor	Frequently present	Infrequent
Characteristics of *HER2*-positive tumors	Intestinal (~30%) more than diffuse (~5%) Esophageal/GEJ (~30%) more than gastric (~20%)	Ductal phenotype
Response to trastuzumab	IHC more predictive of response than FISH	IHC and FISH equally predictive of response

Abbreviation: GEJ, gastroesophageal junction.

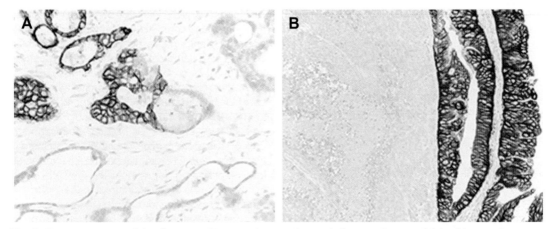

Fig. 6. Heterogeneous staining in upper GI tract adenocarcinoma is frequently seen. (*A*) In this case, heterogeneous HER2 staining is seen with some invasive glands exhibiting 3+ staining and other negative for HER2 overexpression (200×). (*B*) In this gastric adenocarcinoma with intermixed glandular (right half of image) and solid (left half of image) growth patterns, 3+ HER2 protein overexpression was identified by IHC in only the glandular areas (100×), emphasizing the importance of testing multiple areas of morphologically heterogenous carcinomas.

HER2 IN SITU HYBRIDIZATION

In the United States, several commercially available *HER2* gene insitu hybridization testing kits are approved by the FDA (**Table 3**). Some commercially available kits use FISH, such as the PathVysion *HER-2* DNA Probe Kit (Abbott Laboratories) and the *HER2* FISH pharmDX kit (Dako). Other kits use either silver-enhanced in situ hybridization (SISH) (INFORM *HER2* Dual ISH [Ventana]) or chromogenic in situ hybridization (CISH) (*HER2* CISH pharmDX, Dako). The optimal method for evaluating *HER2* gene amplification is not entirely clear and each assay has its benefits. Some arguments in favor of FISH include HER2 screening for the ToGA trial used the *HER2* FISH pharmDx kit,[9] and for this reason FISH can be regarded as the reference in situ hybridization

Table 3
Selected commercially available HER2 in situ hybridization testing kits

Parameter	PathVysion *HER-2* DNA Probe Kit	*HER2* FISH pharmDX	INFORM *HER2* Dual ISH Assay	*HER2* CISH pharmDX
Manufacturer	Abbott	Dako	Ventana	Dako
FDA status	Approved	Approved	Approved	Approved
Assay type	FISH	FISH	SISH	CISH
Methodology	Fluorescent DNA probes to *HER2* gene and Chr17 centromere	Fluorescent DNA probes to *HER2* gene and Chr17 centromere	Labeled *HER2* and Chr17 DNA probes followed by detection with silver-associated antibody	Labeled *HER2* and Chr17 DNA probe followed by detection with alkaline phosphatase-associated antibody
Scoring method	Fluorescence microscopy	Fluorescence microscopy	Brightfield microscopy	Brightfield microscopy
Scoring criteria for amplification	*HER2*:Chr17 ≥2.0	*HER2*:Chr17 ≥2.0	*HER2*:Chr17 ≥2.0 OR >6 *HER2* signals/nuclei[a]	*HER2*:Chr17 ≥2.0 OR >6 *HER2* signals/nuclei[a]

[a] HER2 gene count is recommended by some investigators.[15,39]

test. In addition, *HER2* testing in breast cancer has been standard pathology practice in the United States for decades where most laboratories use FISH to detect *HER2* gene amplification, because it is a well-established assay, having been FDA approved for a much longer period of time than CISH and SISH assays. The use of CISH and SISH is more common in other countries, particularly in Europe, Asia, and Australia, compared with in the United States.[15,39,40] Although CISH and SISH are newer methods of detecting *HER2* gene amplification, they provide some definite benefits compared with FISH. Most importantly, CISH and SISH use conventional brightfield microscopy that is routinely available to practicing pathologists. In contrast, FISH requires expensive special instrumentation and technical expertise more suited to large reference laboratories. The use of conventional brightfield microscopy also allows for better visualization of tumor morphology and easier identification *HER2*-positive foci in a heterogeneous tumor. Finally, CISH and SISH signals are stable, allowing for a permanent archive of the *HER2* test result in contrast to FISH where the fluorescence signals typically fade over time. Regardless of the in situ hybridization assay used, it is important to adhere to the manufacturer's instructions to ensure that the tests are accurate and reliable.

FISH, CISH, and SISH results are expressed as a ratio between the number of copies of the *HER2* gene and the number of copies of Chr17 reference within the nucleus. In most laboratories, the signals for a minimum of 20 tumor cells are counted and an average ratio of *HER2* to Chr17 reference signals is calculated. Some laboratories count a larger number of tumor cell nuclei; in the authors' laboratory, 60 tumor nuclei are evaluated. Regardless of the number of tumor cell nuclei counted, it is vital to screen the tumor for areas of possible *HER2* amplification at a 20× magnification and perform the signal count in these areas. If heterogeneity of the *HER2* copy number is identified, this should be noted in the pathology report. For FISH, the corresponding hematoxylin-eosin–stained section should also be reviewed to ensure that the counting is performed in the area of the tumor. Counts should also be performed in areas with nonoverlapping nuclei, avoiding areas with high nonspecific background and weak, imperceptible signals. In some *HER2*-amplified tumors, identified by FISH, the *HER2* signal is visualized as a confluent nuclear signal where enumeration is not possible. In such instances, the authors typically score these as having greater than 10 *HER2* signals. For CISH and SISH, overlapping signals can form clusters of variable size and the signals cannot be

individually discerned. In this setting, by convention, small clusters (3–5 times the diameter of a single dot) may be counted as 5 or 6 signals whereas large clusters (>5 times the diameter of a single dot) as 10 or 12 signals, depending on which in situ hybridization assay is used.[41] The ToGA investigators defined positive *HER2* gene amplification using a cutpoint of *HER2*:Chr17 ratio of 2.0 or greater. The ASCO/CAP guideline recommendations for breast carcinoma include a FISH equivocal category for cases of *HER2*:Chr17 ratios between 1.8 and 2.2. In such cases of borderline (ratio of 1.8–2.2) *HER2* gene amplification, it is recommended that at least an additional 20 tumor cell nuclei be analyzed to establish the *HER2*:Chr17 ratio.

Evaluating *HER2* gene amplification using *HER2* in situ hybridization may be complicated by issue of Chr17 polysomy or amplification of the Chr17 centromeric reference target. An increased number of centromeric Chr17 signals may indicate an increased number of Chr17 (ie, polysomy) or, alternatively, amplification of the centromeric region of Chr17. In the ToGA study, Chr17 polysomy was defined as 3 or more Chr17 signals on average per nuclei[27] and was reportedly identified in 4.1% of tumors examined.[15] Other investigators have found higher rates (16%) of Chr17 polysomy in gastric carcinoma.[42] Patients with increased *HER2* signals along with increased centromeric Chr17 signals have a *HER2*:Chr17 ratio less than 2.0 and are misclassified as nonamplified, potentially depriving patient eligibility for trastuzumab therapy. Some investigatorss[15,39] advocate using *HER2* gene copy number in addition to the *HER2*:Chr17 ratio in selecting patients for trastuzumab eligibility: average *HER2* signals/nuclei greater than 6 indicate *HER2* amplification, average *HER2* signals/nuclei less than 4 indicate lack of *HER2* amplification, and average *HER2* signals/nuclei between 4 and 6 are equivocal for *HER2* amplification. Although the *HER2* gene count may be useful in identifying *HER2* amplification in the setting of an increased number of centromeric Chr17 signals, it was not used by the ToGA investigators to select patients eligible for trastuzumab therapy and, to the authors' knowledge, has not been validated in a large number of upper GI tract adenocarcinomas. Other investigators[43,44] have demonstrated that, at least for breast carcinoma, alternative Chr17 gene reference probes, such as Smith-Magenis syndrome (*SMS*), retinoic acid receptor alpha (*RARA*), and the p53 (*TP53*) genes, are effective in establishing *HER2* amplification when an increased number of signals with the centromeric Chr17 probe is identified.

Key Features
HER2 ASSESSMENT IN UPPER GASTROINTESTINAL TRACT ADENOCARCINOMA

- The FDA has approved the use of trastuzumab for the treatment of metastatic upper GI tract (gastric, esophageal, and gastroesophageal) adenocarcinomas that meet the ToGA inclusion criteria.

- The European Medicines Agency has approved trastuzumab for IHC 3+ or IHC 2+/FISH-amplified tumors.

- In contrast to breast carcinoma, where there is a high concordance between HER2 assessment in needle core biopsy and subsequent surgical resection, HER2 testing can yield discordant results between biopsy and resections in upper GI tract carcinomas.

- To compensate for heterogeneous HER2 expression, it is recommended that a minimum of 6 to 8 endoscopic biopsy fragments be submitted for HER2 assessment.

- HER2 IHC should be the first-line testing method to select for patients eligible for trastuzumab therapy. With biopsy specimens, all available tumor blocks should be tested by IHC to account for potential heterogenous HER2 protein overexpression. For resection specimens, if a tumor is morphologically heterogeneous, then multiple tumor blocks including different tumor morphologies need to be tested.

ALGORITHMIC APPROACH TO HER2 ASSESSMENT IN UPPER GI TRACT ADENOCARCINOMA

The following algorithmic approach for the assessment of HER2 protein overexpression and gene amplification in upper GI tract adenocarcinoma is suggested, as depicted in **Fig. 7**. The ToGA trial showed evidence of a greater survival benefit for trastuzumab with tumors that expressed higher levels of HER2 protein expression.[9] Thus, HER2 IHC should be the first-line testing method used to select for patients eligible for trastuzumab

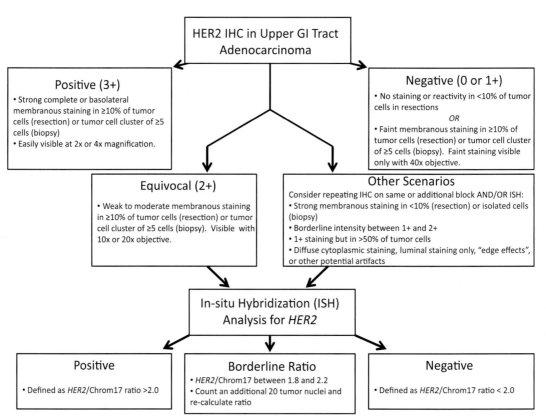

Fig. 7. Algorithm for HER2 testing in upper GI tract adenocarcinoma.

therapy. With biopsy specimens, all available tumor blocks should be tested by IHC to account for potential heterogenous HER2 protein overexpression. For resection specimens, if a tumor is morphologically heterogeneous, then multiple tumor blocks, including different tumor morphologies, need to be tested. The scoring criteria used are different between biopsy and resection specimens. Tumors with 0 or 1+ (negative) staining or 3+ (positive) staining need not be further tested with in situ hybridization analysis. If 2+ HER2 immunohistochemical staining is observed, then in situ hybridization should be performed. If there is any uncertainty in the scoring of the HER2 IHC (eg, diffuse, strong cytoplasmic staining, or significant staining or preservation artifact hindering interpretation), then in situ hybridization should be performed. HER2 in situ hybridization scoring is identical between biopsy and resection specimens. Tumors with borderline in situ hybridization scores (HER2:Chr17 ratio of 1.8–2.2) should be evaluated further by counting additional tumor cell nuclei or potentially testing multiple tumor blocks.

PROGNOSTIC SIGNIFICANCE OF HER2 STATUS

Literature reports have shown conflicting results when evaluating HER2 as a prognostic biomarker. Some reports have shown that HER2 overexpression is associated with worse overall survival[45–48] whereas others have shown that HER2 overexpression is of no prognostic significance.[29,32,49–51] These conflicting data may be due to low prevalence of HER2 in upper GI tract adenocarcinomas and differences in HER2 assessment, particularly with older studies that used different cutpoints to define HER2-positive tumors. Future studies with larger number of patients and using standardized HER2 assessment criteria may help establish the role of HER2 status as a prognostic marker in upper GI tract adenocarcinoma.

QUALITY ASSURANCE

Given the broad availability of IHC, assessment for trastuzumab eligibility is often performed in community-based pathology practices rather than in large, centralized hospital laboratories. In the breast literature, there have been many reports indicating poor correlation between HER2 testing in the community setting and in centralized laboratories.[39,52–54] In the Australian Gastric HER2 Testing Study, however, there was good to very good agreement between laboratories, including community hospitals, for 3+ positive HER2 tumors by IHC.[39] Awareness of the different staining patterns in upper GI tract adenocarcinoma compared with breast carcinoma and of the different scoring schemes depending on specimen type (biopsy vs resection) is also critical. In order to ensure accurate results, stringent internal quality control measures and validation of IHC protocols should be performed. Some investigators have suggested that the initial 25 to 50 cases should be analyzed in parallel using both IHC and in situ hybridization, with an expected concordance rate for 3+ IHC and in situ hybridization amplification between 93% to 98%, depending on which commercially available assay is used.[15] This validation should be performed for upper GI tract adenocarcinomas, even if the assays have been previously validated for HER2 assessment in breast carcinoma. In addition to internal quality control and validation, all hospitals performing HER2 assessment should participate in proficiency testing schemes through external quality assurance programs as they become available in the near future in the United States.

REFERENCES

1. Jemal A, Center MM, DeSantis C, et al. Global patterns of cancer incidence and mortality rates and trends. Cancer Epidemiol Biomarkers Prev 2010; 19(8):1893–907.

2. Jemal A, Siegel R, Xu J, et al. Cancer statistics, 2010. CA Cancer J Clin 2010;60(5):277–300.

3. Parfitt JR, Miladinovic Z, Driman DK. Increasing incidence of adenocarcinoma of the gastroesophageal junction and distal stomach in Canada—an epidemiological study from 1964-2002. Can J Gastroenterol 2006;20(4):271–6.

4. Wagner A. Chemotherapy for advanced gastric cancer. Cochrane Database Syst Rev 2005;(2). CD004064.

5. Gutierrez C, Schiff R. HER2: biology, detection, and clinical implications. Arch Pathol Lab Med 2011; 135(1):55–62.

6. Stern HM. Improving treatment of HER2-positive cancers: opportunities and challenges. Sci Transl Med 2012;4(127):127rv2.

7. King CR, Kraus MH, Aaronson SA. Amplification of a novel v-erbB-related gene in a human mammary carcinoma. Science 1985;229(4717):974–6.

8. Ishikawa T, Kobayashi M, Mai M, et al. Amplification of the c-erbB-2 (HER-2/neu) gene in gastric cancer cells. Detection by fluorescence in situ hybridization. Am J Pathol 1997;151(3):761–8.

9. Bang YJ, Van Cutsem E, Feyereislova A, et al. Trastuzumab in combination with chemotherapy versus chemotherapy alone for treatment of HER2-positive advanced gastric or gastro-oesophageal junction cancer (ToGA): a phase 3, open-label, randomised controlled trial. Lancet 2010;376(9742):687–97.

10. US Food and Drug Administration. Full prescribing information for trastuzumab 2010 [cited August 13, 2011]; Available at: http://www.accessdata.fda.gov/drugsatfda_docs/label/2010/103792s5250lbl.pdf.

11. European Medicines Agency. Committee for medicinal products for human use post-authorisation summary of positive opinion for Herceptin 2009 [cited August 13, 2011]. Available at: www.ema.europa.eu/pdfs/human/opinion/Herceptin_82246709en.pdf.

12. Lee AH, Key HP, Bell JA, et al. Concordance of HER2 status assessed on needle core biopsy and surgical specimens of invasive carcinoma of the breast. Histopathology 2012;60(6):880–4.

13. Chivukula M, Bhargava R, Brufsky A, et al. Clinical importance of HER2 immunohistologic heterogeneous expression in core-needle biopsies vs resection specimens for equivocal (immunohistochemical score 2+) cases. Mod Pathol 2008;21(4):363–8.

14. Lee S, de Boer WB, Fermoyle S, et al. Human epidermal growth factor receptor 2 testing in gastric carcinoma: issues related to heterogeneity in biopsies and resections. Histopathology 2011;59(5):832–40.

15. Ruschoff J, Hanna W, Bilous M, et al. HER2 testing in gastric cancer: a practical approach. Mod Pathol 2012;25(5):637–50.

16. Perrone G, Amato M, Callea M, et al. HER2 amplification status in gastric and gastro-oesophageal junction cancer in routine clinical practice: which sample should be used? Histopathology 2012;61(1):134–5.

17. Negri FV, Bozzetti C, Ardizzoni A, et al. HER-2 discordance between primary gastric carcinoma and paired lymph node metastasis. Hum Pathol 2011;42(6):909–10 [author reply: 10–1].

18. Kim MA, Lee HJ, Yang HK, et al. Heterogeneous amplification of ERBB2 in primary lesions is responsible for the discordant ERBB2 status of primary and metastatic lesions in gastric carcinoma. Histopathology 2011;59(5):822–31.

19. Bozzetti C, Negri FV, Lagrasta CA, et al. Comparison of HER2 status in primary and paired metastatic sites of gastric carcinoma. Br J Cancer 2011;104(9):1372–6.

20. Wolff AC, Hammond ME, Schwartz JN, et al. American Society of Clinical Oncology/College of American Pathologists guideline recommendations for human epidermal growth factor receptor 2 testing in breast cancer. J Clin Oncol 2007;25(1):118–45.

21. Yildiz-Aktas IZ, Dabbs DJ, Cooper KL, et al. The effect of 96-hour formalin fixation on the immunohistochemical evaluation of estrogen receptor, progesterone receptor, and HER2 expression in invasive breast carcinoma. Am J Clin Pathol 2012;137(5):691–8.

22. Tong LC, Nelson N, Tsourigiannis J, et al. The effect of prolonged fixation on the immunohistochemical evaluation of estrogen receptor, progesterone receptor, and HER2 expression in invasive breast cancer: a prospective study. Am J Surg Pathol 2011;35(4):545–52.

23. Moatamed NA, Nanjangud G, Pucci R, et al. Effect of ischemic time, fixation time, and fixative type on HER2/neu immunohistochemical and fluorescence in situ hybridization results in breast cancer. Am J Clin Pathol 2011;136(5):754–61.

24. Cho EY, Srivastava A, Park K, et al. Comparison of four immunohistochemical tests and FISH for measuring HER2 expression in gastric carcinomas [Comparative Study Research Support, Non-U.S. Gov't]. Pathology 2012;44(3):216–20.

25. Boers JE, Meeuwissen H, Methorst N. HER2 status in gastro-oesophageal adenocarcinomas assessed by two rabbit monoclonal antibodies (SP3 and 4B5) and two in situ hybridization methods (FISH and SISH). Histopathology 2011;58(3):383–94.

26. Radu OM, Foxwell T, Cieply K, et al. HER2 amplification in gastroesophageal adenocarcinoma: correlation of two antibodies using gastric cancer scoring criteria, H score, and digital image analysis with fluorescence in situ hybridization. Am J Clin Pathol 2012;137(4):583–94.

27. Hofmann M, Stoss O, Shi D, et al. Assessment of a HER2 scoring system for gastric cancer: results from a validation study. Histopathology 2008;52(7):797–805.

28. Ruschoff J, Dietel M, Baretton G, et al. HER2 diagnostics in gastric cancer-guideline validation and development of standardized immunohistochemical testing. Virchows Arch 2010;457(3):299–307.

29. Kunz PL, Mojtahed A, Fisher GA, et al. HER2 expression in gastric and gastroesophageal junction adenocarcinoma in a US population: clinicopathologic analysis with proposed approach to HER2 assessment. Appl Immunohistochem Mol Morphol 2012;20(1):13–24.

30. Bang Y, Chung H, Xu J, et al. Pathological features of advanced gastric cancer (GC): relationship to human epidermal growth factor receptor 2 (HER2) positivity in the global screening programme of the ToGA trial. J Clin Oncol 2009;27(suppl):15s [abstr 4556].

31. Asioli S, Maletta F, Verdun di Cantogno L, et al. Approaching heterogeneity of human epidermal growth factor receptor 2 in surgical specimens of gastric cancer. Hum Pathol 2012;43(11):2070–9.

32. Grabsch H, Sivakumar S, Gray S, et al. HER2 expression in gastric cancer: rare, heterogeneous and of no prognostic value—conclusions from 924 cases of two independent series. Cell Oncol 2010;32(1–2):57–65.

33. Cottu PH, Asselah J, Lae M, et al. Intratumoral heterogeneity of HER2/neu expression and its consequences for the management of advanced breast cancer. Ann Oncol 2008;19(3):595–7.

34. Brunelli M, Manfrin E, Martignoni G, et al. Genotypic intratumoral heterogeneity in breast carcinoma with HER2/neu amplification: evaluation according to ASCO/CAP criteria. Am J Clin Pathol 2009;131(5):678–82.

35. Wu JM, Halushka MK, Argani P. Intratumoral heterogeneity of HER-2 gene amplification and protein overexpression in breast cancer. Hum Pathol 2010; 41(6):914–7.

36. Apple SK, Lowe AC, Rao PN, et al. Comparison of fluorescent in situ hybridization HER-2/neu results on core needle biopsy and excisional biopsy in primary breast cancer. Mod Pathol 2009;22(9): 1151–9.

37. D'Alfonso T, Liu YF, Monni S, et al. Accurately assessing her-2/neu status in needle core biopsies of breast cancer patients in the era of neoadjuvant therapy: emerging questions and considerations addressed. Am J Surg Pathol 2010;34(4):575–81.

38. Wolff AC, Hammond ME, Schwartz JN, et al. American Society of Clinical Oncology/College of American Pathologists guideline recommendations for human epidermal growth factor receptor 2 testing in breast cancer. Arch Pathol Lab Med 2007; 131(1):18–43.

39. Fox SB, Kumarasinghe MP, Armes JE, et al. Gastric HER2 Testing Study (GaTHER): an evaluation of gastric/gastroesophageal junction cancer testing accuracy in Australia. Am J Surg Pathol 2012; 36(4):577–82.

40. Garcia-Garcia E, Gomez-Martin C, Angulo B, et al. Hybridization for human epidermal growth factor receptor 2 testing in gastric carcinoma: a comparison of fluorescence in-situ hybridization with a novel fully automated dual-colour silver in-situ hybridization method. Histopathology 2011;59(1):8–17.

41. Papouchado BG, Myles J, Lloyd RV, et al. Silver in situ hybridization (SISH) for determination of HER2 gene status in breast carcinoma: comparison with FISH and assessment of interobserver reproducibility. Am J Surg Pathol 2010;34(6):767–76.

42. Liang Z, Zeng X, Gao J, et al. Analysis of EGFR, HER2, and TOP2A gene status and chromosomal polysomy in gastric adenocarcinoma from Chinese patients. BMC Cancer 2008;8:363.

43. Tse CH, Hwang HC, Goldstein LC, et al. Determining true HER2 gene status in breast cancers with polysomy by using alternative chromosome 17 reference genes: implications for anti-HER2 targeted therapy. J Clin Oncol 2011;29(31):4168–74.

44. Troxell ML, Bangs CD, Lawce HJ, et al. Evaluation of Her-2/neu status in carcinomas with amplified chromosome 17 centromere locus. Am J Clin Pathol 2006;126(5):709–16.

45. Garcia I, Vizoso F, Martin A, et al. Clinical significance of the epidermal growth factor receptor and HER2 receptor in resectable gastric cancer. Ann Surg Oncol 2003;10(3):234–41.

46. Yan B, Yau EX, Bte Omar SS, et al. A study of HER2 gene amplification and protein expression in gastric cancer. J Clin Pathol 2010;63(9):839–42.

47. Zhang XL, Yang YS, Xu DP, et al. Comparative study on overexpression of HER2/neu and HER3 in gastric cancer. World J Surg 2009;33(10): 2112–8.

48. Begnami MD, Fukuda E, Fregnani JH, et al. Prognostic implications of altered human epidermal growth factor receptors (HERs) in gastric carcinomas: HER2 and HER3 are predictors of poor outcome. J Clin Oncol 2011;29(22): 3030–6.

49. Barros-Silva JD, Leitao D, Afonso L, et al. Association of ERBB2 gene status with histopathological parameters and disease-specific survival in gastric carcinoma patients. Br J Cancer 2009;100(3): 487–93.

50. Marx AH, Tharun L, Muth J, et al. HER-2 amplification is highly homogenous in gastric cancer. Hum Pathol 2009;40(6):769–77.

51. Yu GZ, Chen Y, Wang JJ. Overexpression of Grb2/ HER2 signaling in Chinese gastric cancer: their relationship with clinicopathological parameters and prognostic significance. J Cancer Res Clin Oncol 2009;135(10):1331–9.

52. Roche PC, Suman VJ, Jenkins RB, et al. Concordance between local and central laboratory HER2 testing in the breast intergroup trial N9831. J Natl Cancer Inst 2002;94(11):855–7.

53. Paik S, Bryant J, Tan-Chiu E, et al. Real-world performance of HER2 testing–National Surgical Adjuvant Breast and Bowel Project experience. J Natl Cancer Inst 2002;94(11):852–4.

54. Zujewski JA. "Build quality in"—HER2 testing in the real world. J Natl Cancer Inst 2002;94(11):788–9.

Lymphomas of the Gastrointestinal Tract: An Update

Lauren B. Smith, MD[a], Eric D. Hsi, MD[b],*

KEYWORDS

• Lymphoma • Non-Hodgkin • Extranodal • Enteropathy-associated • MALT • DLBCL • NK/T
• BCL-U

ABSTRACT

The gastrointestinal tract is the most common extranodal site of non-Hodgkin lymphoma. Certain lymphomas have a predilection for the gastrointestinal tract, including extranodal marginal zone lymphoma of mucosa-associated lymphoid tissue, mantle cell lymphoma, natural killer/T-cell lymphoma, and enteropathy-associated T-cell lymphoma. Follicular lymphoma may also be primary to the gastrointestinal tract. In addition to diagnosing neoplastic conditions, it is important to differentiate lymphomas from atypical reactive proliferations. Recent research relevant to non-Hodgkin lymphomas involving this location is reviewed with an emphasis on novel and evolving areas of classification.

OVERVIEW

Gastrointestinal (GI) lymphomas are the most common type of extranodal lymphoma.[1] They are a diverse group of neoplasms that can affect any portion of the GI tract; however, the most common site is stomach, followed by small bowel and colon. In the past decade, the incidence of GI non-Hodgkin lymphomas has been increasing, with an estimated incidence of 2.7 per 100,000 in a North American population.[2] The classic subtypes of non-Hodgkin lymphoma arising in the GI tract are discussed, with a focus on newer areas of research and classification.

B-CELL NON-HODGKIN LYMPHOMAS

EXTRANODAL MARGINAL ZONE LYMPHOMA OF MUCOSA-ASSOCIATED LYMPHOID TISSUE LYMPHOMA

Gross and Microscopic Features

MALT lymphoma is a B-cell non-Hodgkin lymphoma that commonly arises in the stomach and duodenum. It is highly associated with infection by *Helicobacter pylori*, which sets up the chronic inflammatory milieu that provides abnormal T-cell help to B cells and gives rise to lymphoma.[3] Therefore, a background of chronic or active gastritis is typically seen. Less commonly, there is no evidence of gastritis. Histologically, MALT lymphoma recapitulates normal MALT tissue and is composed of small lymphocytes, which may have monocytoid or centocyte-like morphology, often associated with residual reactive germinal centers that become colonized and overrun by the lymphomatous proliferation. The amount of plasmacytic differentiation is highly variable and can be extensive, mimicking plasma cell neoplasms in rare instances.[4] The immunophenotype of MALT lymphomas by flow cytometry and immunohistochemistry is nonspecific, because they typically lack CD5 and CD10 expression. The diagnostic challenge frequently encountered by pathologists in these cases is differentiating florid gastritis from lymphoma. In establishing the diagnosis, features that favor malignancy include deeply invasive lymphoid infiltrates, monocytoid

Funding: None.
Conflict of Interest: None.
[a] Department of Pathology, University of Michigan Hospital and Health System, M5230 Medical Science I, 1301 Catherine Street, Ann Arbor, MI 48109, USA; [b] Cleveland Clinic Lerner College of Medicine, Cleveland Clinic, L-11, 9500 Euclid Avenue, Cleveland, OH 44195, USA
* Corresponding author.
E-mail address: hsie@ccf.org

Pathologic Key Features

1. Mucosa-associated lymphoid tissue (MALT) lymphoma: lymphoepithelial lesions (LELs), monocytoid lymphocytes, plasmacytic differentiation

2. Primary intestinal follicular lymphoma (PIFL): duodenal/jejunal polyps with abnormal follicles (usually low cytologic grade) within the mucosa

3. Mantle cell lymphoma: numerous polyps, angulated lymphocytes, epithelioid histiocytes, cyclin D1 expression

4. Diffuse large B-cell lymphoma (DLBCL): sheets of large B cells

5. Burkitt lymphoma: terminal ileum mass, intermediate-sized cells, starry-sky pattern, bcl-2 negative, Ki-67 approximately 100%

6. BCL-U: intermediate to large cells, high proliferative fraction, variable morphology, *MYC* rearrangement + *BCL2//IGH* translocation and/or *BCL6* rearrangement

7. Enteropathy-associated T-cell lymphoma (EATL), classic type: pleomorphic intermediate to large cells, necrosis, variably prominent eosinophils, intraepithelial lymphocytes (IELs)

8. EATL type II: small to intermediate-sized cells, CD8 and CD56 expression

9. Natural killer (NK)/T-cell lymphoma: intermediate-sized to large-sized cells, often with angiocentric/destructive lesions, Epstein-Barr virus (EBV)–encoded RNA (EBER) positive

10. NK-cell enteropathy/lymphomatoid gastropathy: superficial lesion, EBER negative

morphology, and well-developed or destructive LELs (**Fig. 1**). Immunophenotyping in paraffin sections may be helpful. CD43, a marker not seen in normal B cells, is expressed in approximately 20% to 30% of cases, and demonstration of coexpression on B cells is an indicator of lymphoma rather than an inflammatory process.[5] The plasma cell component may be light chain restricted in approximately 20% of cases and again indicates a lymphomatous infiltrate.[6] Those laboratories capable of reliably detecting surface immunoglobulin in paraffin sections can also use this to distinguish lymphoma from florid gastritis. B-cell receptor gene rearrangement studies are not routinely recommended because these can be positive in a minority of chronic gastritis cases.[7]

Follow-up biopsies for disease monitoring can be problematic. Scoring systems have been published that are reliable and may help unify terminology.[8,9] In cases of MALT lymphoma, it is prudent to wait at least 8 weeks before repeat biopsy because the infiltrates can persist for an extended period of time.[10] It is also helpful to compare sequential biopsies to evaluate whether the lymphoid infiltrates have increased or decreased in the interval between the biopsies.

Again, use of gene rearrangement studies is not recommended because detectable clones may persist for many months, even in the absence of histologic evidence of lymphoma.[11]

Much work has focused on the genetic alterations found in MALT lymphoma, including characteristic translocations and cytogenetic abnormalities that may be seen. Different locations have different frequencies of cytogenetic translocations. The most common abnormalities found in the stomach include t(11;18)(q21;q21), involving *BIRC3* and *MALT1*[12]; +3; +18; and t(14;18)(q32;q21), involving *IGHV* and *MALT1*.[13,14] In the intestine, the most common abnormalities also include +3, +8, and t(11;18)(q21;q21).[15] A translocation not found in the stomach but found in the intestine is t(1;14)(p22;q32), involving *BCL10* and *IGVH*.[16] Because these abnormalities are not present in every case, the diagnostic utility is limited for classification; however, t(11;18)(q21;q21) in gastric MALT lymphoma has been associated with lack of response to antibiotic therapy (**Fig. 2**).[17]

In terms of therapeutic options besides antibiotic therapy, low-dose external beam radiation has been used with excellent overall and relapse-free survival in patients who do not respond to *H pylori* therapy.[18]

Fig. 1. MALT lymphoma. (*A*) H&E section of stomach, 100× original magnification. (*B*) H&E section LEL, 400× original magnification.

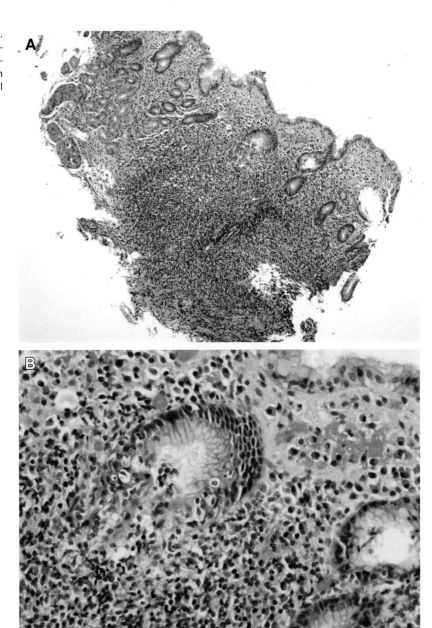

Differential Diagnosis

The differential diagnosis includes other B-cell non-Hodgkin lymphomas. In the GI tract, it is essential to exclude mantle cell lymphoma, because these typically behave aggressively. CD5 and cyclin D1 immunohistochemistry are often used to exclude mantle cell lymphoma, although CD5 can be negative.[19] If suspicion exists for mantle cell lymphoma, cyclin D1 is the most reliable and specific immunohistochemical study. Other B-cell lymphomas composed of small cells should also be considered, including follicular lymphoma and chronic lymphocytic leukemia/small lymphocytic lymphoma. Morphologically, diffuse follicular lymphoma can mimic marginal zone lymphoma, because both can be composed of cells

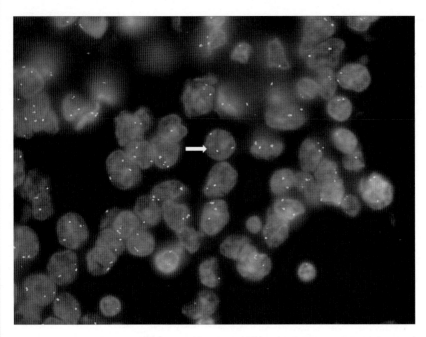

Fig. 2. FISH showing t(11;18)(q21aq21) *API2/MALT1* using break-apart probe. The *arrow* shows a cell with the translocation. (*Courtesy of* Dr Bryan Betz, PhD, Ann Arbor.)

with the appearance of centrocytes. Chronic lymphocytic leukemia/small lymphocytic lymphoma may show proliferation centers and, immunophentypically, the B cells often coexpress CD5 and CD43. Review of the peripheral blood demonstrates a lymphocytosis in a majority of cases.[20]

DLBCL can arise from low-grade MALT lymphoma and should be diagnosed with large aggregates or sheets of transformed large cells are present. As with low-grade MALT lymphomas, a search for *H pylori* should be performed. Recent studies have shown that early-stage DLBCL that are *H pylori* positive respond frequently to Helicobacter eradication therapy alone.[21]

FOLLICULAR LYMPHOMA (SYSTEMIC AND PRIMARY INTESTINAL)

Gross and Microscopic Features

Follicular lymphoma involving the GI tract may present as a manifestation of systemic disease, or, alternatively, may be the sole site of disease. Follicular lymphoma is uncommon and comprises only 1% to 3% of GI lymphomas.[22] An entity, now recognized as a variant of follicular lymphoma in the 2008 edition of the WHO Classification of Tumors of the Haematopoietic and Lympid Tissues, is primary intestinal follicular lymphoma (PIFL).[23] It has a predilection for the second portion of the duodenum and jejunum and typically presents as nodular or polypoid lesions or, occasionally, patches or plaques.[24,25] A majority of patients with duodenal involvement also have jejunal or ileal

lesions. PIFL may also involve other sites, including the ileum and, less commonly, the colon.[22] Demographically, it occurs more often in female patients. A less-favorable outcome has been found in male patients, patients with abdominal symptoms, and patients without duodenal disease.[25]

Histologically, PIFL manifests as nodular infiltrates within the superficial mucosa. As in systemic follicular lymphoma, the neoplastic B cells typically express CD10, BCL6, and bcl-2 (**Fig. 3**). BLC2 expression is typically intense. Like nodal follicular lymphomas, the *IGH/BCL2* fusion is present.[26–28] As opposed to nodal follicular lymphoma, intestinal disease often shows follicular dendritic cell meshwork at the periphery of the abnormal follicles.[25]

Prognosis

Follicular lymphoma can be classified as primary intestinal only if other sites of disease have been excluded. In these cases, patients have excellent survival, even without therapy.[23,27] If other sites of disease exist, the term, primary intestinal, should not be used, although the prognosis may be better than follicular lymphoma that does not involve the GI tract. Because many studies have included both types of follicular lymphoma, it is difficult to know whether the prognosis is related to stage or subtype.

Differential Diagnosis

In a GI location, it is important to consider reactive conditions in the differential diagnosis. Prominent

Fig. 3. PIFL. (*A*) H&E section, 20× original magnification. (*B*) H&E, 200× original magnification.

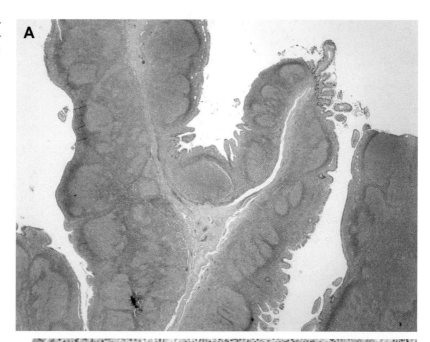

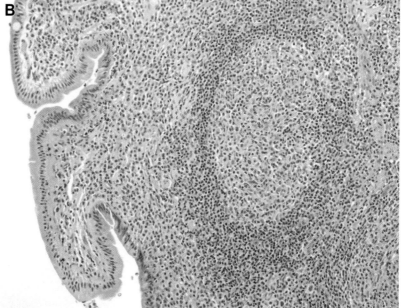

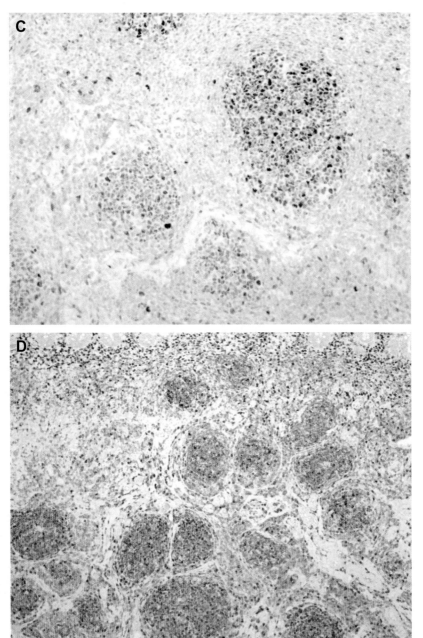

Fig. 3. (*C*) BCL6 immuno-histochemical stain, 200× original magnification. (*D*) bcl-2 immunohisto-chemical stain, 100× orig-inal magnification.

lymphoid aggregates, often seen on biopsy of the ileocecal valve, can mimic follicular lymphoma because they can be markedly disrupted and difficult to identify on hematoxylin-eosin (H&E) sections. Immunohistochemical studies for CD10, BCL6, and bcl-2 can be helpful adjuncts if suspicion for lymphoma exists. The prominent lymphoid aggregates are CD10 and BCL6 positive and bcl-2 negative.

MANTLE CELL LYMPHOMA

Gross and Microscopic Features

Mantle cell lymphoma often involves the GI tract in a pattern commonly termed, *lymphomatous polyposis*. Patients commonly present with abdominal pain and GI bleeding. The colon may be carpeted with polyps that can be seen by an endoscopist. Other presentations include ulcerative or infiltrative lesions (**Fig. 4**).[29]

Microscopically, the polyps are composed of lymphoid proliferations within the mucosa and submucosa. Occasionally, these can be a transmural proliferation. Histologically, mantle cell lymphoma is characterized by angulated small to intermediate-sized lymphocytes (**Fig. 5**). Often, there are admixed epithelioid histiocytes and hyalinized vessels. Different architectural patterns

occur, including mantle zone expansions and diffuse or nodular proliferations. In situ mantle cell lymphoma has been recently described with a normal-appearing mantle zone that is cyclin D1 positive. The clinical significance of this finding is unclear, because it often occurs in patients with more typical morphologic features elsewhere. These rarely reported in situ cases seem to occur as incidental findings in lymph node biopsies and have an indolent course, although further study and longer follow-up are needed to truly assess risk of progression.[30] The authors are aware of only a single case report occurring in the colon, which was identified retrospectively 2 years after an overt systemic mantle cell lymphoma diagnosis.[31]

The more aggressive morphologic variants include the blastoid and pleomorphic types. The blastoid variant has cells with dispersed chromatin resembling myeloid or lymphoid blasts and a high mitotic rate. The pleomorphic variant resembles DLBCL.

Using immunohistochemical studies, the neoplastic B-cells in mantle cell lymphoma typically express CD20, CD5, and cyclin D1. Cytogenetic and fluorescence in situ hybridization (FISH) studies on mantle cell lymphoma demonstrate t(11;14)(q13;q32) in the vast majority of cases. In rare cases that are negative for cyclin D1, cyclin

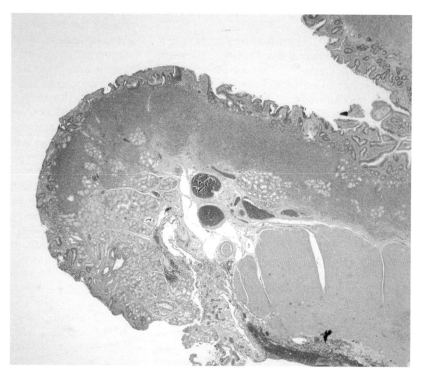

Fig. 4. Mantle cell lymphoma. Infiltrative lesion in a stomach removed for gastric adenocarcinoma. H&E section, 20× original magnification.

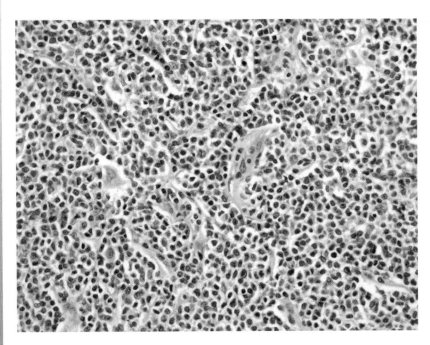

Fig. 5. Mantle cell lymphoma composed of angulated lymphocytes and epithelioid histiocytes. H&E section, 400× original magnification.

D2/D3 may be involved but testing for this is difficult because other types of lymphoma express these markers.[32] SOX11, a member of the SOX C group of transcription factors, is expressed in the great majority of mantle cell lymphoma and can be useful in identifying cases of cyclin D1–negative mantle cell lymphoma of typical and blastoid variant types.[33,34]

Recent research has focused on the cases that have an indolent clinical course, which comprise 10% to 15% of cases.[35,36] Although some studies have suggested that SOX11-positive cases are typically more indolent that SOX11-negative cases, other studies have found that this is not predictive of clinical behavior. In a multivariate analysis in one recent study, which included age, Eastern Cooperative Oncology Group score, lactate dehydrogenase, p53, and SOX11, the SOX11 status was not found an independent predictor of clinical behavior.[37] In many studies, indolent cases have been associated with non-nodal disease.[36,38]

DIFFUSE LARGE B-CELL LYMPHOMA

DLBCL is commonly seen in the GI tract. It can involve any site but often occurs in the stomach and large intestine. Histologically, it is characterized by sheets of large cells with variable pleomorphism and mitotic activity (**Fig. 6**). The immunophenotype is variable but pan B-cell markers, such as CD19, CD20, and CD79a, are typically expressed. CD5 is rarely expressed and CD10 is variably expressed. When confronted with a DLBCL in the GI tract, evidence of a low-grade lymphoma, such as a MALT-type lymphoma or follicular lymphoma, should be sought to exclude a transformation of one of these lymphomas. In the stomach, DLBCLs may contain LELs composed of large cells; however, the appropriate diagnosis is DLBCL. The differential diagnosis includes Burkitt lymphoma, especially in pediatric cases, and B-cell lymphoma, unclassifiable (BCL-U) with features intermediate between DLBCL and Burkitt lymphoma. This differential diagnosis is discussed in detail.

DLBCL has been subtyped into activated B-cell (ABC) and germinal center B-cell (GCB) types based on gene expression array studies.[39] The first immunohistochemical algorithm that was used to classify the cases is now known as the Hans classifier.[40] Subsequent studies suggested that this approach was not adequate for differentiating GCB from ABC based on gene expression results; however, in high-quality laboratories, this can be done with reasonable (>80%) accuracy. Subsequently, additional algorithms were developed using FOXP3 and GCET[41] or LMO2[42] in an attempt classify these cases more accurately. Studies suggest, however, that these may be equivalent with concordance in the 86% to 87% range.[43,44]

Fig. 6. DLBCL in stomach. (*A*) H&E section, 400× original magnification. (*B*) CD20 immunohisto-chemical stain, 200× original magnification.

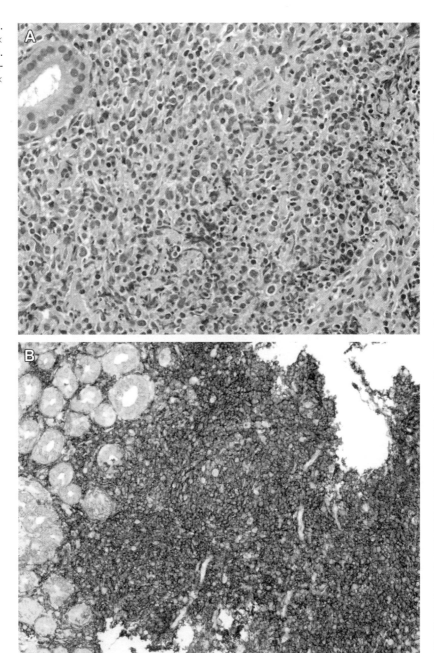

BURKITT LYMPHOMA AND RELATED ENTITIES

Gross and Microscopic Features

Classic Burkitt lymphoma is more commonly found in children and typically presents as a mass in the terminal ileum. Histologically, it is characterized by sheets of intermediate-sized cells with inconspicuous nucleoli. The cells typically have a homogeneous appearance with numerous mitoses and admixed tingible body macrophages reflecting the high proliferative rate (**Fig. 7A, B**). On review of touch preparations, the cells may have numerous cytoplasmic vacuoles.

The immunophenotype of Burkitt lymphoma includes expression of CD10, CD20, and surface immunoglobulin light chains. bcl-2 is negative, as are blast markers, such as TdT and CD34. The proliferative fraction should approach 100% using

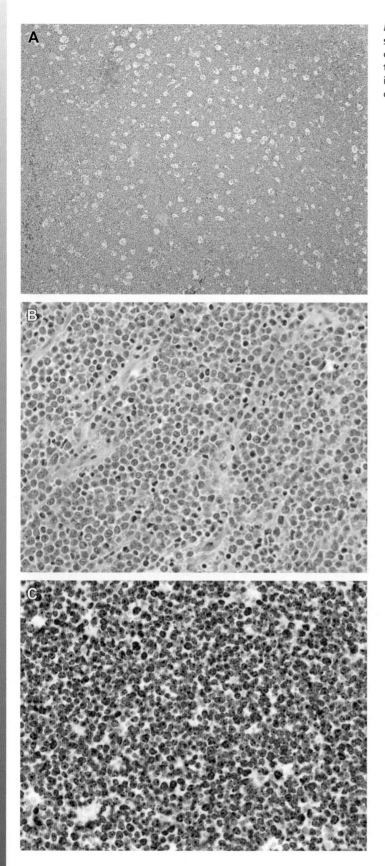

Fig. 7. Burkitt lymphoma. (*A*) Starry-sky appearance, H&E section, 100× original magnification. (*B*) H&E section, 400× magnification. (*C*) Ki-67 immuohistochemical stain, 400× original magnification.

Ki-67 immunohistochemistry (**Fig. 7C**). Although not specific, *MYC* protein is highly expressed and can serve as a clue that a *MYC* translocation might be present. Conventional cytogenetic studies typically show a simple karyotype with a *MYC* translocation involving an immunoglobulin gene (heavy or light chain genes) as the partner gene.[45] FISH studies may also be performed to demonstrate *MYC* rearrangement. The differential diagnosis includes B lymphoblastic lymphoma, which also typically shows a starry-sky pattern and expresses TdT and/or CD34; DLBCL with a high proliferative fraction; and a new entity in the 2008 World Health Organization (WHO) classification, BCL-U, with features intermediate between DLBCL and Burkitt lymphoma.

Differential Diagnosis

In some instances, cases seem to have overlapping features between Burkitt lymphoma and DLBCL. BCL-U is a new category in the WHO 2008 classification and has been an active area of research since its introduction.[46] This category was created because it became evident that there is a subset of cases previously classified as either DLBCL or atypical Burkitt lymphoma and that have a more aggressive clinical course and molecular features intermediate between follicular lymphoma and DLBCL.[47,48]

Cases of BCL-U typically occur in adults in at least the sixth decade of life. Some studies have shown that the most common extranodal sites for these lymphomas are the head and neck region and GI tract.[49] A subset of the cases of BCL-U, arguably the most diagnostically defined group, has a complex karyotype with *MYC* rearrangements and either *BCL6* rearrangements and/or *BCL2/IGH* translocations. These cases have been termed, *double-hit* or *triple-hit*, to reflect the presence of these molecular abnormalities.

Immunophenotypically, the double-hit lymphomas with *BCL2/IGH* translocation with *MYC* rearrangement typically express CD10 and the proliferative rate is variable but is greater than 75% in the majority of cases; however, the morphology often does not resemble Burkitt lymphoma (**Fig. 8**).[50] In a recent study, cases of *BCL6* and *MYC* rearrangement were more likely ABC type (CD10 negative); however, because these did not have an immunophenotype resembling Burkitt, it is difficult to classify them as BCL-U[49] based on the WHO definition. Although bcl-2 is negative in classic Burkitt lymphoma, many of the BCL-U cases are bcl-2 positive, and some arise in patients with a history of follicular lymphoma.[50] Although there is no standard chemotherapeutic regimen

that is used for this type of lymphoma, many centers are using a more-aggressive approach than standard R-CHOP, such as R-EPOCH. BCL2 and aurora A kinase small molecule inhibitors may have utility in these patients based on preliminary studies.[51]

Diagnostic difficulty arises in these cases because there are no definitive diagnostic criteria that separate these cases from DLBCL. The proliferative fraction can overlap with traditional DLBCL. These cases were initially identified based on gene expression array data that are not available in a clinical setting; therefore, definitive diagnosis in routine practice can be challenging and somewhat arbitrary. At this time, they are not limited strictly to the double-hit or triple-hit cases, although this may change as the diagnostic criteria are refined. In the future, this designation may be limited to cases of *MYC* rearrangement and *BCL2/IGH* translocation and/or *BCL6* rearrangement.

NK-CELL AND PERIPHERAL T-CELL LYMPHOMAS AND RELATED REACTIVE ENTITIES

ENTEROPATHY-ASSOCIATED T-CELL LYMPHOMA

Overview

EATL lymphoma is a rare lymphoma that typically involves the small intestine and, in some cases, is associated with celiac disease. There are currently 2 types of EATL, as defined by the WHO 2008 classification:

1. The classic type occurs more commonly in white populations and typically occurs in patients with celiac disease. An association has been established in certain HLA types (HLA-DQ2 and HLA-DQ8).[52]
2. EATL type II differs in that it is more likely to affect all ethnicities and does not have an established association with celiac disease.

The immunophenotype also differs between the 2 subtypes. Because these entities are rare, research is limited. There has been more inquiry, however, into EATL type II recently, which sheds some light on the pathophysiology of this rare entity.

Diagnosis

Classic-type EATL is morphologically characterized by large, pleomorphic cells with a marked inflammatory infiltrate, often including eosinophilic abscesses and prominent necrosis (**Fig. 9**).[53] The immunophenotype is somewhat variable, but the cells typically express CD3, CD7, CD103, and

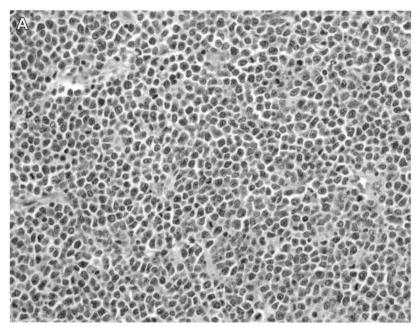

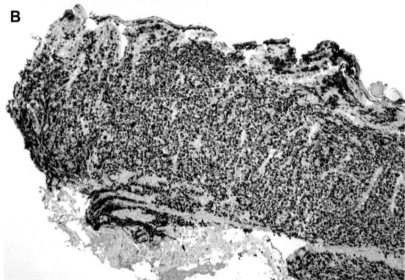

Fig. 8. BCL-U. (*A*) H&E section showing variably sized cells, 400× original magnification. (*B*) Ki-67 immunohistochemical stain showing a high proliferative fraction, 100× original magnification.

GzB and lack CD5 and CD56. The cells are believed to arise from native intraepithelial T-lymphocytes.[52] CD4 and CD8 are often negative.

Patients who develop the classic type of EATL often have a history of refractory celiac disease/sprue, a condition in which a gluten-free diet does not ameliorate the symptoms or histologic findings. Refractory sprue is a serious condition with a high mortality rate secondary to malabsorption and a high incidence of lymphoma.[54]

In patients with refractory sprue who develop lymphoma at a later time, evidence of immunophenotypic T-cell aberrancies and identical T-cell receptor gene rearrangements often are found in both the sprue biopsies and the lymphoma specimen.[55] Aberrant IEL immunophenotype is termed, *type 2 refractory sprue*, not to be confused with type II EATL.

Type II EATL is characterized by a monomorphic infiltrate of small to intermediate-sized cells with a

Fig. 9. Classic EATL. (*A*) H&E section showing pleomorphic cells, 400× original magnification. (*B*) H&E section showing prominent eosinophilia, 400× original magnification. (*Courtesy of* Dr David Arps, MD, Ann Arbor.)

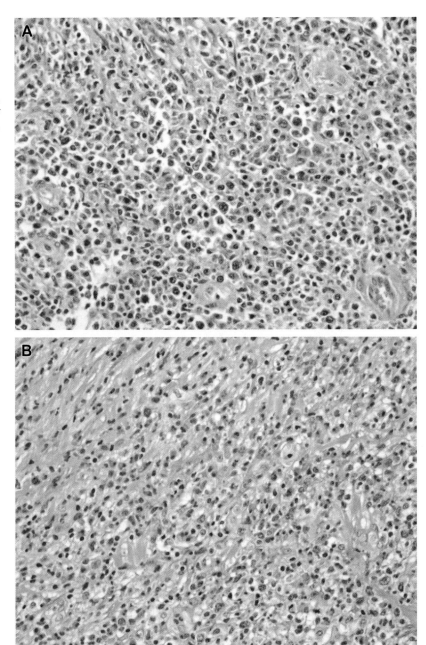

less prominent inflammatory infiltrate (**Fig. 10**). Although necrosis is not typical, prominent mitotic activity is present. These cases often express CD56 (**Fig. 11**) and CD8, unlike classic-type EATL. As in the classic type, CD5 is typically negative.

Two series have focused on EATL in Asian populations where celiac disease is virtually nonexistent.[56,57] By focusing on this population of patients, the investigators attempted to clarify the clinical, histopathologic, and immunophenotypic findings in type II EATL. Similar to the classic-type EATL, patients in these series also showed a male predominance and older age at presentation. Intestinal perforation and high-stage disease were also common consistent with an aggressive clinical course. Chan and colleagues[56] also showed that the neoplastic T cells were more likely to be of gamma-delta type,

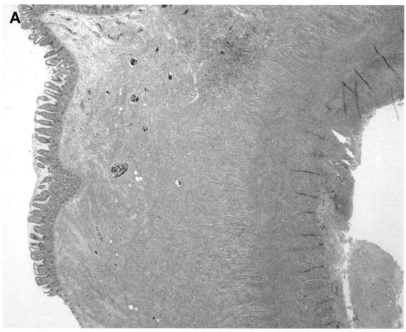

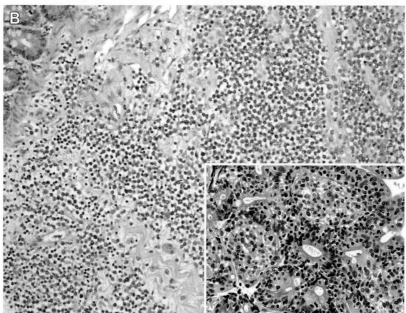

Fig. 10. EATL type II in a specimen resected after perforation. (*A*) H&E section, 20× original magnification. (*B*) H&E section, 200× original magnification. (*Inset*) H&E section, 400× original magnification. Increased intraepithelial lymphocytes.

rather than alpha-beta, suggesting that these may be better defined as gamma-delta T-cell lymphomas. Both studies showed some variability in terms of CD56 and CD8 expression. Although both types of EATL are believed to arise from intraepithelial T-cells, these studies suggest that there may be a good argument for separating

them as 2 distinct entities. Chan and colleagues[56] suggest the term, *monomorphic intestinal T-cell lymphoma*.

Conflicting data exist regarding the IELs present in both entities. Although it is clear that the IELs in the classic type share the same immunophenotype as the tumor and are thought of as a dysplastic

Fig. 11. EATL type II. CD56 immunohistochemical stain, 200× original magnification.

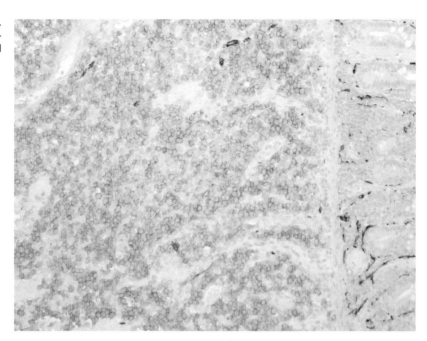

precursor lesion, often presenting in patients with refractory sprue, the situation is not as clear in type II EATL. Some studies have shown that the lymphocytes do not have the same immunophenotype as the tumor; Chan and colleagues[56] showed that some cases are concordant whereas others are discordant.

NK/T-CELL LYMPHOMA

Gross and Microscopic Features

The GI tract is the most common extranasal site of extranodal NK/T-cell lymphoma. This lymphoma is more common in Asian countries and is encountered less frequently in the United States. The tumor is often ulcerated and is composed of small to large cells with marked necrosis and frequently an angiocentric growth pattern. A recent study showed that the vast majority (92%) had necrosis, whereas more than half, but not all, were angiodestructive (69%).[58]

Immunophenotypically, this neoplasm typically expresses CD2, cytoplasmic CD3ε, CD56, cytotoxic molecules, and, less commonly, CD7 or CD30. In situ hybridization for EBER is always positive (**Fig. 12**).[59] Although T-cell receptor gene rearrangement studies are typically germline, rare cases show a clonal gene rearrangement, because a small proportion of cases are of cytotoxic T-cell origin.

Prognosis

Patients with extranasal disease have a poorer prognosis than those with disease limited to the sinonasal area.[60] A recent study showed cell size and CD30 expression as possible adverse prognostic factors, with larger cell size worse.[61] Effective treatment regimens combine one or more therapies, including radiation with chemotherapy, stem cell transplant, and immunotherapy.[62]

NK-CELL ENTEROPATHY/LYMPHOMATOID GASTROPATHY

Gross and Microscopic Features

NK-cell enteropathy, also known as lymphomatoid gastropathy, is a recently described benign condition that can mimic extranodal NK/T-cell lymphoma and occurs in the GI tract. Approximately 18 cases have been described in the literature.[63–65] These patients present clinically with vague abdominal complaints. Biopsies reveal ulcerated mucosa in the stomach, small intestine, and colon. Histologically, the findings consist of a superficial infiltrate of intermediate to large-sized cells, typically with intact muscularis mucosae. The cells may focally obliterate the normal architecture or the architecture may be preserved. The cells are homogeneous and lack prominent nucleoli. Immunophenotypically, they express cCD3, CD56, and

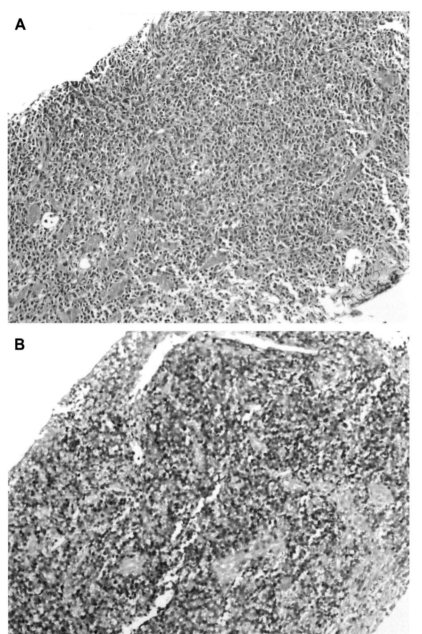

Fig. 12. Extranodal NK/T-cell lymphoma involving liver. (*A*) H&E section, 200× original magnification. (*B*) In situ hybridization for Epstein-Barr virus encoded RNA (EBER), 200× original magnification.

variable CD2. In situ hybridization for EBER is negative.

These proliferations are of unknown cause; however, it is postulated that this may be an unusual inflammatory condition, because NK cells are involved in adaptive immunity.[66] To avoid misdiagnosing these cases as NK/T-cell lymphoma, several features are helpful. The cells do not show the angiodestructive and angioinvasive features of NK/T-cell lymphomas. Necrosis is not present, although there may be individual cell apoptosis. T-cell receptor gene rearrangement studies are negative. Perhaps most importantly, EBV is not expressed. Finally, the superficial nature of the infiltrate is also an important feature. These lesions can recur and persist over months to years without progression. None of the patients described in the largest series has died from disease.

△△ **Differential Diagnosis**
of **GI Lymphomas—Reactive Mimics**

1. Florid *H pylori* gastritis
2. Prominent lymphoid aggregate (particularly involving ileocecal valve)
3. Peyer patches
4. Indolent NK-cell proliferations

Differential Diagnosis and Prognosis

The differential diagnosis includes extranodal NK/T-cell lymphoma, which often involves the GI tract, EATL, and peripheral T-cell lymphoma not otherwise specified. Because the original series of patients only included 8 cases with a median follow-up of 30 months, this is a new and evolving area in the realm of hematopathology.[65]

△△ **Differential Diagnosis**
of **GI Lymphomas—Histologic Features**

Lymphoma Type	Cells	Immunophenotype	Clinical Behavior
Extranodal marginal zone lymphoma of MALT lymphoma	Small monocytoid or centrocyte-like morphology, ± plasma cells	CD20+, CD5−, CD10−, CD43±	Indolent, often responds to antibiotic therapy
PIFL	Small centrocytes admixed with larger centroblasts	CD20+, CD10+, BCL6+, bcl-2+	Indolent behavior if limited to GI tract; may not require treatment
Mantle cell	Typically small to intermediate-sized, angulated lymphocytes; may be blastoid or pleomorphic (large)	CD20+, CD5+, CD43+, cyclin D1+, FMC7+	Typically more aggressive than other B-cell non-Hodgkin lymphomas of small cells; indolent cases exist
DLBCL	Sheets of large cells	GCB: CD20+, CD10+, BCL6+, GCET+, LMO2+ ABC: CD20+, BCL6±, CD10−, MUM-1+,	Aggressive but may be cured with chemotherapy
Burkitt lymphoma	Homogeneous, intermediate-sized cells, inconspicuous nucleoli	CD20+, CD10+, bcl-2−, Ki-67 ∼100%	Aggressive but may be cured with chemotherapy
BCL-U	Variable morphology, intermediate to large cells	CD20+, CD10+, Ki-67 varies, typically >80%, bcl-2±	Very aggressive
EATL, classic type	Large pleomorphic cells	CD3+, CD5−CD4−, CD7+, CD8±, CD103+	Aggressive
EATL type II	Small to intermediate-sized cells	CD3+, CD5−, CD7+, CD8+, CD56+	Aggressive
Extrandodal NK/T-cell lymphoma, nasal type	Intermediate-sized to large-sized cells	CD2+, CD3ε+, CD7±, CD56+, EBER+	Aggressive if widespread (extranasal)
NK-cell enteropathy/ lymphomatoid gastropathy	Intermediate-sized to large-sized cells	CD2+, CD3ε+, CD56+, EBER−	Indolent (not neoplastic)

Pitfalls

! Rebiopsy for MALT lymphoma after diagnosis should not be done too soon, because it takes time for the lymphoid infiltrates to resolve. Biopsies should not be performed before 8 weeks after diagnosis.

! Mantle cell lymphoma may be CD5 negative. In cases of lymphomatous polyposis clinically, it is important to do a cyclin D1 immunostain to exclude mantle cell lymphoma.

! DLBCL can be difficult to differentiate from BCL-U. In cases of high proliferative rate or *MYC* protein, cases that are CD10 positive may benefit from FISH studies for *MYC, BCL2//IGH* translocation, and *BCL6* rearrangement.

! EATL may express CD30 and be misdiagnosed as anaplastic large cell lymphoma. Anaplastic large cell lymphoma should have diffuse and uniform expression of CD30. It is often more focal in EATL.

! NK-cell enteropathy/lymphomatoid gastropathy may be misdiagnosed as NK/T-cell lymphoma. EBER should be positive in NK/T-cell lymphoma and negative in NK-cell enteropathy/lymphomatoid gastropathy.

SUMMARY

The GI tract is an important site of extranodal non-Hodgkin lymphoma. The entities reviewed are either classically or commonly seen in this location. Although many of these entities are well established, such as MALT lymphoma, DLBCL, and NK/T-cell lymphoma, others are evolving. BCL-U is an area of active research into the proper diagnostic criteria and therapeutic interventions. EATL type II and NK-cell enteropathy are rare entities that require additional study.

REFERENCES

1. Cirillo M, Federico M, Curci G, et al. Primary gastrointestinal lymphoma: a clinicopathological study of 58 cases. Haematologica 1992;77:156–61.

2. Howell JM, Auer-Grzesiak I, Zhang J, et al. Increasing incidence rates, distribution and histological characteristics of primary gastrointestinal non-Hodgkin lymphoma in a North American population. Can J Gastroenterol 2012;26:452–6.

3. Bhandari A, Crowe SE. Helicobacter pylori in gastric malignancies. Curr Gastroenterol Rep 2012;14:489–96.

4. Wohrer S, Troch M, Streubel B, et al. Pathology and clinical course of MALT lymphoma with plasmacytic differentiation. Ann Oncol 2007;18:2020–4.

5. Lai R, Weiss LM, Chang KL, et al. Frequency of CD43 expression in non-Hodgkin lymphoma. A survey of 742 cases and further characterization of rare CD43+ follicular lymphoma. Am J Clin Pathol 1999;111:488–94.

6. Inagaki H, Nonaka M, Nagaya S, et al. Monoclonality in gastric lymphoma detected in formalin-fixed, paraffin-embedded endoscopic biopsy specimens using immunohistochemistry, in situ hybridization, and polymerase chain reaction. Diagn Mol Pathol 1995;4:32–8.

7. Hsi ED, Greenson JK, Singleton TP, et al. Detection of immunoglobulin heavy chain gene rearrangement by polymerase chain reaction in chronic active gastritis associated with *helicobacter pylori*. Hum Pathol 1996;27:290–6.

8. Copie-Bergman C, Wotherspoon AC, Capella C, et al. Gela histological scoring system for post-treatment biopsies of patients with gastric MALT lymphoma is feasible and reliable in routine practice. Br J Hematol 2013;160:47–52.

9. Wotherspoon AC, Doglioni C, Diss TC, et al. Regression of primary low-grade B-cell gastric lymphoma of mucosa-associated lymphoid tissue type after eradicatin of *Helicobacter pylori*. Lancet 1993;342:575–7.

10. Cavalli F, Isaacson PG, Gascoyne RD, et al. MALT lymphomas. Hematology 2001;2001:241–58.

11. Montalban C, Santon A, Boixeda C, et al. Treatment of low grade gastric mucosa-associated lymphoid tissue lymphoma in stage I with Helicobacter pylori eradication. Long-term results after sequential histologic and molecular follow-up. Haematologica 2001;86:609–17.

12. Auer IA, Gascoyne RD, Conners JM, et al. t(11;18)(q21;21) is the most common translocation in MALT lymphomas. Ann Oncol 1997;8:979–85.

13. Streubel B, Lamprecht A, Dierlamm J, et al. t(14;18)(q32;q21) involving IGH and MALT1 is a frequent chromosomal aberration in MALT lymphoma. Blood 2003;101:2335–9.

14. Sanchez-Izquierdo D, Buchonnet G, Siebert R, et al. MALT1 is deregulated by both chromosomal

translocation and amplification in B-cell non-Hodgkin lymphoma. Blood 2003;101:4539–46.

15. Remstein ED, Dogan A, Einerson RR, et al. The incidence and anatomic site specificity of chromosomal translocations in primary extranodal marginal zone B-cell lymphoma of mucosa-associated lymphoid tissue (MALT lymphoma) in North America. Am J Surg Pathol 2006;30:1546–53.

16. Willis TG, Jadayel DM, Du MQ, et al. Bcl10 is involved in t(1;14)(p22;q32) of MALT B cell lymphoma and mutated in multiple tumor types. Cell 1999;96:35–45.

17. Liu H, Ruskon-Fourmestraux A, Lavergne-Slove A, et al. Resistance of t(11;18) positive gastric mucosa-associated lymphoid tissue to Helicobacter pylori eradication therapy. Lancet 2001;357:39–40.

18. Okada H, Takemoto M, Kawahara Y, et al. A prospective analysis of the efficacy and long-term outcome of radiation therapy for gastric mucosa-associated lymphoid tissue lymphoma. Digestion 2012;86:179–86.

19. Liu Z, Dong HY, Gorczyca W, et al. CD5- mantle cell lymphoma. Am J Clin Pathol 2002;118:216–24.

20. Muller-Hermelink HK, Montserrat E, Catovsky D, et al. Chronic lymphocytic leukemia/small lymphocytic lymphoma. In: Swerdlow SH, Campo E, Harris NL, et al, editors. WHO classification of tumours of the haematopoietic and lymphoid tissues. 4th edition. Lyon (France): IARC; 2008. p. 180–2.

21. Kuo SH, Yeh KH, Wu MS, et al. Helicobacter pylori eradication therapy is effective in the treatment of early-stage H. pylori-positive gastric diffuse large B-cell lymphomas. Blood 2012;119:4838–44.

22. Misdraji J, Harris NL, Hasserjian RP, et al. Primary follicular lymphoma of the gastrointestinal tract. Am J Surg Pathol 2011;35:1255–63.

23. Harris NL, Swerdlow SH, Jaffe ES, et al. Follicular lymphoma. In: Swerdlow SH, Campo E, Harris NL, et al, editors. WHO classification of tumours of the haematopoietic and lymphoid tissues. 4th edition. Lyon (France): IARC; 2008. p. 220–6.

24. Yoshino T, Myake K, Ichimura K, et al. Increased incidence of follicular lymphoma in the duodenum. Am J Surg Pathol 2000;24:688–93.

25. Takata K, Sato Y, Nakamura N, et al. Duodenal and nodal follicular lymphomas are distinct: the former lacks activation-induced cytadine deaminase and follicular dendritic cells despite ongoing somatic hypermutation. Mod Pathol 2009;22:940–9.

26. Damaj G, Verkarre V, Delmer A, et al. Primary follicular lymphoma of the gastrointestinal tract: a study of 25 cases and a literature review. Ann Oncol 2003;14:623–9.

27. Mori M, Kobayashi Y, Maeshima AM, et al. The indolent course and high incidence of t(14;18) in primary duodenal follicular lymphoma. Ann Oncol 2010;21:1500–5.

28. Shia J, Teruya-Feldstein J, Pan D, et al. Primary follicular lymphoma of the gastrointestinal tract: a clinical and pathologic study of 26 cases. Am J Surg Pathol 2002;26:216–24.

29. Kim JH, Jung HW, Kang KJ, et al. Endoscopic findings in mantle cell lymphoma with gastrointestinal tract involvement. Acta Haematol 2012;127:129–34.

30. Carvajal-Cuenca A, Sua LF, Silva NM, et al. In situ mantle cell lymphoma: clinical implications of an incidental finding with indolent clinical behavior. Haematologica 2012;97:270–8.

31. Neto AG, Oroszi G, Protiva P, et al. Colonic in situ mantle cell lymphoma. Ann Diagn Pathol 2012;16:508–14.

32. Mozos A, Royo C, Hartmann E, et al. SOX11 expression is highly specific for mantle cell lymphoma and identifies the cyclin D1-negative subtype. Haematologica 2009;94:1555–62.

33. Ek S, Dictor M, Jerkeman M, et al. Nuclear expression of the non B-cell lineage SOX11 transcription factor identifies mantle cell lymphoma. Blood 2008;11:800–5.

34. Zeng W, Fu K, Guintanilla-Fend L, et al. Cyclin D1-negative blastoid mantle cell lymphoma identified by SOX11 expression. Am J Surg Pathol 2012;36:214–9.

35. Fernandez V, Salamero O, Espinet B, et al. Genomic and gene expression profiling defines indolent forms of mantle cell lymphoma. Cancer Res 2010;70:1408–18.

36. Ondrejka SL, Lai R, Smith SD, et al. Indolent mantle cell leukemia: a clinicopathological variant characterized by isolated lymphocytosis, interstitial bone marrow involvement, kappa light chain restriction, and good prognosis. Haematologica 2011;96:1121–7.

37. Nygren L, Wennerhold SB, Klimkowska M, et al. Prognostic role of SOX11 in a population-based cohort of mantle cell lymphoma. Blood 2012;119:4215–23.

38. Orchard J, Garand R, Davis Z, et al. A subset of t(11;14) lymphoma with mantle cell features displays mutated IgVH genes and includes patients with good prognosis, nonnodal disease. Blood 2003;101:4975–81.

39. Wright G, Tan B, Rosenwald A, et al. A gene expression-based method to diagnose clinically distinct subgroups of diffuse large B-cell lymphoma. Proc Natl Acad Sci U S A 2003;100:9991–6.

40. Hans CP, Weisenburger DD, Greiner TC, et al. Confirmation of the molecular classification of diffuse large B-cell lymphoma by immunohistochemistry using a tissue microarray. Blood 2004;103:275–82.

41. Choi WW, Weisenburger DD, Greiner TC, et al. A new immunostain algorithm classifies diffuse large

B-cell lymphoma into molecular subtypes with high accuracy. Clin Cancer Res 2009;15:5494–502.

42. Natkunam Y, Farinha P, Hsi ED, et al. LMO2 protein expression predicts survival in patients with diffuse large B-cell lymphoma treated with anthracycline-based chemotherapy with and without rituximab. J Clin Oncol 2008;26:447–54.

43. Meyer PN, Fu K, Greiner TC, et al. Immunohisto-chemical methods for predicting cell of origin and survival in patients with diffuse large B-cell lymphoma treated with rituximab. J Clin Oncol 2011; 29:200–7.

44. Said JW. Aggressive B-cell lymphomas: how many categories do we need? Mod Pathol 2013; 26(Suppl 1):S42–56.

45. Seegmiller AC, Garcia R, Huang R, et al. Simple karyotype and bcl-6 expression predict a diagnosis of Burkitt lymphoma and better survival in IG-MYC rearranged high grade B-cell lymphomas. Mod Pathol 2010;23:909–20.

46. Kluin PM, Harris NL, Stein H, et al. B-cell lymphoma, unclassifiable, with features intermediate between diffuse large B-cell lymphoma and Burkitt lymphoma. In: Swerdlow SH, Campo E, Harris NL, et al, editors. WHO classification of tumours of the haematopoietic and lymphoid tissues. 4th edition. Lyon (France): IARC; 2008. p. 265–6.

47. Dave SS, Fu K, Wright GW, et al. Molecular diagnosis of Burkitt's lymphoma. N Engl J Med 2006; 354:2431–42.

48. Hummel M, Bentink S, Berger H, et al. A biologic definition of Burkitt's lymphoma from transcriptional and genomic profiling. N Engl J Med 2006;354:2419–30.

49. Mationg-Kalaw E, Tan LH, Tay K, et al. Does the proliferation fraction help identify mature B cell lymphomas with double- and triple-hit translocations? Histopathology 2012;61:1214–8.

50. Li S, Fayad LE, Lennon PA, et al. B-cell lymphomas with MYC/8q24 rearrangements and IGH@BCL2/t(14;18)(q32;q21): an aggressive disease with heterogeneous histology, germinal center B-cell immunophenotype and poor outcome. Mod Pathol 2012; 25:145–56.

51. Friedberg JW. Double-hit diffuse large B-cell lymphoma. J Clin Oncol 2012;28:3439–43.

52. Isaacson PG, Chott A, Ott G, et al. Enteropathy-associated T-cell lymphoma. In: Swerdlow SH, Campo E, Harris NL, et al, editors. WHO classification of tumours of the haematopoietic and lymphoid tissues. 4th edition. Lyon (France): IARC; 2008. p. 289–91.

53. Chott A, Haedicke WW, Mosberger I, et al. Most CD56+ intestinal lymphomas are CD8+ CD5- T-cell lymphomas of monomorphic small to medium size histology. Am J Pathol 1998;153:1483–90.

54. Rubio-Tapia A, Murray JA. Classification and management of refractory coeliac disease. Gut 2010; 59:547–57.

55. de Mascarel A, Belleannee G, Stanislas S, et al. Mucosal intraepithelial T-lymphocytes in refractory celiac disease: a neoplastic population with a variable CD8 phenotype. Am J Surg Pathol 2008;32: 744–51.

56. Chan JK, Chan AC, Cheuk W, et al. Type II enteropathy-associated T-cell lymphoma: A distinct aggressive lymphoma with frequent γδ T-cell receptor expression. Am J Surg Pathol 2011;35:1557–69.

57. Tse E, Gill H, Loong F, et al. Type II enteropathy-associated T-cell lymphoma: a multicenter analysis from the Asia Lymphoma Study Group. Am J Hematol 2012;87:663–8.

58. Li S, Feng X, Li T, et al. Extranodal NK/T-cell lymphoma, nasal type: a report of 73 cases at MD Anderson Cancer Center. Am J Surg Pathol 2013;37: 14–23.

59. Chan JK, Quintanilla-Martinez L, Ferry JA, et al. Extranodal NK/T-cell lymphoma, nasal type. In: Swerdlow SH, Campo E, Harris NL, et al, editors. WHO classification of tumours of the haematopoietic and lymphoid tissues. 4th edition. Lyon (France): IARC; 2008. p. 285–8.

60. Au WY, Weisenburger DD, Intragumtornchai T, et al. Clinical differences between nasal and extranasal natural killer/T-cell lymphoma: a study of 136 cases from the International Peripheral T-cell Lymphoma Project. Blood 2009;113:3931–7.

61. Hong J, Park S, Baek HL, et al. Tumor cell nuclear diameter and CD30 expression as potential prognostic parameters in patients with extranodal NK/T-cell lymphoma, nasal-type. Int J Clin Exp Pathol 2012;5:939–47.

62. Lee J, Cho SG, Chung SM, et al. Retrospective analysis of treatment outcomes for extranodal NK/T-cell lymphoma (ENKL), nasal type, stage I-IIE: single institute experience of combined modality treatment for early localized nasal extranodal NK/T-cell lymphoma (ENKL). Ann Hematol 2013; 92(3):333–43.

63. Tanaka T, Megahed N, Takata K, et al. A case of lymphomatoid gastropathy: an indolent CD56-positive atypical gastric lymphoid proliferation, mimicking aggressive NK/T cell lymphomas. Pathol Res Pract 2011;207:786–9.

64. Takeuchi K, Yokoyama M, Ishizawa S, et al. Lymphomatoid gastropathy: a distinct clinicopathologic entity of self-limited pseudomalignant NK-cell proliferation. Blood 2010;116:5631–7.

65. Mansoor A, Pittaluga S, Beck PL, et al. NK-cell enteropathy: a benign NK-cell lymphoproliferative disease mimicking intestinal lymphoma: Clinicopathologic features and follow-up in a unique case series. Blood 2011;117:1447–52.

66. Vivier E, Tomasello E, Baratin M, et al. Functions of natural killer cells. Nat Immunol 2008;9(5): 503–10.

Mesenchymal Tumors of the Gastrointestinal Tract Other than GIST

Leona A. Doyle, MD, Jason L. Hornick, MD, PhD*

KEYWORDS

- Mesenchymal tumor • GIST • Gastrointestinal tract • Sarcoma

ABSTRACT

Mesenchymal tumors involve the gastrointestinal (GI) tract more frequently than other visceral organs. Many such tumors are small and benign, and are increasingly being detected incidentally during colonoscopic screening. Some tumors show distinctive features at this site, such as schwannoma and clear cell sarcoma–like tumor of the GI tract. Without knowledge of these features, recognition of these tumor types can be difficult. This review addresses recent developments and diagnostic features of mesenchymal tumors of the GI tract other than gastrointestinal stromal tumor (GIST).

OVERVIEW

Two groups of benign mesenchymal lesions frequently encountered in biopsy specimens from the gastrointestinal (GI) tract are lipomas and vascular lesions. Lipomas may arise at any site in the GI tract but are particularly common in the right colon, where they may be either mucosal or submucosal, and predominantly occur in elderly female patients.[1,2] Lipoma consists of a well-circumscribed proliferation of mature adipocytes (**Fig. 1**). The overlying epithelium may show mild regenerative changes, potentially mimicking a hyperplastic polyp. Rarely, patients develop multiple lipomas throughout the GI tract, so-called lipomatous polyposis.[3]

Vascular proliferations, including hemangiomas, vascular malformations, and lymphangiomas, are most common in the small and large intestines. Lymphangioma consists of discrete dilated thin-walled lymphatics that usually involve the mucosa and submucosa and may occasionally extend into the muscularis propria (**Fig. 2**). Vascular malformations are congenital lesions that consist of thin- and thick-walled veins and arteries of variable caliber. Angiodysplasia is an acquired lesion that occurs mainly in elderly patients and is typically found in the submucosa of the right colon.[4] It consists of a discrete cluster of dilated, tortuous veins and venules. The distinction between a hemangioma and angiodysplasia is somewhat arbitrary.

The diagnosis of lipoma and vascular lesions involving the GI tract is usually straightforward; as such, they are not discussed in further detail in this review.

One of the most commonly encountered mesenchymal tumors of the GI tract in surgical pathology practice is gastrointestinal stromal tumor (GIST). Over the past decade, great progress has been made in improving recognition of this tumor, understanding its molecular pathogenesis, and in the development of effective targeted systemic therapies. Recent developments in the understanding of GIST pathogenesis have included the identification of defects in the succinate dehydrogenase enzyme complex in a clinically and pathologically distinctive subset of GIST wild type for *KIT* and *PDGFRA* mutations,[5–9] and the identification of *BRAF* mutations in approximately 10% of wild-type GISTs.[10–13] The purpose of this review is to address recent developments and diagnostic features of non-GIST mesenchymal tumors that involve the GI tract. Many of these tumors fall into the morphologic differential diagnosis with GIST; thus, recognition of these tumors is essential in the evaluation of any suspected mesenchymal neoplasm occurring in the GI tract.

Department of Pathology, Brigham and Women's Hospital, Harvard Medical School, 75 Francis Street, Boston, MA 02115, USA

* Corresponding author.
E-mail address: jhornick@partners.org

Surgical Pathology 6 (2013) 425–473
http://dx.doi.org/10.1016/j.path.2013.05.003
1875-9181/13/$ – see front matter © 2013 Elsevier Inc. All rights reserved.

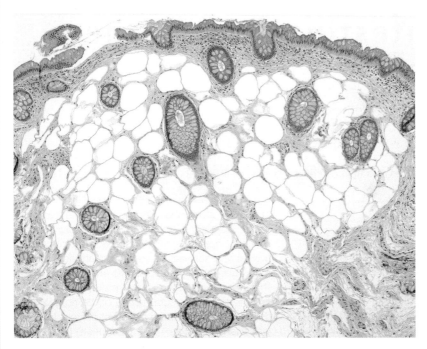

Fig. 1. Mucosal lipoma composed of mature fat surrounding colonic crypts.

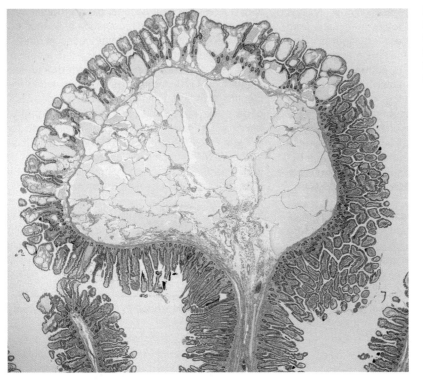

Fig. 2. Lymphangioma of the small intestine consisting of variably sized dilated lymphatics within the mucosa and submucosa.

SMOOTH MUSCLE TUMORS—LEIOMYOMA

OVERVIEW

Leiomyoma, a benign pure smooth muscle tumor, is the second most common mesenchymal tumor of the GI tract after GIST. Leiomyoma is the most common spindle cell neoplasm of the esophagus. Leiomyoma occurs less frequently, however, at other sites in the GI tract, and, after the esophagus, the most commonly involved site is the colorectum. Involvement of the stomach and small intestine is rare, unlike GIST which occurs most often at these sites. Diffuse leiomyomatosis is rare and may arise sporadically or as part of a familial syndrome, such as Alport syndrome; children and young adults are most often affected.[14,15]

In the esophagus, leiomyomas are most common in young adults, with a median patient age of 35 years.[16] There is a slight male predilection. The distal segment is involved in approximately 80% of cases, followed by the mid and proximal segments. The most common presenting symptom is dysphagia, with occasional cases identified as incidental findings. In the colon and rectum, patients are usually older, with a median age of 62 years, and there is a marked male predominance.[17] Leiomyomas of the colon and rectum are usually small, and are therefore more often identified incidentally, during colonoscopic screening, but they may present with lower GI bleeding. Tumors arise most often in the rectum and sigmoid (75% of cases), followed by the descending and transverse colon.[17]

Key Features
LEIOMYOMA

- Benign smooth muscle neoplasm
- Commonest mesenchymal tumor of esophagus and colon
- Well-circumscribed fascicles of smooth muscle
- Diffuse expression of smooth muscle actin (SMA) and desmin

GROSS FEATURES

Leiomyomas are well circumscribed and have a firm, white, often lobulated, cut surface, resembling uterine leiomyoma. In the esophagus, the median tumor size is 5 cm, with a range of less than 1 cm to 18 cm.[16] In the colon and rectum, leiomyomas are significantly smaller, with a median size of 0.4 cm and a range of 0.1 cm to 2 cm.[17]

MICROSCOPIC FEATURES

Leiomyomas of the esophagus arise within the muscularis propria,[16] whereas those of the colon and rectum involve the muscularis mucosae, with only rare cases occurring within the muscularis propria.[18] The tumors are well circumscribed and composed of bland, well-differentiated smooth muscle cells and, as such, show a fascicular growth pattern of spindle cells with brightly eosinophilic cytoplasm and blunt-ended, cigar-shaped nuclei with fine chromatin (**Fig. 3**). There is at most minimal cytologic atypia and mitotic activity is absent or low. Tumor necrosis is not seen. Occasional tumors may show nuclear atypia and, without any other worrisome histologic features, are considered analogous to so-called symplastic leiomyoma, lacking potential for an adverse outcome.[17] Scattered admixed eosinophils and mast cells are frequently present. In most cases, the overlying epithelium is intact.

Leiomyomas show diffuse expression of SMA, desmin, and caldesmon in all cases and are negative for S100, CD34, and KIT (see **Fig. 3**).[16] Care must be taken to avoid overinterpretation of KIT positivity in mast cells, which may be abundant in leiomyoma and, therefore, to avoid an erroneous diagnosis of GIST, which is rare in the esophagus.

DIAGNOSIS AND DIFFERENTIAL DIAGNOSIS

In most cases, the diagnosis of leiomyoma is straightforward. In small biopsies, however, the differential diagnosis of GIST may be considered. As discussed previously, GIST involving the esophagus is rare, but the finding of KIT expression in mast cells in leiomyoma is a diagnostic pitfall in this regard. The spindled cells of GIST have tapering nuclei and pale cytoplasm, in contrast to the blunt-ended nuclei and brightly eosinophilic cytoplasm of leiomyoma. The vast majority of GISTs are positive for KIT, DOG1, and CD34, all of which are negative in leiomyoma.[19,20]

Leiomyosarcoma may be a diagnostic consideration, and, in small biopsies, distinguishing between leiomyoma and well-differentiated leiomyosarcoma may not be possible. In such cases, examination of the excision specimen usually allows for distinction between the two, as leiomyosarcoma shows infiltrative growth, atypia, pleomorphism, necrosis, and high mitotic activity.

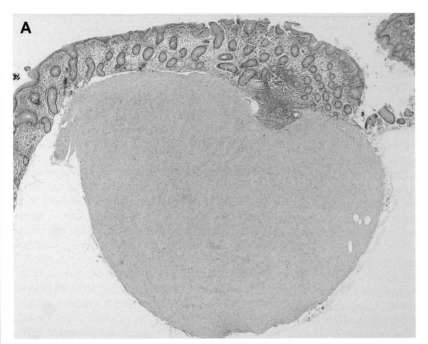

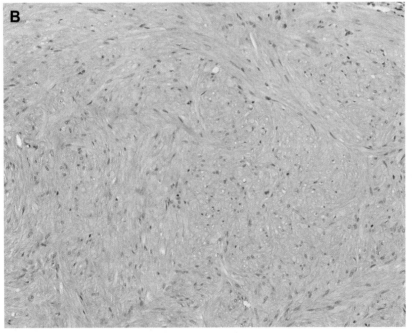

Fig. 3. Leiomyoma associated with the muscularis mucosae of the colon, showing sharp circumscription (*A*) and fascicles of bland spindle cells with abundant eosinophilic cytoplasm and blunt-ended nuclei (*B*).

Fig. 3. Tumor cells are diffusely and strongly positive for SMA (*C*) and desmin (*D*).

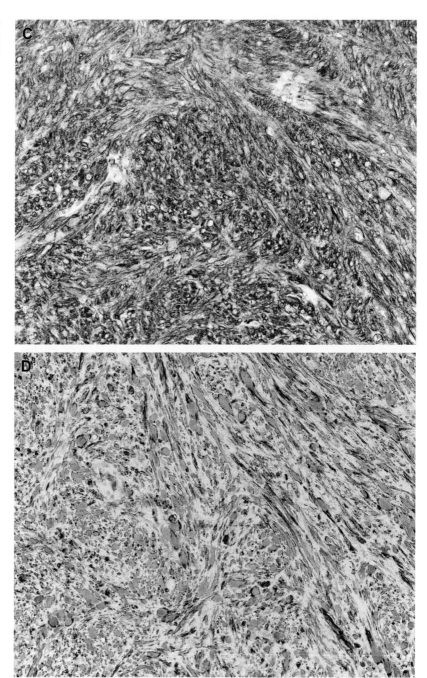

PROGNOSIS

Leiomyomas are benign tumors. Recurrence is rare; thus, complete excision (or enucleation) is curative in the majority of cases.

> ### Pitfalls
> LEIOMYOMA
>
> ! Abundant KIT-positive mast cells in esophageal leiomyoma may lead to an erroneous diagnosis of GIST
>
> ! Leiomyoma may be difficult or impossible to distinguish from well-differentiated leiomyosarcoma in small biopsies

SMOOTH MUSCLE TUMORS—LEIOMYOSARCOMA

OVERVIEW

Primary leiomyosarcoma of the GI tract is rare. Prior to its recognition, many GISTs were thought to represent leiomyosarcoma. Among spindle cell neoplasms of the stomach and small and large intestines, GIST is far more common than leiomyosarcoma.[18] When occurring in the GI tract, leiomyosarcoma arises most frequently in the colon, followed by small intestine and esophagus. Patients are usually middle-aged to elderly adults, with a median age of 60 years.[21] No apparent gender predilection is seen. Presenting symptoms are related to a mass lesion and depend on the anatomic site of involvement, and, therefore, include upper or lower GI bleeding, dysphagia, or obstruction. In the colon, leiomyosarcoma seems to arise in the right colon more often than the left.[21]

> ### Key Features
> LEIOMYOSARCOMA
>
> - Extremely rare tumor of the GI tract
> - Most cases arise in the colon or small intestine
> - Fascicles of smooth muscle cells with varying degrees of atypia, pleomorphism, necrosis, and mitotic activity
> - Diffuse expression of SMA and variable expression of desmin and caldesmon
> - Aggressive tumor with a poor prognosis

GROSS FEATURES

Leiomyosarcomas are usually large, ranging from 3 cm to 19 cm, with an average size of 6 cm. Tumors are variably circumscribed and/or infiltrative and are predominantly centered in the muscularis propria. Extension through serosa and into mucosa occurs occasionally. In many cases of colonic leiomyosarcoma, the tumor forms a polypoid intraluminal mass. The cut surface is variably tan, white, and firm, and necrosis may be present.

MICROSCOPIC FEATURES

The morphologic appearance of GI leiomyosarcoma is similar to leiomyosarcoma occurring at other sites. Tumors are composed of fascicles of spindle cells showing varying degrees of smooth muscle differentiation, with brightly eosinophilic cytoplasm and blunt-ended nuclei. In contrast to leiomyoma, leiomyosarcoma shows nuclear atypia, cytologic pleomorphism, high cellularity, tumor necrosis, and high mitotic activity (**Fig. 4**). Depending on the tumor grade, the degree of all these features may vary. Ulceration of overlying mucosa is common, and, rarely, infiltration of tumor between crypts or glands is present.

Consistent with its line of differentiation, the tumor cells of leiomyosarcoma show expression of SMA, usually in a multifocal or diffuse pattern. Desmin is less frequently positive, with expression seen in 70% to 80% of cases. Caldesmon shows variable expression in leiomyosarcoma, present in approximately 50% of cases. CD34, KIT, and S100 are usually negative, but focal CD34 expression is occasionally present.[18,21] Cytokeratin expression is found in 30% to 40% of leiomyosarcomas.[22,23]

DIAGNOSIS AND DIFFERENTIAL DIAGNOSIS

When approaching a smooth muscle neoplasm of the GI tract, the most common differential diagnosis is with GIST, particularly because GIST is more common than leiomyosarcoma, but also because both tumors may show morphologic overlap and GIST often shows expression of SMA and, less commonly, desmin. In contrast to leiomyosarcoma, however, the tumor cells of GIST have palely eosinophilic and syncytial cytoplasm, and the nuclei have a more slender and tapering appearance. Immunohistochemistry can readily distinguish the two: the vast majority of GISTs are positive for KIT and DOG1, both of which are negative in leiomyosarcoma.[19,20]

Another consideration when approaching an apparently malignant smooth muscle neoplasm in an intra-abdominal location is smooth muscle

Fig. 4. Jejunal leiomyo-sarcoma composed of fascicles of spindle cells with cytologic atypia and pleomorphism; the brightly eosinophilic cytoplasm and blunt-ended nuclei suggest smooth muscle differen-tiation (*A*). Nuclear aty-pia and scattered pleomorphic cells are also present (*B*).

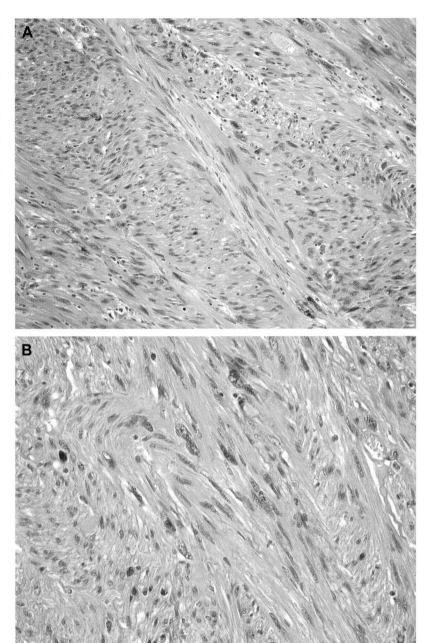

differentiation in dedifferentiated liposarcoma. This is especially so if the mass is predominantly centered on the serosa and appears to be invading from outside the bowel wall. In such cases, evaluation for overexpression or amplification of MDM2 and CDK4, characteristic of dedifferentiated liposarcoma, by immunohisto-chemistry and/or fluorescence in situ hybridiza-tion (FISH), respectively, can resolve this differential diagnosis.

Differential Diagnosis
LEIOMYOSARCOMA

- GIST: pale indistinct cytoplasm, tapering nuclei, positive for KIT and DOG1
- Inflammatory myofibroblastic tumor (IMT): tapering nuclei, prominent inflammatory infiltrate, ALK expression in 50%
- Dedifferentiated liposarcoma: predominantly extramural involvement, MDM2 and CDK4 positive

PROGNOSIS

Due to the rarity of primary leiomyosarcoma of the GI tract, data regarding prognosis are limited, but most patients have an aggressive clinical course, with death from disease occurring in the majority of patients.[16,21]

Pitfalls
LEIOMYOSARCOMA

! Cytokeratin expression in 30% to 40% of tumors

! Heterologous smooth muscle differentiation can occur in dedifferentiated liposarcoma

---

PECOMA FAMILY OF TUMORS

OVERVIEW

Perivascular epithelioid cell tumors (PEComas) are an unusual family of neoplasms that show dual smooth muscle and melanocytic differentiation. They can arise at any site, including soft tissues of extremities, visceral soft tissue (clear cell, sugar' tumor, lymphangioleiomyomatosis), kidney (angiomyolipoma), gynecologic tract, and urinary tract, as well as liver, pancreas, and GI tract.[24] Most PEComas occurring in the liver with classic appearances of angiomyolipoma are still referred to as angiomyolipoma.[25] A sclerosing variant exists and occurs virtually always in retroperitoneal soft tissue.[26] Limited data exist on PEComas occurring in the GI tract, but a majority of cases seem to occur in the colon.[27–29] In general, PEComas of visceral sites show a female predilection and typically occur in middle-aged adults, with a median patient age of 46 years.[30] Presenting

Key Features
PECOMA

- Dual smooth muscle and melanocytic differentiation
- Female predilection
- Loss of *TSC1* and *TSC2* result in up-regulation of the mTOR pathway
- Nests, sheets, or fascicles of epithelioid and/or spindled cells with abundant clear, granular, and palely eosinophilic cytoplasm
- Malignant forms of PEComa exist
- Prediction of behavior is difficult, but most malignant forms show striking atypia, high mitotic activity, ± necrosis

symptoms of PEComas involving the GI tract may include abdominal pain, GI bleeding, and obstructive symptoms. Although angiomyolipomas are often associated with tuberous sclerosis, GI PEComas are usually sporadic; in a series of 4 colonic PEComas, no patient showed evidence of this syndrome.[28] However, regardless of the presence or absence of the clinical syndrome, most PEComas show loss of *TSC1* and *TSC2*, resulting in up-regulation of the mTOR pathway, which can be targeted with mTOR inhibitors such as sirolimus.[31,32] Less frequently, translocations involving the *TFE3* gene are present.[33]

GROSS FEATURES

Tumors are usually reasonably well circumscribed but unencapsulated. The cut surface is usually white and solid and may show areas of hemorrhage. Tumor size ranges from 3 cm to 6 cm.

MICROSCOPIC FEATURES

The tumor cells of PEComa typically grow in nests, sheets, or short fascicles, and show a characteristic radial arrangement around blood vessels. The cells are variably epithelioid and/or spindled with abundant clear, granular, and palely eosinophilic cytoplasm and round vesicular nuclei with small nucleoli (**Fig. 5**). The cells may also take on a myoid appearance, having less cytoplasm and a spindled morphology. Atypia is variable within tumors; malignant forms of PEComa may show striking cytologic atypia. Mitotic activity is also variable, with malignant tumors often showing high mitotic rates, as well as necrosis.[30] The vascular network is usually prominent and composed of capillaries and small medium-sized thin-walled vessels.

Fig. 5. PEComa of the pancreas with a sheet-like and focally whorled growth pattern (*A*). Epithelioid tumor cells of a PEComa with abundant clear and granular eosinophilic cytoplasm and arrangement around a blood vessel (*B*). A spindled or myoid appearance is also common (*C*).

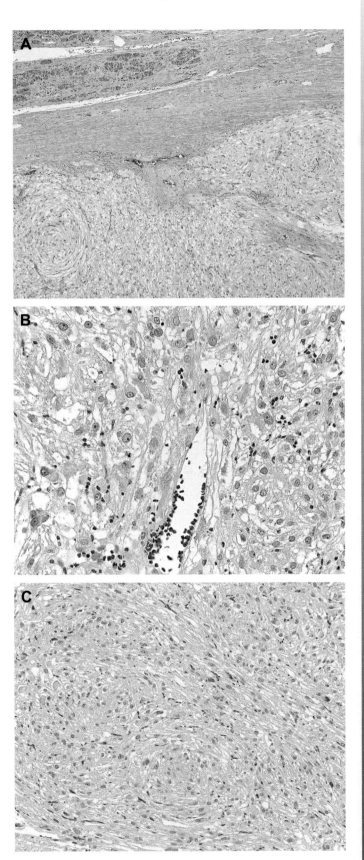

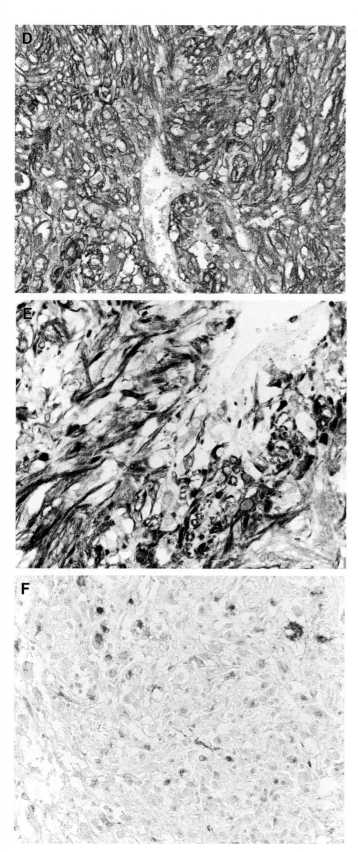

Fig. 5. Tumor cells are positive for SMA (*D*), desmin (*E*), HMB45 (*F*), and melan-A (*G*).

Fig. 5.

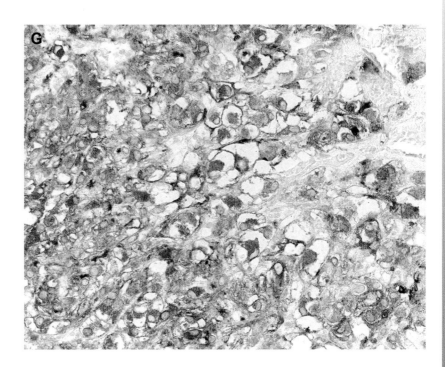

Angiomyolipoma of the liver consists of thick walled vessels, admixed epithelioid or spindled tumor cells, and variable amounts of mature fat.

Given the potentially wide differential diagnosis for these tumors, immunohistochemistry is usually needed to confirm a diagnosis of PEComa. PEComa shows immunohistochemical evidence of both myoid and melanocytic differentiation. Smooth muscle markers (alpha-isoform actin, muscle-specific actin, desmin, caldesmon, calponin, and smooth-muscle myosin) are variably expressed in terms of intensity and extent; expression of just 1 muscle marker may be seen.[34] Similarly, markers of melanocytic differentiation (HMB-45, MART-1, tyrosinase, and microphthalmia transcription factor [MiTF]) are also variably expressed (see **Fig. 5**). HMB-45 is the most frequently positive melanocytic marker. S-100 protein expression is uncommon in PEComa.[26] TFE3 protein is present in a subset of PEComas with *TFE3* gene fusions, and the presence of TFE3 expression in PEComa is generally mutually exclusive with MiTF expression.[33] KIT, keratin, and CD34 expression is typically absent.[30]

DIAGNOSIS AND DIFFERENTIAL DIAGNOSIS

The main differential diagnostic considerations of PEComa of the GI tract include pure smooth muscle tumors, epithelioid GIST, clear-cell sarcoma, paraganglioma, metastatic renal cell carcinoma, and metastatic melanoma.

Pure smooth muscle tumors of the GI tract include both leiomyoma and leiomyosarcoma. In some cases, distinction from PEComa may be impossible morphologically, particularly if the epithelioid cells of PEComa are absent. Smooth muscle tumors lack expression of HMB45, melanA/MART1, and TFE3, and thus immunohistochemistry can often readily distinguish the two.

Epithelioid GIST may also mimic PEComa; however, the tumor cells of GIST lack the granular quality of the cytoplasm and the intimate association with blood vessels typically present in PEComa. PEComa is generally negative for KIT and DOG1, whereas GIST is negative for melanocytic markers but may show focal SMA and desmin expression.

Clear cell sarcoma (CCS)-like tumor of the GI tract may occasionally mimic PEComa, given that both may be composed of spindled and epithelioid cells and that PEComa may show focal expression of S100.[26] However, CCS-like tumors lack an intimate association with blood vessels and frequently contain osteoclast-like giant cells and pseudoglandular areas. The tumor cells of CCS-like tumors show strong diffuse S100 positivity but are negative for SMA, desmin, and

Differential Diagnosis
PECOMA

- Metastatic renal cell carcinoma: PAX8 and EMA positive

- Metastatic melanoma: diffuse S100 expression, negative for SMA and desmin

- Pure smooth muscle tumors: negative for HMB-45 and melan A

- CCS-like tumor of the GI tract: S100 positive, negative for HMB-45 and melan A

- Epithelioid GIST: less cytoplasmic granularity, KIT and DOG1 positive

- Paraganglioma: synaptophysin and chromogranin positive

Pitfalls
PECOMA

! S100 expression in 10% to 20% of cases, usually focal

! Focal KIT and DOG1 expression occasionally present

melanocytic markers (unlike conventional CCS of somatic soft tissue). If doubt still exists, molecular studies to evaluate for *EWSR1* rearrangement can help confirm a diagnosis of CCS-like tumor.

Paraganglioma mimics PEComa by showing a strikingly nested growth pattern, prominent vascular network, and lesional cells that have abundant clear cytoplasm. The cells of paraganglioma express synaptophysin and chromogranin, however, and are negative for smooth muscle and melanocytic markers.

Perhaps the most common mimics of PEComa are metastatic tumors, in particular renal cell carcinoma and metastatic melanoma. Both may show a nested growth pattern, an admixture of epithelioid and spindled cells with variable amounts of clear or palely eosinophilic cytoplasm, and a prominent vascular network among tumor cells. Knowledge of the patient's clinical history is crucial, but immunohistochemistry is also invaluable. Renal cell carcinoma is positive for paired box gene 8 (PAX8) and epithelial membrane antigen (EMA), unlike PEComa. Melanoma shows more immunohistochemical variability but may show diffuse S100 positivity, variable expression of secondary melanocytic markers or may be negative for all. Melanoma is usually negative for SMA and desmin.

PROGNOSIS

PEComas are tumors of variable and somewhat unpredictable biologic potential. In most cases, they pursue a benign course, but in deep visceral soft tissues, these lesions show a range of clinical behavior ranging from benign to very aggressive; aggressive behavior may be suggested by the presence of marked atypia, high mitotic activity, or necrosis.

GLOMUS TUMOR

OVERVIEW

Glomus tumor is a mesenchymal neoplasm composed of perivascular modified smooth muscle cells. Although occurring far more commonly in peripheral soft tissues,[35] glomus tumors are well recognized to arise in the GI tract, virtually always in the stomach[36,37] but with occasional reported cases occurring in the small intestine[38,39] and colon.[37,40] In the stomach, tumors involve the antrum more frequently than the gastric corpus.[37]

GI glomus tumors occur over a broad patient age range but nearly always arise in adults, with a mean age of approximately 53 years.[37] There may be a slight female predilection for this tumor type.[37] The most common presenting symptoms are related to upper GI bleeding (melena, anemia, and rarely hematemesis) and abdominal pain or reflux-type symptoms. Patients may also present with obstruction or perforation, and some tumors are incidental findings at the time of endoscopy or surgery for other reasons.

Key Features
GLOMUS TUMOR

- Virtually all GI cases arise in the wall of stomach, antrum more than corpus

- Middle-aged adults

- Multiple nodules of cells with clear or palely eosinophilic cytoplasm and sharply defined cell borders

- Prominent dilated hemangiopericytoma-like blood vessels; tumor cells are intimately associated with the vessel walls

- Diffuse SMA expression, focal caldesmon expression; negative for desmin

- Malignant forms of gastric glomus tumor exist but are rare

GROSS FEATURES

Tumors are usually well-circumscribed intramural masses, many of which are multinodular. Tumor size is variable, ranging from 1 cm to 9 cm, with an average of 2 cm to 3 cm. The tumors may extend into the mucosal or serosal surfaces, and overlying mucosal ulceration may be present. The cut surface of glomus tumor is variably white to pink, red to brown, or rubbery in texture and may show hemorrhage. Cystic change and calcifications may be present.[37]

MICROSCOPIC FEATURES

Glomus tumor involving the GI tract is typically composed of multiple nodules of tumor cells that splay the smooth muscle of the muscularis propria apart. Within the nodules, variably dilated hemangiopericytoma-like blood vessels are present, and the tumor cells are intimately associated with the vessel walls (**Fig. 6**). The tumor cells may form solid sheets, nests, or occasionally trabeculae.[36,37] The tumors often contain variably hyalinized or collagenous stroma. Myxoid change, calcification, and metaplastic bone are occasionally seen.[37] The glomus tumor cells are round, with moderate amount of clear or palely eosinophilic cytoplasm, sharply defined cell borders, which is often the most striking feature of this tumor, and central round nuclei with fine chromatin and inconspicuous nucleoli (see **Fig. 6**). Occasionally, oncocytic change may be present, and rarely the tumor cells have a spindled morphology. Vascular invasion is present in approximately 35% of cases[37] and may represent a pattern of local growth of tumor rather than a predictor of distant metastasis. In general, nuclear atypia and necrosis are not seen, and mitotic activity is low, usually less than 1 per 50 high-power fields [HPFs].[37] Malignant forms of gastric glomus tumor exist but are rare, and may be identified by large tumor size (usually greater than 5 cm), nuclear atypia, spindled morphology, and high mitotic activity.[37,41] However, the criteria for malignancy that have been used in peripheral glomus tumors[41] do not seem to apply to GI glomus tumors, particularly size criteria, as the majority of glomus tumors greater than 2 cm in size have pursued a benign clinical course.

The immunohistochemical features of glomus tumor are consistent and reflect their modified smooth muscle nature. Diffuse or multifocal expression of SMA is present in virtually all cases and highlights the cell membranes of the tumor cells. Caldesmon positivity is found in approximately 60% of cases and is typically variable in extent (see **Fig. 6**). CD34 expression is found in 25% of cases, usually in a small subset of cells. Weak staining for synaptophysin may be found in up to 20% of gastric glomus tumors, which can lead to an erroneous diagnosis of carcinoid tumor; however, glomus tumor cells are consistently negative for chromogranin.[37] Interestingly, expression of synaptophysin does not appear to occur in glomus tumors arising at peripheral sites. Also negative are KIT, DOG1, S100, desmin, CD20, CD45, and cytokeratins.

DIAGNOSIS AND DIFFERENTIAL DIAGNOSIS

Glomus tumors may mimic carcinoid tumors, epithelioid GIST, or, less frequently lymphoma. Similar to glomus tumor, carcinoid tumor is composed of round epithelioid cells, with a variably solid, nested, or trabecular growth pattern. The finding of focal synaptophysin positivity in glomus tumor may also contribute to difficulty distinguishing the two.[37] However, carcinoid tumor is centered in the mucosa and submucosa in most cases, and the tumor cells have less-prominent cell borders and coarser nuclear chromatin than glomus tumor cells. Furthermore, unlike carcinoid tumors, glomus tumor cells are negative for chromogranin and cytokeratins.

Epithelioid GIST may mimic glomus tumor, given the similar cytomorphologic features and the possibility of multinodular growth in a subset of GIST, *succinate dehydrogenase–deficient* GIST.[6,42] The tumor cells of epithelioid GIST tend to be somewhat larger in size than those of glomus tumor, have less prominent cell borders and more abundant palely eosinophilic syncytial cytoplasm, and lack the intimate association with blood vessels seen in glomus tumor. Immunohistochemistry can readily differentiate these 2 tumor types: epithelioid GIST is usually positive for DOG1 and often expresses KIT (although staining may be weak or focal) and CD34,[6,42,43] in contrast to glomus tumor, which shows just focal positivity for CD34 in 10% to 20% of cases and is negative for KIT and DOG1. Epithelioid GIST may show expression of SMA but lacks the strong, diffuse membranous pattern seen in glomus tumor.

Less commonly, glomus tumor may resemble lymphoma, in particular extranodal marginal zone B-cell lymphoma (mucosa-associated lymphoid tissue [MALT] lymphoma). The cohesive growth pattern, prominent cell borders, and fine chromatin of glomus tumor are helpful morphologic features to distinguish the two. If doubt remains, immunohistochemistry is helpful, as glomus tumor cells are negative for CD45 and CD20, and lymphoma is negative for SMA.[37]

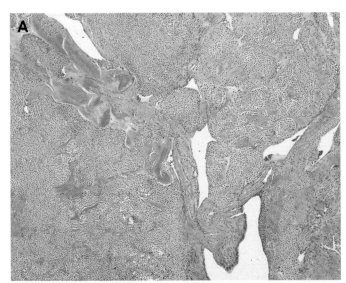

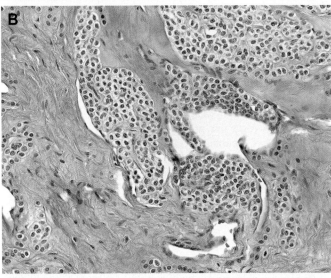

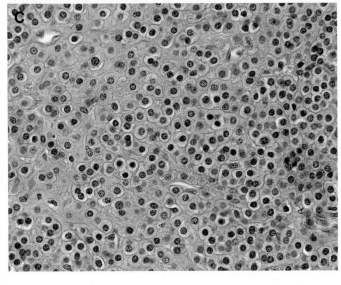

Fig. 6. Glomus tumor of the stomach showing a nested and trabecular proliferation (*A*) of round cells, which are intimately associated with vessels (*B*). The tumor cells characteristically have prominent cell borders and small, central round nuclei (*C*).

Fig. 6. Diffuse expression of SMA is seen in all cases (*D*), and focal expression of caldesmon is also frequently present (*E*).

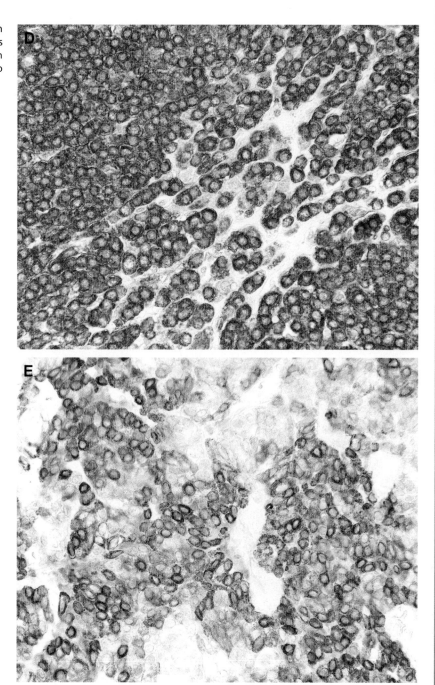

Differential Diagnosis
GLOMUS TUMOR

- Epithelioid GIST: less-prominent cell borders, KIT and DOG1 positive
- Carcinoid tumor: synaptophysin and chromogranin positive
- MALT lymphoma: less cohesive cells, positive for CD45 and CD20

PROGNOSIS

In the vast majority of cases, glomus tumor is benign and complete resection by wedge or segmental resection or partial gastrectomy is curative. However, there are at least 2 cases in the literature, however, of gastric glomus tumors that metastasized to liver and resulted in patient death. Both of those tumors were greater than 5 cm in size, and 1 showed mild atypia, spindle cell foci, and vascular invasion, but had very low mitotic activity (less than 1 per 50 HPFs).[37,41]

Pitfalls
GLOMUS TUMOR

! Synaptophysin expression in 20% of gastric glomus tumors may lead to an erroneous diagnosis of carcinoid tumor

! Difficult to predict behavior in cases with atypical histologic features

INFLAMMATORY FIBROID POLYP

OVERVIEW

Inflammatory fibroid polyps are frequently encountered mesenchymal lesions in the GI tract. Originally described by Vanek in 1949[44] as 'gastric submucosal granuloma with eosinophilic infiltration' and thought to represent a reactive process, this benign, usually solitary, polypoid lesion is now known to represent a true neoplastic process, characterized by mutations in platelet-derived growth factor receptor-alpha (*PDGFRA*).[45] Inflammatory fibroid polyps occur over a wide age range, with cases reportedly occurring in patients from ages 1 to 93 years,[46,47] with a median age of 56

Key Features
INFLAMMATORY FIBROID POLYP

- Most common in stomach, in particular, the antrum
- Characterized by mutations in *PDGFRA*
- Bland fibroblastic/myofibroblastic cells in a loose edematous myxoid and collagenous stroma
- Perivascular onionskin fibrosis
- Eosinophil-rich inflammatory infiltrate
- CD34 expression in 80%, SMA in 20%

to 66 years. There is no apparent gender predilection. The stomach and small intestine are the most commonly involved sites; the colon and esophagus are rarely affected.[46–48] Within the stomach, tumors occur most frequently in the antrum. Presenting symptoms are related to the anatomic site of involvement, but the most frequently encountered symptoms are GI bleeding, abdominal pain, and obstruction. Incidentally detected inflammatory fibroid polyps are uncommon, probably due to their large size at presentation compared with other polypoid lesions of the GI tract.[47]

GROSS FEATURES

The average size of an inflammatory fibroid polyp is 3 cm to 4 cm, with a range of 0.4 cm to 30 cm. The tumors are usually fairly well circumscribed, unencapsulated, and show a soft or firm white, yellow, or gray appearance. Tumors predominantly involve the submucosa but may extend into muscularis propria or into overlying mucosa and result in ulceration.

MICROSCOPIC FEATURES

Inflammatory fibroid polyp is composed of bland spindled and stellate cells set within a variably loose edematous myxoid and collagenous stroma containing an eosinophil-rich inflammatory infiltrate (**Fig. 7**). The lesion is centered in the submucosa but may involve mucosa or infiltrate into muscularis propria. The spindled cells are believed to be fibroblastic/myofibroblastic in nature and, as such, have small amounts of palely eosinophilic cytoplasm, slender ovoid or stellate nuclei with fine chromatin, and usually inconspicuous nucleoli. The cells tend to be loosely

Fig.   7. Inflammatory fibroid polyp frequently shows ulceration of the overlying mucosa and can mimic granulation tissue (*A*). The spindle cells are set in a loosely collagenous stroma with prominent small to medium-sized blood vessels (*B*).

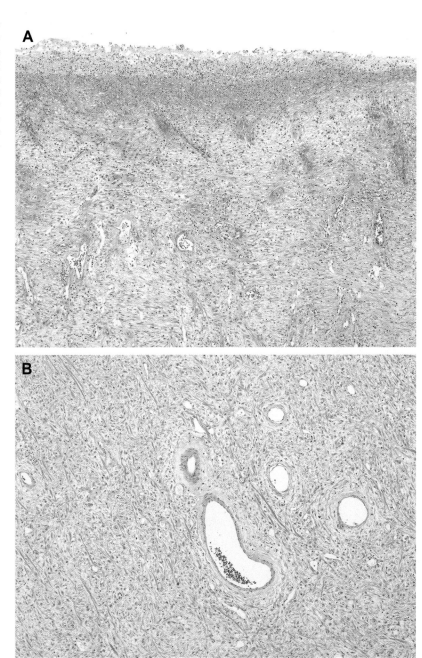

distributed in the stroma, which is usually edematous. An 'onion-skin' pattern of perivascular fibrosis is typical. There is no significant atypia or necrosis and mitotic activity is low, usually less than 2 mitoses per 50 HPFs.[46,47] Inflammatory fibroid polyp has a prominent vascular network, consisting of capillaries and thin-walled and thick-walled medium-sized blood vessels. Occlusion of some of these vessels is present in approximately 25% of cases.[47] The inflammatory infiltrate typically consists of predominantly eosinophils with some admixed lymphocytes, whereas plasma cells and neutrophils are usually not seen.

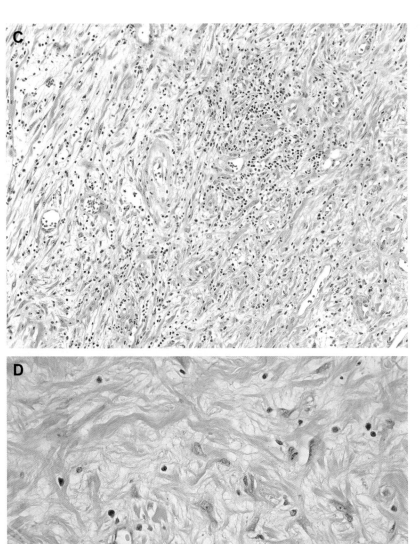

Fig. 7. Perivascular fibrosis is often present, as is a mixed inflammatory infiltrate (C). The lesional cells are bland and spindled to stellate in shape, and the inflammatory infiltrate is usually eosinophil-rich (D).

Consistent with fibroblastic/myofibroblastic differentiation, the tumor cells express CD34 in approximately 80% of cases, SMA in approximately 20% of cases, and desmin in 5%. S100, KIT, DOG1, and cytokeratins are negative.[47–50] Recent studies have documented activating PDGFRA mutations in up to 60% of inflammatory fibroid polyps occurring in exons 12, 14, and 18, similar to those seen in a subset of GISTs.[50–52] More specifically, exon 12 mutations have been found to occur more commonly in small intestinal inflammatory fibroid polyps, whereas exon 18 mutations are most often found in gastric tumors.[52] Expression of PDGFRA is seen in 95% of cases.[50]

DIAGNOSIS AND DIFFERENTIAL DIAGNOSIS

Differential diagnostic considerations for inflammatory fibroid polyp include IMT, smooth muscle tumors, and plexiform fibromyxoma as well as a reactive process.

Similar to inflammatory fibroid polyp, IMT may arise in the wall of the GI tract, is composed of spindled myofibroblastic cells, and contains a prominent admixed inflammatory infiltrate. However, in contrast to inflammatory fibroid polyp, IMT occurs in a younger age group, tends to be more infiltrative and often more cellular with a fascicular architecture, and lacks a prominent vascular network. The inflammatory infiltrate is rich in plasma cells, unlike inflammatory fibroid polyp. The spindle cells of IMT express SMA and desmin in approximately 90% and 60% of cases, respectively, and ALK expression is seen in up to 60% of cases.[53–55]

Smooth muscle tumors of the GI tract may mimic inflammatory fibroid polyp, particularly if they undergo torsion and become edematous. The presence of brightly eosinophilic cytoplasm and cigar-shaped nuclei suggest a diagnosis of smooth muscle tumor. Smooth muscle tumors also lack the eosinophilic infiltrate of inflammatory fibroid polyp. Virtually all smooth muscle tumors express SMA, desmin, and caldesmon to varying degrees and less often show CD34 positivity as compared to inflammatory fibroid polyp.

Similar to inflammatory fibroid polyp, plexiform fibromyxoma also occurs most commonly in the gastric antrum, but is predominantly intramural in location.[56,57] Plexiform fibromyxoma grows in a characteristic multinodular or plexiform pattern and is composed of bland spindle cells embedded within a variably myxoid, collagenous, and fibromyxoid stroma. In addition, the characteristic inflammatory infiltrate of inflammatory fibroid polyp is not present in plexiform fibromyxoma, and the cells of plexiform fibromyxoma are typically negative for CD34.

The appearances of inflammatory fibroid polyp often resemble granulation tissue with an associated reactive myofibroblastic proliferation. Helpful features that favor a diagnosis of inflammatory fibroid polyp over granulation tissue include condensation of the spindled cells around vessels, perivascular fibrosis, and prominent eosinophils. Clinical history is often informative. Immunohistochemical staining for PDGFRA may be useful to support a diagnosis of inflammatory fibroid polyp.

> ◭◭ **Differential Diagnosis**
> **INFLAMMATORY FIBROID POLYP**
>
> - Plexiform fibromyxoma: multinodular or plexiform growth, negative for CD34
> - IMT: more infiltrative, fascicular, and cellular; SMA positive in 90% and ALK in 50%
> - Smooth muscle tumors of the GI tract: SMA and desmin positive
> - Non-neoplastic granulation tissue

PROGNOSIS

Inflammatory fibroid polyp is a benign tumor. Local recurrences after complete resection and distant metastasis have not been described.

PLEXIFORM FIBROMYXOMA

OVERVIEW

Plexiform fibromyxoma is a morphologically distinct benign mesenchymal tumor that occurs predominantly in the stomach.[56–58] Also referred to as 'plexiform angiomyxoid myofibroblastic tumor',[56] the subsequent recognition of a significant fibrous or collagenous component in some of these tumors has led to the current designation of plexiform fibromyxoma.[57,59] Within the stomach, virtually all tumors arise in the gastric antrum, where they may extend into surrounding soft tissues or into the pylorus and duodenum. Rarely, plexiform fibromyxoma arises in the small intestine (Hornick JL, personal communication, 2010). Plexiform fibromyxoma has been reported to occur in patients of all ages, including children, but most commonly arises in the fifth decade. No gender predilection is seen. Presenting symptoms include

> **Key Features**
> **PLEXIFORM FIBROMYXOMA**
>
> - Virtually all tumors arise in the gastric antrum
> - Characteristic multinodular and plexiform pattern within muscularis propria
> - Composed of bland oval to spindled tumor cells in a myxoid, collagenous, and fibromyxoid stroma
> - Prominent vascular network
> - SMA positive in spindle cells

abdominal pain, upper or lower GI bleeding, anemia, gastric outlet obstruction, and, rarely, gastric perforation.

GROSS FEATURES

Tumors typically range in size from 2 cm to 15 cm, with a mean size of 4 cm to 5 cm, and appear as an intramural mass, which may extend into the gastric lumen or bulge externally and involve the serosal surface. Occasionally, multiple discrete subserosal nodules are present. Tumors are lobulated and variably circumscribed and the cut surface may be gray-red, tan, white, gelatinous, and glistening.

MICROSCOPIC FEATURES

Plexiform fibromyxoma arises within the muscularis propria of the stomach and shows a multinodular and plexiform growth pattern that splays the smooth muscle fibers of the muscularis propria apart (**Fig. 8**). The nodules are composed of a paucicellular or moderately cellular proliferation of bland oval to spindled tumor cells with indistinct cytoplasm, small nuclei, and inconspicuous nucleoli, embedded within a variably myxoid, collagenous, or fibromyxoid stroma. A prominent capillary proliferation is frequently present.[56,57] The tumor cells have minimal, if any, nuclear atypia. Mitotic activity is typically low, usually less than 5 per 50 HPFs.[57] Ulceration of the overlying mucosa is common. Extension of tumor into the mucosa may also occur, as may extension into the subserosa or serosa, often in the form of subserosal/serosal nodules and cellular, solid non-plexiform spindle cell proliferations. Vascular invasion was noted in 33% of tumors in 1 study but is of no apparent clinical significance.[57] Tumor necrosis is rare.

Immunohistochemically, the tumor cells are positive for α-SMA, which may be diffuse or multifocal in extent, and are virtually always negative for KIT, DOG1, CD34, and S100 protein.[56–58] However, it has been reported that some tumors show focal desmin or caldesmon expression and may correspondingly show histologic features suggestive of smooth muscle differentiation.[56,59] KIT or PDGFRA mutations are not found in plexiform fibromyxoma.[56,57]

DIAGNOSIS AND DIFFERENTIAL DIAGNOSIS

The most frequent differential diagnoses encountered with this tumor are with other neoplasms, namely, the rare myxoid variant of GIST, inflammatory fibroid polyp, myxoid variant of soft tissue perineurioma, and desmoid fibromatosis, but also with non-neoplastic reactive myofibroblastic proliferations.

Myxoid variant of GIST is uncommon and is composed of a uniform, often fascicular, proliferation of spindled or epithelioid tumor cells, without the plexiform growth pattern seen in plexiform fibromyxoma.[60] Tumor cells are positive for KIT, DOG1, and CD34, unlike those of plexiform fibromyxoma. Importantly, however, a subset of GIST, the 'succinate-dehydrogenase deficient' type, also shows a plexiform growth pattern but tends to have at least a minor component of epithelioid tumor cell morphology and is more cellular than plexiform fibromyxoma.[6,42] Succinate dehydrogenase–deficient GIST can be easily distinguished from plexiform fibromyxoma using immunohistochemistry, as the tumor cells are positive for KIT, DOG1, and CD34, similar to conventional GISTs. Additional immunohistochemistry for SDHB and SDHA can then be used to confirm a diagnosis of succinate dehydrogenase–deficient GIST.[5–9]

Inflammatory fibroid polyp also arises most commonly in the gastric antrum but is predominantly submucosal in location, unlike plexiform fibromyxoma, which is predominantly intramural.[46,47] Inflammatory fibroid polyp is also composed of bland spindle cells, but these cells characteristically form an 'onion-skin' condensation around blood vessels, and the tumor does not show a plexiform growth pattern. Furthermore, the characteristic inflammatory infiltrate, especially eosinophils, associated with inflammatory fibroid polyp is not present in plexiform fibromyxoma.

Myxoid soft tissue perineurioma is rare in the stomach but may mimic plexiform fibromyxoma histologically, and could be considered if a tumor is predominantly based outside the stomach. Soft tissue perineurioma consists of bland elongated spindle cells with delicate cytoplasmic processes, within a myxoid and variably fibrous stroma.[61] The tumor cells are typically positive for EMA, CD34, and, variably, for claudin-1, all of which highlight the long cytoplasmic processes and help distinguish it from plexiform fibromyxoma.

In needle biopsies, the differential diagnosis with desmoid fibromatosis may be encountered. Desmoid fibromatosis is characterized by long sweeping fascicles of bland spindled cells with small nucleoli and variable amounts of palely eosinophilic cytoplasm. Recognition of this pattern should allow for distinction of these two entities, and immunohistochemistry for β-catenin, which is positive in the nuclei in approximately 70% of desmoid fibromatosis cases, may also be a useful tool.[62]

Fig. 8. Plexiform fibromyxoma within the muscularis propria of the stomach, showing a multinodular and plexiform growth pattern (*A*). A prominent capillary proliferation is present within the nodules (*B*). Bland oval to spindled tumor cells with indistinct cytoplasm, small nuclei, and inconspicuous nucleoli are embedded within a myxoid stroma (*C*).

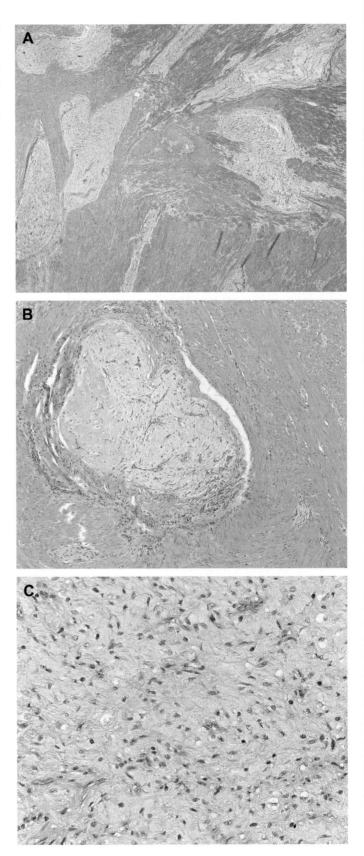

Differential Diagnosis
PLEXIFORM FIBROMYXOMA

- Myxoid GIST: KIT and DOG1 positive
- Inflammatory fibroid polyp: not plexiform/multinodular, CD34 positive
- Perineurioma: slender tapering nuclei with elongated cytoplasmic processes; EMA, claudin-1, CD34 positive
- Desmoid fibromatosis: long sweeping fascicles of spindle cells, nuclear β-catenin in 70%

Key Features
INFLAMMATORY MYOFIBROBLASTIC TUMOR

- Most common in young patients
- In the GI tract, colon and small intestine most frequently involved
- Fascicular spindle cell neoplasm composed of myofibroblastic cells
- Prominent inflammatory infiltrate composed chiefly of plasma cells and lymphocytes
- SMA positive in 90% and ALK in 50%
- Approximately 50% of IMTs show clonal rearrangements of the *ALK* gene
- Tendency to recur locally, but metastasis is rare
- Epithelioid inflammatory myofibroblastic sarcoma is a distinctive aggressive variant

Distinguishing plexiform fibromyxoma from a reactive myofibroblastic proliferation may be difficult in some cases. The presence of a predominantly intramural based process with the characteristic plexiform growth pattern favors plexiform fibromyxoma rather than a reactive process. In both cases, the lesional spindled cells may be positive for SMA, and reactive myofibroblasts may also show variable expression of desmin.

PROGNOSIS

Plexiform fibromyxoma is a benign tumor. Complete resection is typically curative, and local recurrences or metastasis have not been described. The presence of vascular invasion does not seem to be associated with an adverse outcome.

Pitfalls
PLEXIFORM FIBROMYXOMA

! Satellite nodules in serosal tissues

! Vascular invasion in one-third of tumors of no apparent clinical significance

INFLAMMATORY MYOFIBROBLASTIC TUMOR

OVERVIEW

IMT is a mesenchymal neoplasm of intermediate biologic potential that in the past was encompassed under the broad terms of *inflammatory pseudotumor* and *inflammatory fibrosarcoma*. IMT most often arises in lung or abdominal soft tissues of children and young adults, although a wide age range and anatomic distribution has been documented.[53] In the GI tract, tumors involve the colon and small intestine most frequently, followed by stomach and esophagus.[47] The average age of patients with IMT of the GI tract is 43 years, but like IMT occurring elsewhere, the range is extremely wide, spanning 9 months to 84 years in the largest study of IMT involving the GI tract to date.[47] Presenting symptoms include abdominal pain and mass lesion, and a subset of patients develops constitutional symptoms such as fever and weight loss. Abnormalities in serologic inflammatory markers, including elevated erythrocyte sedimentation rate and hypergammaglobulinemia, may be found and typically resolve after tumor resection.

Epithelioid inflammatory myofibroblastic sarcoma, a clinicopathologically distinct aggressive variant of IMT, is an intra-abdominal sarcoma with a predilection for male patients, which shows nuclear membrane or perinuclear anaplastic lymphoma kinase (ALK) expression, due to a *RANBP2-ALK* fusion that is commonly identified in this variant.[63]

GROSS FEATURES

IMT is usually infiltrative, and the average tumor size is 6 cm to 7 cm. The cut surface has a white-tan, fibrous, myxoid, or fleshy cut surface. In the GI tract, the tumor may appear to arise from the serosal aspect, may extend into the bowel wall to produce a polypoid lesion, or may be centered within the muscularis propria or submucosa.

MICROSCOPIC FEATURES

IMT is a fascicular spindle cell neoplasm, composed of myofibroblastic cells with slender tapering nuclei, small nucleoli, and variable amounts of pale indistinct cytoplasm. The tumor cells are set in a myxoid or collagenous stroma with a prominent inflammatory infiltrate composed chiefly of plasma cells and lymphocytes, and occasionally eosinophils (**Fig. 9**). There is at most mild cytologic atypia. Mitotic activity is low in IMT. Some cases show marked stromal sclerosis, resembling desmoid fibromatosis.[64] Atypical morphologic features in IMT inconsistently associated with an increased risk for adverse outcome include hypercellularity, necrosis, abundant large ganglion-like cells, multinucleated or anaplastic giant cells, pleomorphism, atypical mitoses, and necrosis.[55]

Immunohistochemically, the tumor cells of IMT show variable expression of SMA in 80% to 90% of cases and HHF-35 and desmin in up to 60% each. Approximately one-third of cases may show focal positivity for cytokeratins AE1/AE3 and CAM5.2.[53,64] S100, myogenin/myf4, MyoD1, and KIT are negative in IMT.[64] MDM2 expression is common in IMT; therefore, care should be taken in the evaluation of this marker, because the differential diagnosis of IMT with inflammatory liposarcoma may be a consideration, particularly in intra-abdominal tumors.[65] Approximately 50% of IMTs show clonal rearrangements of the *ALK* gene, a receptor tyrosine kinase, located on chromosome 2 at band 2p23, and show corresponding overexpression at the protein level, which can be detected immunohistochemically (see **Fig. 9**).[66] A variety of gene partners can be fused to *ALK* in IMT as a result of various chromosomal rearrangements, including tropomyosin 3, tropomyosin 4, CLTC, RANBP2, CARS, ATIC, and SEC31L1.

Unlike conventional IMT, epithelioid inflammatory myofibroblastic sarcoma typically contains abundant myxoid stroma with prominent admixed neutrophils. In addition to ALK, tumor cells of this variant of IMT usually express desmin and CD30 (the latter typically weak) and SMA in 50%. Tumors are negative for myogenin/myf4, caldesmon, keratins, EMA, and S100. Expression of desmin and negativity for EMA is helpful in distinguishing this tumor from anaplastic large cell lymphoma.

DIAGNOSIS AND DIFFERENTIAL DIAGNOSIS

The differential diagnosis of IMT includes, but is not limited to, GIST, desmoid fibromatosis, nodular fasciitis, and dedifferentiated liposarcoma. Depending on the degree of atypia and anatomic site, the differential diagnosis may also include other myxoid and spindle cell neoplasms.

Differential Diagnosis
INFLAMMATORY MYOFIBROBLASTIC TUMOR

- GIST: lacks significant inflammatory infiltrate, KIT and DOG1 positive
- Desmoid fibromatosis: long sweeping fascicles of spindle cells, nuclear β-catenin in 70%
- Dedifferentiated liposarcoma: greater cytology atypia, positive for MDM2 and CDK4
- Nodular fasciitis: does not occur in the GI tract

GIST shows a uniform fascicular, whorled, or occasionally sheet-like growth pattern and lacks the prominent inflammatory infiltrate of IMT. The tumor cells of GIST express KIT and DOG1, unlike those of IMT. Although the cytomorphology of desmoid fibromatosis may mimic that of IMT, desmoid fibromatosis is distinguished by its long sweeping fascicles and expression of nuclear β-catenin in up to 70% of cases. Nodular fasciitis does not occur at intra-abdominal sites; thus, clinical context is the most helpful consideration with this morphologic differential diagnosis. Inflammatory well-differentiated liposarcoma, or dedifferentiated liposarcoma, may mimic IMT. Helpful features to support a diagnosis of liposarcoma include the presence of marked nuclear atypia in the spindle cells, a component of adipocytic well-differentiated liposarcoma, expression of both MDM2 and CDK4, and negativity for ALK. As discussed previously, however, a subset of IMT expresses MDM2, and 50% of IMT are negative for ALK; in selected cases, FISH for 12q13-15 amplification, which is found in well-differentiated/dedifferentiated liposarcoma but not IMT, may be useful.

PROGNOSIS

IMT is considered a neoplasm of intermediate biologic potential; it shows a tendency to recur

---

Pitfalls
INFLAMMATORY MYOFIBROBLASTIC TUMOR

! May be positive for MDM2

! Occasionally can show nuclear atypia

! Epithelioid inflammatory myofibroblastic sarcoma has round cell morphology and expresses CD30

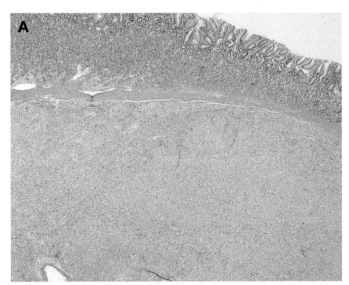

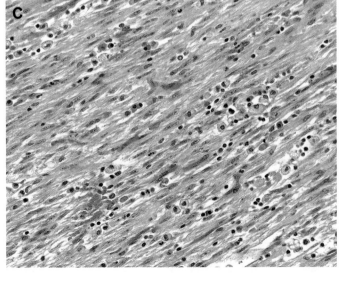

Fig. 9. IMT of the stomach forming a circumscribed mass (*A*). The tumor is composed of fascicles of myofibroblastic spindle cells with minimal atypia and an admixed inflammatory infiltrate composed of plasma cells and lymphocytes (*B, C*).

Fig. 9. The tumor cells are positive for SMA (*D*) and ALK (*E*).

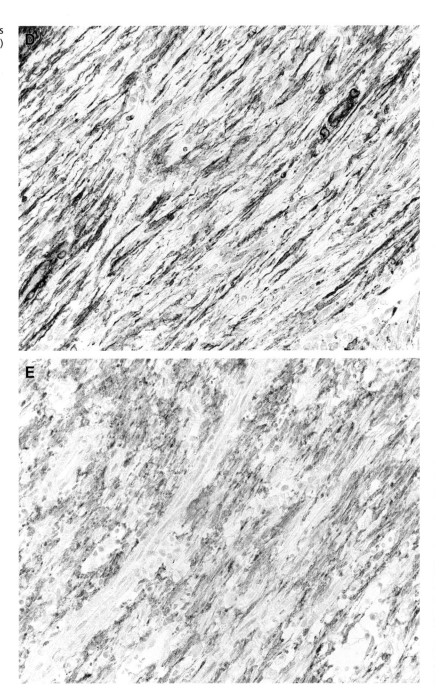

locally, but metastasis occurs in less than 5% of cases.[55] IMT arising in the abdomen or pelvis has the greatest rate of recurrence, occurring in approximately 25% of cases.[64,67]

In contrast, epithelioid inflammatory myofibroblastic sarcoma pursues an aggressive course with rapid local recurrences and frequent death due to disease.[63]

SCHWANNOMA

OVERVIEW

Schwannoma is a benign peripheral nerve sheath tumor, commonly found in somatic soft tissues, but which rarely arises in the GI tract. Within the GI tract, schwannomas occur most

Key Features
SCHWANNOMA

- A majority of GI cases arise in stomach, predominantly in the corpus

- Distinctive features include peripheral lymphoid cuff, lack of a capsule, and uniform cellularity

- Diffuse nuclear and cytoplasmic S100 expression and variable GFAP expression

frequently in the stomach, followed by the colorectum.[68–70] Within the stomach, tumors most often involve the gastric corpus[69,70] and within the colon the cecum is most often involved.[68] Schwannomas of the small intestine and esophagus are exceedingly rare.

Schwannomas involving the GI tract occur over a wide age range, with a peak incidence in older adults in the sixth and seventh decades. For gastric schwannomas, there is a marked female predominance,[70,71] but there is no apparent gender predilection for colorectal schwannomas.[68] Presenting symptoms depend on the anatomic site of involvement and include upper or lower GI bleeding, abdominal pain, or symptoms of obstruction; in some cases, tumors are detected incidentally by radiologic imaging or endoscopy. Isolated schwannoma of the GI tract has no known association with neurofibromatosis type 1 (NF1) or type 2.[68–71]

GROSS FEATURES

Tumors are typically located within the submucosa or muscularis propria, but may extend into overlying mucosa to protrude into the gastric/colonic lumen or may bulge into the serosal surface. The average size is approximately 3 cm, with a range of 0.5 cm to 11 cm reported. On cut surface, the tumors are well circumscribed, may be vaguely lobulated, and have a yellow fleshy appearance. Cystic chance is occasionally seen.

MICROSCOPIC FEATURES

Schwannomas occurring in the GI tract show several distinct features compared with schwannomas occurring outside the GI tract. They are well circumscribed but unencapsulated and thus lack the EMA-positive perineurial capsule seen in other schwannomas. They also

characteristically have a peripheral lymphoid cuff, often with germinal center formation (**Fig. 10**). Thick-walled or hyaline vessels are less conspicuous in schwannoma of the GI tract, and nuclear palisading and Verocay bodies are not seen. Finally, they lack the variably cellular Antoni A and B patterns, and instead tend to be uniformly cellular.[68–71] Regardless of anatomic site, however, schwannomas are composed exclusively of Schwann cells. The growth pattern of GI tract schwannomas is variably fascicular or whorled but may also show a sheet-like or trabecular growth pattern. One tumor arising in the colon was reported to have a strikingly plexiform growth pattern.[68] The tumor cells in most cases are spindled with tapering nuclei, uniform fine chromatin with a single small nucleolus and indistinct palely eosinophilic cytoplasm. Scattered cells with nuclear enlargement and degenerative pleomorphism are common. Several tumors occurring in the colon have been described as having a predominantly epithelioid cytomorphology.[68] Mitotic activity is typically low, less than 5 per 50 HPFs in the majority of cases. Necrosis is not found.

The tumor stroma is usually collagenous and may show patchy myxoid change. Admixed inflammatory cells, predominantly lymphocytes with fewer plasma cells, are often present, and aggregates of foamy histiocytes may also be seen.[70]

The immunohistochemical profile of schwannoma reflects its pure composition of Schwann cells, with diffuse nuclear and cytoplasmic S100 expression and variable glial fibrillary acidic protein (GFAP) expression (see **Fig. 10**).[71] Scattered CD34-positive cells may also be present.[68,71] The tumor cells are negative for KIT, DOG1, desmin, SMA, HMB45, and cytokeratins.

In contrast to soft tissue schwannomas, which commonly show monosomy of chromosome 22, this finding has not been found in gastric schwannomas, which instead have been found to show polysomy of chromosomes 22, 2, and 18, suggesting that the underlying pathogenetic mechanisms may differ between these tumor types.[71]

DIAGNOSIS AND DIFFERENTIAL DIAGNOSIS

Particularly in small biopsies, the morphologic differential diagnosis of schwannoma includes GIST. GIST also arises in the muscularis propria but lacks a peripheral lymphoid cuff. The tumor cells may be spindled or epithelioid, as in schwannoma, but are usually more monotonous in their

Fig. 10. Gastric schwannoma is well circumscribed and surrounded by a lymphoid cuff (*A*). This type of schwannoma is composed of a uniform fascicular proliferation of spindled cells with tapering nuclei and mild atypia (*B*) that show diffuse strong expression of S100 protein (*C*).

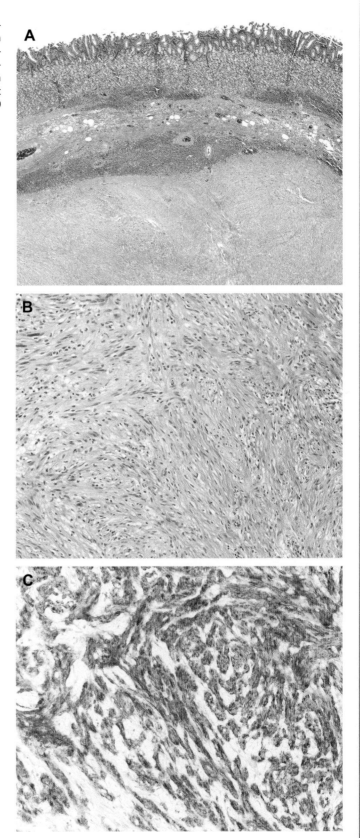

appearance. Immunohistochemistry is helpful in this differential; the tumor cells of GIST are positive for KIT and DOG1 in greater than 90% of cases.[43,72,73]

IMT is also a diagnostic consideration, given its fascicular growth pattern of spindled cells with minimal atypia and a prominent inflammatory infiltrate. Most IMTs occur in a younger patient age group than schwannomas of the GI tract. Furthermore, they are usually less circumscribed and lack a peripheral lymphoid cuff, and the tumor cells variably express SMA, desmin, and ALK, unlike those of schwannoma.[53,54]

Metastatic melanoma frequently involves the GI tract and may appear as a well-circumscribed nodule, but is frequently intramucosal. Similarly, tumor cells of both lesions may have diffuse expression of S100. In contrast to schwannoma, melanoma usually shows a greater degree of cytologic pleomorphism and nuclear atypia, including macronucleoli, and higher mitotic activity and lacks a peripheral lymphoid cuff. Immunohistochemical stains with second-line melanocytic markers, such as HMB45 and melanA/MART1, can further help in the differential diagnosis, because both are negative in schwannoma.

CCS-like tumor of the GI tract may occasionally be mistaken for gastric schwannoma, particularly given that both show diffuse S100 expression. Morphologically, however, the former tumor has a more nested and infiltrative architecture, occasionally with pseudoglandular features, shows greater cytologic atypia, and lacks a peripheral lymphoid cuff. Schwannoma often coexpresses GFAP and lacks *EWSR1* gene rearrangement.

PROGNOSIS

Schwannomas are benign tumors, and complete excision is curative; local recurrences or metastases have not been reported.[68–71]

> **Pitfall**
> SCHWANNOMA
>
> ! Diffuse S100 expression may lead to erroneous diagnosis of metastatic melanoma or CCS-like tumor of the GI tract

PERINEURIOMA

OVERVIEW

Perineurioma is a benign nerve sheath tumor composed of perineurial cells. In the GI tract, most perineuriomas present as a small mucosal polyp, but occasionally may occur as a submucosal mass; the latter tumors are indistinguishable from soft tissue perineuriomas.[74,75] It is now recognized that a majority of polyps previously classified as benign fibroblastic polyp[76] represent mucosal perineurioma, due to both their virtually indistinguishable morphologic appearances and demonstration of variable expression of EMA in some lesions formerly classified as benign fibroblastic polyp.[75,77]

Mucosal perineurioma occurs with greatest frequency in the left colon, in particular the rectosigmoid region. Perineuriomas of soft tissue type rarely arise in the small intestine.[74] Patients tend to be middle aged, with a median occurrence in the 6th decade. There is no gender predilection

---

△△ **Differential Diagnosis**
SCHWANNOMA

- GIST: lacks a peripheral lymphoid cuff, tumor cells are monotonous in appearance and positive for KIT, DOG1, and CD34

- IMT: younger age group, less circumscribed, S100 negative

- Metastatic melanoma: greater pleomorphism, may express second-line melanocytic markers

- CCS-like tumor of the GI tract: nested, ± pseudoglandular areas, greater cytologic atypia, *EWSR1* gene rearrangement

---

 Key Features
MUCOSAL PERINEURIOMA

- Usually presents as a mucosal polyp in the rectosigmoid region

- Whorls of bland spindle cells with ovoid/slender nuclei and delicate elongated cytoplasmic processes, entrapping colonic crypts

- Hyperplastic or serrated epithelial changes in 70% of cases, associated with *BRAF* mutations

- Positive for EMA, claudin-1, and less often CD34

for these lesions.[75] Most cases are detected incidentally during screening colonoscopy, but occasional patients may present with lower GI tract bleeding, abdominal pain, or, rarely, an obstructive mass-forming lesion.[74]

GROSS FEATURES

The majority of lesions present as small sessile polyps limited to the mucosa, with a median size of 0.3 cm to 0.4 cm. Rarely, intestinal perineurioma may occur as a large well-circumscribed submucosal mass, in the range of 3 cm to 5 cm, with a fibrous or myxoid cut surface.[74]

MICROSCOPIC FEATURES

The morphologic appearances of mucosal perineurioma are distinctive. The lesions are composed of bland spindle cells with ovoid or slender nuclei and indistinct eosinophilic cytoplasm (**Fig. 11**). In some cases, delicate elongated cytoplasmic processes may be appreciated. The cells grow in a whorled pattern, entrapping colonic crypts and often condensing around preexisting crypts. The intervening stroma usually has a finely collagenous appearance. Necrosis and atypia are not seen, and mitotic activity is minimal or absent.

Adjacent serrated crypts are present in 70% to 80% of cases, often indistinguishable from an otherwise conventional hyperplastic polyp (or occasionally a sessile serrated adenoma/polyp). *BRAF* mutations have been found in the epithelial component in the majority of such cases, suggesting that at least a subset of mucosal perineuriomas exist as hybrid lesions with hyperplastic polyps; the perineurial component in such examples may in fact be reactive in nature.[78]

Immunohistochemically, the spindle cells show features of perineurial differentiation, with consistent expression of EMA and staining for claudin-1 in approximately 50% of lesions; CD34 is positive in occasional cases (see **Fig. 11**). It is important to note that EMA expression is often only weak in intensity and distribution. Examination under high power may be required to appreciate positive staining, which usually highlights the elongated cytoplasmic processes of the lesional cells. The cells are consistently negative for S100, GFAP, neurofilament protein, KIT, pan-keratin, SMA, and desmin.[74]

Electron microscopic studies have consistently demonstrated features of perineurial differentiation within these tumors (i.e., elongated cell processes with prominent pinocytotic vesicles and scattered tight junctions).[75]

DIAGNOSIS AND DIFFERENTIAL DIAGNOSIS

The morphologic differential diagnosis of perineurioma includes mucosal Schwann cell hamartoma, ganglioneuroma, neurofibroma, and leiomyoma.

Schwann cell hamartoma may closely mimic mucosal perineurioma. Both are intramucosal lesions that have a somewhat infiltrative growth pattern and are composed of spindle cells that entrap colonic crypts. The cells of Schwann cell hamartoma tend to be plumper with more brightly eosinophilic cytoplasm than those of perineurioma and lack the delicate elongated cytoplasmic processes of perineurial cells. Schwann cell hamartoma is composed exclusively of Schwann cells and is, therefore, diffusely positive for S100.[79]

Ganglioneuroma of the GI tract occurs in 3 forms:

1. Solitary polypoid ganglioneuroma, which has no known syndromic associations and predominantly involves the mucosa
2. Ganglioneuromatous polyposis, which may be associated with Cowden syndrome (PTEN hamartoma syndrome) and also predominantly involves the mucosa
3. Diffuse ganglioneuromatosis, which occurs in patients with NF1 or multiple endocrine neoplasia type 2b (MEN2B) and involves the myenteric plexus and extends through the wall of the intestine[80]

Similar to perineurioma, polypoid ganglioneuroma is poorly circumscribed and shows entrapment of colonic crypts but lacks an associated serrated polyp. Ganglioneuromas are composed of a mixed population of S100-positive Schwann cells, neurofilament protein–positive axons, and ganglion cells, unlike perineurioma, which lacks

---

△△ *Differential Diagnosis*
MUCOSAL PERINEURIOMA

- Schwann cell hamartoma: plumper spindled cells without elongated cytoplasmic processes, diffusely positive for S100 and negative for EMA

- Ganglioneuroma: mixed population of S100-positive Schwann cells, neurofilament protein–positive axons, and ganglion cells

- Neurofibroma: rare in the GI tract, mural mass, usually associated with NF1, mixed population of Schwann cell, perineurial cells, fibroblasts, and axons

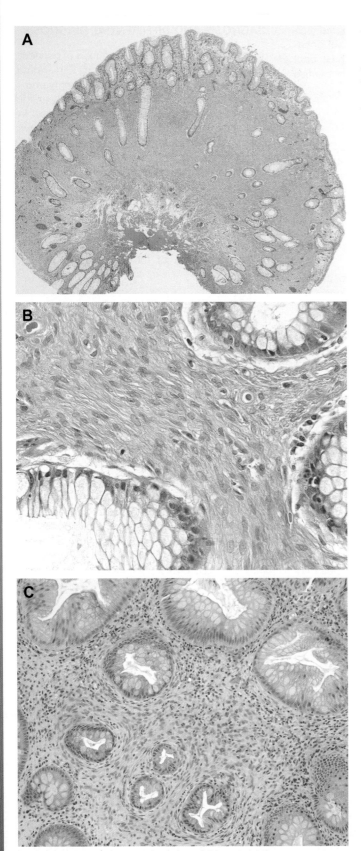

Fig. 11. Mucosal perineurioma presenting as a polypoid lesion in the colon (*A*) and composed of slender spindle cells with elongated palely eosinophilic cytoplasmic processes that surround existing crypts (*B*). Associated hyperplastic changes in the surrounding crypts are often present (*C*).

Fig. 11. The tumor cells show expression of EMA (*D*) and variable reactivity for claudin-1 (*E*).

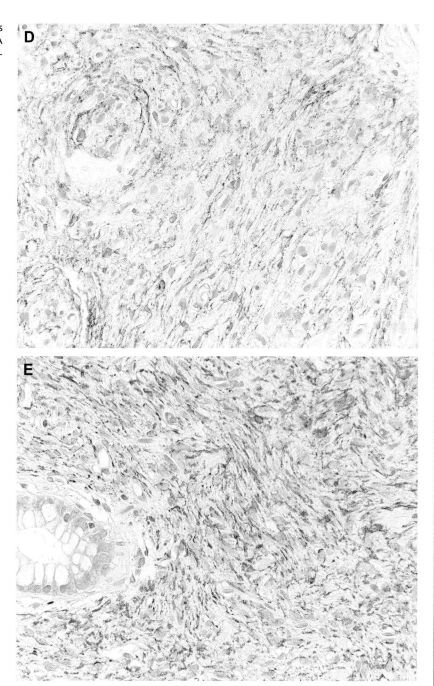

these cell types and is therefore negative for S100 and neurofilament protein (NFP).

Neurofibroma of the GI tract is rare. Most small mucosal lesions previously classified as neurofibroma likely represent Schwann cell hamartomas. When occurring in the GI tract, neurofibroma is highly associated with NF1.[81,82] The tumor is composed of a mixed population of Schwann cell, perineurial cells, fibroblasts, and axons, and this mixed composition is reflected in the immunoprofile, with expression of S100, NFP, and EMA to varying degrees.

In contrast to perineurioma, leiomyoma is usually well circumscribed, and the tumor cells have brightly eosinophilic cytoplasm and blunt cigar-shaped nuclei. The tumor cells of leiomyoma express SMA, desmin, and caldesmon, unlike those of perineurioma.

PROGNOSIS

Perineuriomas are benign; no local recurrences have been reported.[74,75]

MUCOSAL SCHWANN CELL HAMARTOMA

OVERVIEW

Mucosal Schwann cell hamartoma is a benign intramucosal Schwann cell proliferation that was recently described by Gibson et al[79] who helped clarify the classification of benign neural lesions of the GI tract. Many of the cases in the original series had been previously diagnosed as neurofibroma or neuroma, both of which carry significant syndromic implications for NF1 and MEN2B, respectively. In contrast, no syndromic associations have been found for mucosal Schwann cell hamartoma.

> ### Key Features
> #### MUCOSAL SCHWANN CELL HAMARTOMA
>
> - Benign intramucosal Schwann cell proliferation
>
> - Many cases probably previously diagnosed as neurofibroma or neuroma
>
> - Usually presents as a mucosal polyp in the rectosigmoid region
>
> - Variably circumscribed proliferation of bland spindle cells with tapering or wavy nuclei, entrapping colonic crypts
>
> - Diffusely positive for S100

Mucosal Schwann cell hamartoma typically occurs in middle-aged to older adults, and the median patient age is 62 years. There is a slight female predominance. These lesions arise in the colon, by far most commonly in the left colon and particularly in the rectosigmoid region.[79] The majority of cases are detected incidentally as polyps during screening colonoscopy.

GROSS FEATURES

Endoscopically, mucosal Schwann cell hamartoma appears as a small polypoid lesion. Virtually all lesions are less than 1 cm; the mean size is 0.25 cm.[79]

MICROSCOPIC FEATURES

Mucosal Schwann cell hamartoma is a variably circumscribed, intramucosal, uniformly cellular proliferation of bland spindle cells (**Fig. 12**). The spindle cells have tapering or wavy nuclei with inconspicuous nucleoli, abundant eosinophilic cytoplasm, and indistinct cell borders. There is no nuclear atypia or pleomorphism, and mitotic activity is usually absent. As the lesion expands in the lamina propria, it tends to trap the colonic crypts within the proliferation.

Immunohistochemically, the spindle cells show diffuse expression of S100, consistent with Schwannian differentiation (see **Fig. 12**). Epithelial membrane antigen, CD34, claudin-1, SMA, and KIT are consistently negative.

DIAGNOSIS AND DIFFERENTIAL DIAGNOSIS

Mucosal perineurioma may mimic Schwann cell hamartoma. Both are intramucosal nerve sheath lesions that have a somewhat infiltrative growth pattern and are composed of spindle cells. Morphologically, however, the spindle cells of perineurioma tend to be more slender than those of Schwann cell hamartoma and have delicate elongated cytoplasmic processes.[74] The cytoplasmic processes are highlighted by variable EMA and claudin-1 expression, both of which are negative in Schwann cell hamartoma. Furthermore, perineurioma lacks expression of S100.[74]

Mucosal neuroma, a lesion typically found in patients with MEN2B, may be confused with Schwann cell hamartoma, more so because many Schwann cell hamartomas were previously classified as neuroma, despite their clinical and pathologic differences to those occurring in the setting of MEN2B. Mucosal neuroma of MEN2B classically occurs in the oral cavity or on the lips or tongue and is rare in the GI tract proper.[83] Histologically, mucosal neuroma is composed of hyperplastic bundles of nerve fibers with frequent axons, which can be highlighted by stains for neurofilament protein.

Neurofibroma of the GI tract is highly associated with NF1.[81,82] Many cases of Schwann cell hamartoma were previously classified as neurofibroma, but there are several morphologic and immunohistochemical features that help distinguish between the two, thus allowing for appropriate clinical management. Neurofibroma is composed of a mixed population of Schwann cells, perineurial-like cells, fibroblasts, and axons. This mixed population is reflected in the heterogeneous staining pattern of neurofibroma, with expression of S100 seen in a subset of cells, in

Fig. 12. Mucosal Schwann cell hamartoma of the colon has somewhat irregular borders (*A*) and is composed of plump ovoid to spindled cells with palely eosinophilic cytoplasm (*B*).

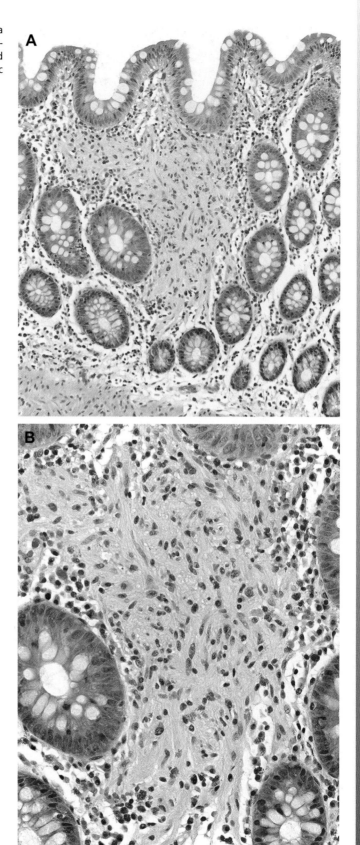

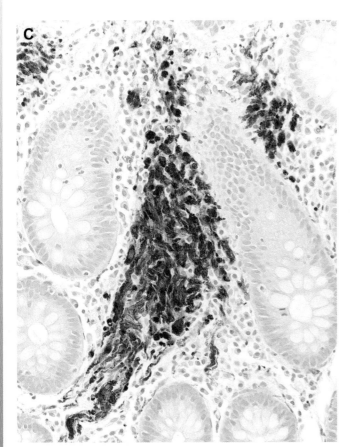

Fig. 12. The cells are diffusely positive for S100 (*C*).

contrast to the strong, diffuse pattern seen in Schwann cell hamartoma. EMA and NFP may show expression in perineurial-like cells and axons, respectively, in neurofibroma. Most neurofibromas of the GI tract are mural mass lesions centered in the submucosa or muscularis propria, secondarily extending into the overlying mucosa.

Ganglioneuroma of the GI tract is classified into 3 groups: solitary polypoid ganglioneuroma, ganglioneuromatous polyposis, and diffuse ganglioneuromatosis.[80] All 3 types of ganglioneuroma are composed of a mixed population of Schwann cells, axons, and ganglion cells, and may, therefore, mimic Schwann cell hamartoma, because there is usually a predominance of Schwann cells. Identification of ganglion cells, however, which are not seen in Schwann cell hamartoma, distinguish between these two entities.

A similar and likely related lesion to Schwann cell hamartoma, mucosal benign epithelioid nerve sheath tumor, has been described by Lewin and colleagues.[84] Similar to Schwann cell hamartoma, these tumors are composed of a pure population of Schwann cells entrapping colonic crypts but, unlike Schwann cell hamartoma, the lesional cells have an epithelioid cytomorphology.

The relationship between Schwann cell hamartoma and GI schwannoma is unclear, although histologic features favor classification as distinct entities. While both lesions are composed of a pure population of Schwann cells, Schwann cell hamartoma lacks the circumscription, peritumoral lymphoid aggregates, dense collagenous stroma, and nuclear heterogeneity of GI schwannomas.

Differential Diagnosis
MUCOSAL SCHWANN CELL HAMARTOMA

- Mucosal perineurioma: slender spindle cells, positive for EMA, ± claudin-1 and CD34

- Mucosal neuroma: rare in GI tract, associated with MEN2B, hyperplastic bundles of nerve fibers with frequent axons, positive for NFP

- Ganglioneuroma: mixed population of S100-positive Schwann cells, neurofilament protein–positive axons, and ganglion cells

- Neurofibroma: rare in the GI tract; usually associated with NF1, mixed population of Schwann cell, perineurial cells, fibroblasts, and axons

PROGNOSIS

Mucosal Schwann cell hamartoma is benign, and there are no known syndromic associations and no apparent increased risk of developing other neural lesions.

Pitfall
MUCOSAL SCHWANN CELL HAMARTOMA

! Some cases were previously called neuromas or neurofibromas, which are strongly associated with MEN2B and NF1, respectively; Schwann cell hamartoma has no syndromic implications

CLEAR CELL SARCOMA–LIKE TUMOR OF THE GASTROINTESTINAL TRACT

OVERVIEW

Clear cell sarcoma (CCS)-like tumor of the GI tract has distinctive pathologic and genetic features from conventional CCS of tendons and aponeuroses.[85,86] The alternative designation of 'malignant GI neuroectodermal tumor' was recently proposed for these tumors,[87] which previously were also referred to as 'osteoclast-rich tumors of the GI tract with features resembling CCS of soft parts'.[88] In contrast to conventional CCS, these tumors usually show a sheet-like and less nested growth pattern, contain osteoclast-like giant cells, and, most significantly, lack evidence of melanocytic differentiation

Key Features
CLEAR CELL SARCOMA–LIKE TUMOR OF THE GI TRACT

- Differs from conventional CCS by predominantly sheet-like growth pattern, osteoclastic-like giant cells, and lack of melanocytic differentiation ultrastructurally and immunohistochemically

- Sheets and nests of epithelioid and spindle cells with palely eosinophilic cytoplasm; focal pseudoglandular/alveolar architecture

- S100 positive; negative for HMB45 and other melanocytic markers

- EWSR1-ATF1 and EWSR1-CREB1 fusion genes found in approximately 90% of tumors

- Aggressive clinical course

ultrastructurally and immunohistochemically, being consistently negative for HMB45 and other secondary melanocytic markers.[86–88] They both, however, express S100 and often harbor the EWSR1-ATF1 (or EWSR1-CREB1) fusion gene.[87,89,90]

Tumors arise most often in the small intestine, followed by stomach and colon. The mean patient age is 42 years (range 17–77 years), and patients are usually young to middle-aged adults. There is no apparent gender predilection. In a study of 16 cases, 69% had nodal metastases at the time of diagnosis, and 44% had liver metastases.[87] Presenting symptoms include abdominal pain, intestinal obstruction, weight loss, anemia, and fever.

GROSS FEATURES

Grossly, tumors are usually centered in the submucosa and muscularis propria. Tumor size is variable, but most measure between 2 cm and 15 cm, with an average size of 5 cm. Tumors are usually solid and firm, and the cut surface is tan-white and lobulated, with focal hemorrhage and/or necrosis and occasional cystic change. Occasionally, tumors grow as exophytic masses that protrude into the lumen of the bowel and may also grow as circumferential masses that mimic carcinoma or lymphoma. Overlying mucosal ulceration is frequently present.

MICROSCOPIC FEATURES

Tumors primarily involve the submucosa and muscularis propria, but occasionally extend into mucosa. The tumors are usually composed of sheets of round to epithelioid cells, often with a focally nested growth pattern (**Fig. 13**). In some tumors, ovoid to spindled cells predominate. The epithelioid cells have small amounts of palely eosinophilic cytoplasm and round to oval nuclei with vesicular chromatin and small but distinct nucleoli. Mitotic activity is variable, ranging from 0 to 20 mitoses per 10 HPFs. The nuclei of the spindled cells have similar appearances. It is common to see a mixed growth pattern, with focal areas of pseudoglandular/alveolar, pseudopapillary, microcystic, and fascicular architecture. Scattered osteoclast-like giant cells are present in approximately 50% of cases.[87]

Immunohistochemistry demonstrates S100 positivity in all cases, usually with a strong and diffuse pattern (see **Fig. 13**). SOX10, a neuroectodermal marker, has also been found to be positive in all cases examined. The melanocytic markers, HMB45, melan A, MiTF, and tyrosinase, are negative.[86,87] KIT, DOG1, CD34, GFAP, cytokeratins, desmin, SMA, and CD99 are also consistently

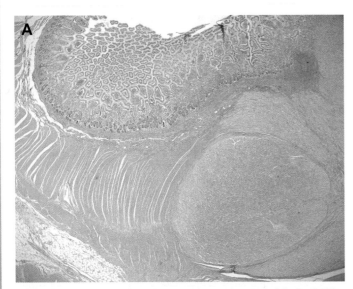

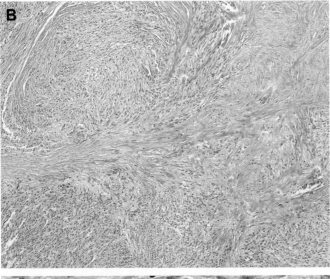

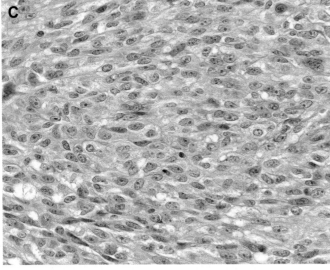

Fig. 13. CCS-like tumor of the GI tract involving the muscularis propria of the small intestine with a nodular growth pattern (*A*). Infiltrative areas are usually present (*B*). The tumor cells are variably spindled or epithelioid with round to oval nuclei and small distinct nucleoli (*C*).

Fig. 13. Pseudoglandular areas may be present (*D*). Multinucleated giant cells are frequently present (*E*). Diffuse expression of S100 protein (*F*) in the absence of HMB-45 expression (*G*) is a consistent finding.

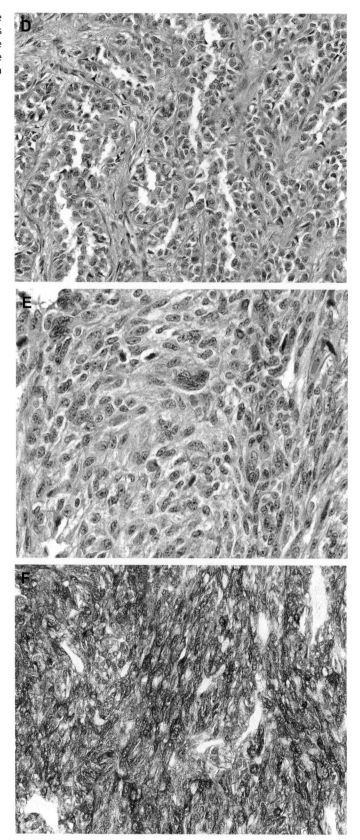

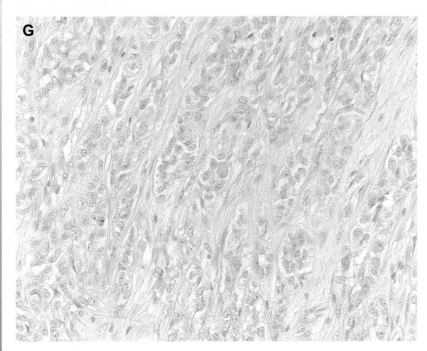

Fig. 13.

negative. Expression of synaptophysin and NSE is found in approximately 50% of cases.[87] Ultrastructural studies do not show evidence of melanocytic differentiation, but instead some features of neural differentiation have been described, including interdigitating cell processes containing dense-core granules and clear vesicles resembling synaptic bulbs,[87] leading investigators to suggest that these tumors may arise from components of the autonomic nervous system.

EWSR1-ATF1 and *EWSR1-CREB1* fusion genes are found in approximately 90% of tumors, resulting from t(12;22)(q13;q12) or t(2;22)(q34;q12), respectively.[86,87] FISH for *EWSR1* rearrangement and/or polymerase chain reaction–based methods to look for the common translocations of this tumor are therefore useful diagnostic adjuncts to exclude a diagnosis of melanoma.

DIAGNOSIS AND DIFFERENTIAL DIAGNOSIS

The differential diagnostic considerations when encountered with a possible CCS-like tumor of the GI tract include conventional CCS, metastatic melanoma, GIST, and monophasic synovial sarcoma.

CCS formerly was thought to represent a primary soft tissue counterpart of cutaneous malignant melanoma. Nonetheless, it is now known that CCS exhibits a consistent and characteristic t(12;22)(q13;q12) chromosomal translocation that is not shared by melanocytic lesions of the skin.[89,90] CCS typically involves tendons or aponeuroses of the extremities of young adults, but rarely involves the GI tract, and, at the latter location, is less common than CCS-like tumor of the GI tract. CCS is characterized by epithelioid and/or spindle-shaped tumor cells with clear or palely eosinophilic cytoplasm, in a nested or fascicular growth pattern with a delicate fibrovascular stroma.[91] Melanin pigmentation is rarely observed on hematoxylin-eosin stained sections. The immunohistochemical features of CCS largely mirror those of melanoma, with reactivity for S100 protein, tyrosinase, MART-1, HMB-45, and microphthalmia transcription factor.[92] A helpful clue to the diagnosis of CCS is the presence of HMB45 positivity that is stronger and more diffuse than S100 positivity, a finding that is unusual in melanoma.

The small intestine is a common site for metastatic melanoma, which is much more common than CCS-like tumor. Given the diffuse expression of S100 in both tumor types, CCS-like tumor may easily be mistaken for metastatic melanoma. Clinical correlation to determine if there is a history of melanoma at other sites is helpful; molecular/cytogenetic studies to demonstrate the presence of *EWSR1* rearrangement can be used to confirm the diagnosis of CCS-like tumor.

Monophasic synovial sarcoma may rarely arise in the GI tract, particularly in the stomach, where it may resemble CCS-like tumor. The tumor cells in synovial sarcoma typically have less cytoplasm

Differential Diagnosis
CLEAR CELL SARCOMA-LIKE
TUMOR OF THE GI TRACT

- Conventional CCS: more uniformly nested, prominent nucleoli, positive for HMB-45 and melan A

- Metastatic melanoma: more nuclear atypia and pleomorphism with macronucleoli, absence of *EWSR1* rearrangement

- Monophasic synovial sarcoma: positive for TLE1, keratin, and EMA, *SS18 (SYT)* gene rearrangement

- GIST: lacks pseudoglandular areas, positive for KIT, DOG1, and CD34

and overlapping nuclei. In addition, cytokeratin and EMA positivity, as well as nuclear expression of TLE1, are all seen in the majority of synovial sarcomas, and demonstration of *SS18 (SYT)* rearrangement due to the presence of t(X;18) can help confirm the diagnosis in difficult cases.

GIST may also fall into the differential diagnosis with CCS-like tumor of the GI tract, given that it can also have mixed epithelioid and spindled cell morphology. Pseudoglandular areas and osteoclast-like giant cells, however, are rarely seen in GIST. Furthermore, although the tumor cells of GIST may show focal S100 expression in a small subset of cases (most often in the duodenum), most tumors are diffusely positive for KIT, DOG1, and CD34, in contrast to CCS-like tumor.

PROGNOSIS

The clinical course of CCS-like tumor of the GI tract is aggressive in most cases, and the prognosis is poor. In a recent study reporting clinical follow-up of 12 patients with CCS-like tumor of the GI tract, 50% of patients had died of disease, with a mean survival of 32 months, and 4 patients were alive with metastatic disease at up to 36 months.[87]

Pitfalls
CLEAR CELL SARCOMA-LIKE
TUMOR OF THE GI TRACT

! Pseudoglandular architecture may mimic adenocarcinoma

! May be difficult to distinguish from metastatic melanoma

FOLLICULAR DENDRITIC CELL SARCOMA

OVERVIEW

Follicular dendritic cell (FDC) sarcoma is a neoplasm composed of FDCs, which are normal components of the humoral immune response system and act as antigen-presenting cells, and which reside in primary and secondary lymphoid follicles. Most FDC sarcomas arise in lymph nodes or lymphoid-rich tissues, such as the tonsil or spleen, but extranodal tissues are occasionally involved, including the GI tract. The most common sites of involvement within the GI tract are the stomach and colon,[93,94] but cases have also been described in the small intestine.[95] Most patients are middle-aged adults (median age of 40 years) but the age range is wide, and occasional cases occur in children. Rarely, FDC sarcoma arises in association with hyaline-vascular Castleman disease.[95]

Key Features
FOLLICULAR DENDRITIC CELL
SARCOMA

- Monotonous population of plump ovoid to spindled cells with syncytial, eosinophilic cytoplasm and prominent admixed lymphocytes

- The tumor cells express CD35, CD21, and variable CD23

GROSS FEATURES

FDC sarcoma is usually well circumscribed with a fleshy cut surface. Tumor size of extranodal FDC sarcomas ranges from 1 cm to 20 cm, with an average of 6 cm.

MICROSCOPIC FEATURES

FDC sarcoma is composed of a monotonous population of plump ovoid to spindled cells with syncytial, eosinophilic cytoplasm, arranged in sheets, fascicles, and whorls and with a storiform growth pattern (**Fig. 14**). The nuclei usually have smooth nuclear contours, small nucleoli, and dispersed chromatin.[95,96] The tumor cells are characteristically admixed with small lymphocytes, usually B cells. FDC sarcomas arising in the liver tend to have a plasma cell predominant infiltrate.[93] Most cases have mild to moderate nuclear atypia, but occasional cases show more striking pleomorphism.

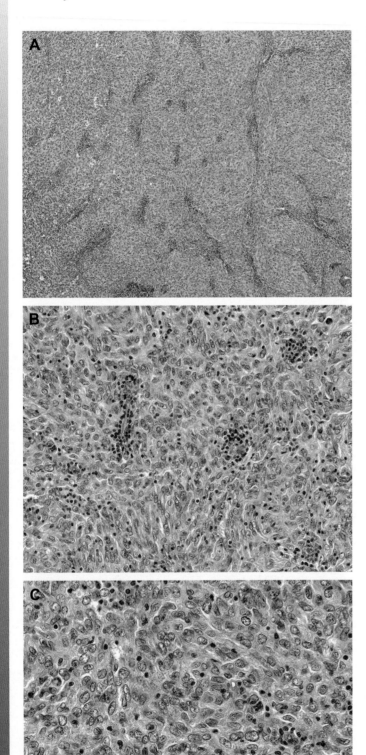

Fig. 14. FDC sarcoma is composed of sheets, fascicles, and whorls (*A*) of monotonous plump ovoid to spindled cells with syncytial, eosinophilic cytoplasm and scattered small lymphocytes (*B*). The nuclei have mildly irregular nuclear contours, dispersed chromatin, and small nucleoli (*C*).

Fig. 14. The tumor cells express CD35 (*D*) and CD21 (*E*).

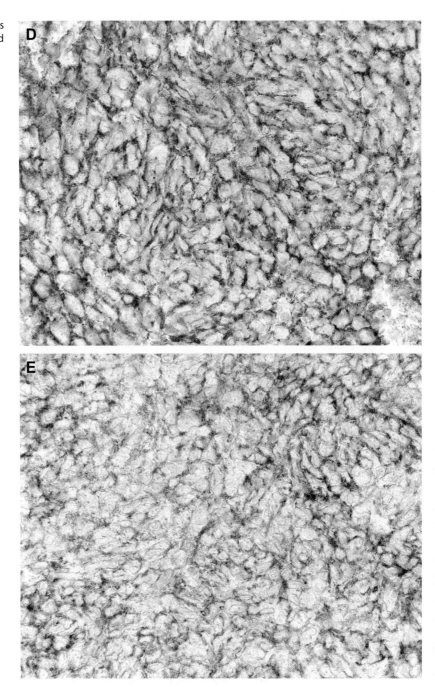

The mitotic rate is highly variable, with a median of 3 per 10 HPFs[93]; 30% of tumors show necrosis.

The tumor cells of FDC sarcoma express CD35, CD21, and variably CD23, all antigens of normal FDCs (see **Fig. 14**).[96,97] Less-specific markers that may also be positive include clusterin, fascin, and D2-40 (podoplanin).[98,99] EMA is commonly positive, and occasionally S100 expression is found. Cytokeratins, desmin, and CD1a are consistently negative.

DIAGNOSIS AND DIFFERENTIAL DIAGNOSIS

Particularly in the stomach, FDC sarcoma may resemble schwannoma. Both are composed of spindled or ovoid cells with mild atypia arranged

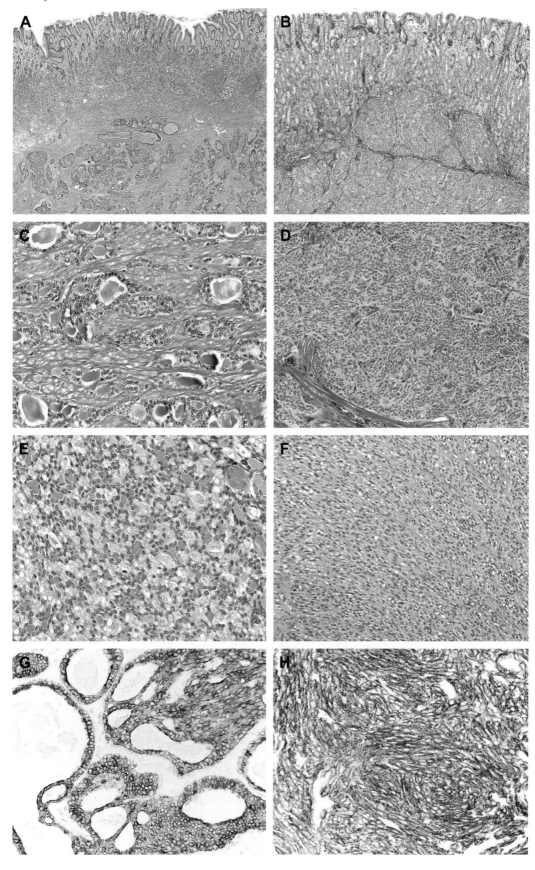

△△ *Differential Diagnosis*
FOLLICULAR DENDRITIC CELL
SARCOMA

- Schwannoma: more elongated spindle cells, collagenous stroma, S100 positive

- GIST: KIT and DOG1 positive

in fascicles, with an admixed inflammatory infiltrate. However, the inflammatory infiltrate in FDC sarcoma is often more pronounced, and the nuclei of the lesional cells tend to be predominantly plump and ovoid and surrounded by amphophilic cytoplasm that merges to produce a syncytial appearance. Most FDC sarcomas do not have a peripheral lymphoid cuff like that seen in schwannoma. Immunohistochemistry is useful to distinguish the two; FDC sarcoma does not show diffuse S100 protein expression like that seen in schwannoma and instead expresses CD35 and CD21.

GIST, in particular the epithelioid type, can show some similarity to FDC sarcoma, in that it often grows in sheets composed of monotonous tumor cells with indistinct borders and a syncytial appearance; admixed lymphocytes are occasionally present. FDC sarcoma is usually less fascicular, however, and has a more prominent inflammatory cell component. In addition, GIST expresses KIT, DOG1, and CD34, whereas FDC sarcoma expresses CD35 and CD21.[97]

Carcinoma may also mimic FDC sarcoma,[100] but FDC sarcoma tends, to be more monotonous in appearance than carcinoma and lacks expression of cytokeratins.

PROGNOSIS

FDC sarcoma carries a significant risk for both local recurrence and metastasis.[95] Extranodal location, large tumor size, and high mitotic rate have been associated with more aggressive clinical behavior.

GASTROBLASTOMA

OVERVIEW

Gastroblastoma is a recently described biphasic/mixed epithelial-mesenchymal tumor.[101] To date, all reported cases have arisen in the stomach,[101–103] apart from 1 probable primary duodenal tumor.[104] This tumor type appears to be very rare, with just 6 cases reported in the literature to date; however, the authors have now seen 2 such cases. Of the 6 reported cases, 2 patients were female and 4 male, ranging in age from 9 to 30 years. Presenting symptoms include abdominal pain, symptoms of upper GI bleeding (melena or anemia) or a palpable mass.

Key Features
GASTROBLASTOMA

- Rare biphasic/mixed epithelial-mesenchymal tumor

- Virtually all cases arise in the stomach

- Spindle cell component is positive for CD10; epithelial component is positive for cytokeratins

GROSS FEATURES

Tumors range in size from 3 cm to 15 cm and involve the gastric wall. Extension into subserosa and/or overlying mucosa may be present. Gastroblastoma may be solid or solid and cystic and is typically at least partially circumscribed and multinodular or lobulated. The cut surface varies from tan to gray-fleshy to white in appearance and may show focal hemorrhage or friability.

MICROSCOPIC FEATURES

The defining feature of gastroblastoma is a biphasic population of epithelial cells and spindled cells, the latter representing the mesenchymal component (**Fig. 15**). The mesenchymal

Fig. 15. Gastroblastoma with a predominant epithelial component involving the gastric wall (*A*). Extension of tumor into mucosa may occur (*B*). Patterns of epithelial differentiation include gland formation with luminal eosinophilic secretions (*C*), pseudorosette formation (*D*), and primitive cells with intracellular and extracellular mucin production (*E*). The mesenchymal component consists of uniform ovoid to spindle-shaped cells with small nuclei with minimal nuclear atypia and inconspicuous nucleoli (*F*). The epithelial component is positive for cytokeratins, such as AE1/AE3 (*G*), whereas the spindle cell component is positive for CD10 (*H*).

component typically predominates and consists of uniform ovoid to spindle-shaped cells with blunt-ended nuclei, minimal to mild nuclear atypia, inconspicuous nucleoli, and variable mitotic activity (ranging from less than 1 to up to 30 mitoses per 50 HPFs).[101] The growth pattern of this component varies from loose and reticular to more compact whorls or fascicles. The epithelial component tends to merge with the spindle cell component and may show variable morphologies within the same tumor. Appearances include sheets, nests, or cords of epithelioid cells, with variable amounts of cytoplasm and round to oval nuclei with at most mild nuclear atypia. Nucleoli are usually inconspicuous, and nuclear grooves may be seen. Gland formation is often found, and in some cases luminal eosinophilic secretions and/or mucin are abundant.[101,103] Hyaline extracellular globules may also be seen. Rosette formation has been described.[102,103] The tumor stroma is usually collagenous.

Electron microscopy performed in 1 case revealed desmosomes and microvilli, consistent with true epithelial differentiation within the tumor.[102]

Immunohistochemically, the spindle cell component shows expression of CD10, whereas the epithelial component shows expression of cytokeratins AE1/AE3, CK18, and focal expression of CK7 in some cases (see **Fig. 15**). CK20 and EMA are typically negative, but 1 case has shown EMA expression.[102] Both components are typically negative for CD34, CD99, desmin, SMA, S100, calretinin, p63, synaptophysin, chromogranin, TTF-1, and CDX2, although 1 reported case showed expression of CD99 in both the epithelial and spindle cell components of the tumor and expression of desmin and SMA in the spindle cell component.[104] KIT expression has been reported in the epithelial component of 2 tumors.[102,103] *KIT* mutations have not been identified in this tumor,[102] and all examined cases have been negative for *SS18* (*SYT*) gene rearrangement.[101,104] One tumor was reported to show cytoplasmic dot-like positivity for DOG1 in the spindle cell component and luminal positivity in the epithelial component.[101]

DIAGNOSIS AND DIFFERENTIAL DIAGNOSIS

The exceedingly rare gastric carcinosarcoma falls into the differential diagnosis with gastroblastoma. In contrast to gastroblastoma, gastric carcinosarcoma occurs in an older age group, has a poor prognosis with an aggressive clinical course, and histologically is composed of highly atypical cells showing squamous, adenocarcinomatous, or undifferentiated pleomorphic cytomorphology.[101]

Gastroblastoma may mimic biphasic synovial sarcoma, particularly because the epithelial components of both tumors are often cytologically bland. Synovial sarcoma is rare in the GI tract, where it shows a predilection for the stomach and is usually monophasic in type.[105] The epithelial component of synovial sarcoma tends to show a more abrupt transition with the spindle cell component than seen in gastroblastoma. Immunohistochemically, the epithelial component, and, to a lesser degree the spindle cell component, demonstrates positivity for cytokeratins and EMA, and both components show nuclear staining for TLE1 in approximately 90% of cases.[106,107] Furthermore, gastroblastoma lacks the *SS18* gene rearrangement.

Myoepithelial tumors of the GI tract are rare but may also have a biphasic morphology. Myoepithelial tumors have variable morphologic appearances and can show cords, nests, or trabeculae of epithelial cells, often in a myxoid stroma, along with a bland spindle cell component.[108] The tumor cells show a myoepithelial immunophenotype and thus demonstrate variable expression of S100, GFAP, EMA, cytokeratins, and p63, which helps in the distinction from gastroblastoma.[108]

The mesenchymal component of gastroblastoma may mimic GIST, particularly given the reported finding of KIT or DOG1 expression in several cases. Unlike GIST, however, gastroblastoma contains an epithelial component, and diffuse staining for KIT or DOG1 is not found.[101]

△△ *Differential Diagnosis*
      GASTROBLASTOMA

- Biphasic synovial sarcoma: positive for TLE1, keratin/EMA-positive cells in spindle cell component, *SS18* (*SYT*) gene rearrangement

- Gastric carcinosarcoma: older age, greater cytologic atypia

- Myoepithelial tumors: variable expression of S100, GFAP, EMA, cytokeratins, and p63

- GIST: lacks glandular structures, positive for KIT, DOG1, and CD34

PROGNOSIS

In the original series reported by Miettinen and colleagues,[101] all 3 patients showed no evidence of recurrence or metastasis and were alive without disease at 3.5, 5, and 14 years. Other cases seem to have a similar indolent clinical course, but 1 recently reported case of gastroblastoma arising in a 28-year-old man showed evidence of disseminated peritoneal disease and lymph node metastasis at the time of presentation. In that case, the tumor had a predominantly epithelial morphology but had low mitotic activity.[103]

REFERENCES

1. Hancock BJ, Vajcner A. Lipomas of the colon: a clinicopathologic review. Can J Surg 1988;31:178–81.
2. Siegal A, Witz M. Gastrointestinal lipoma and malignancies. J Surg Oncol 1991;47:170–4.
3. Santos-Briz A, Garcia JP, Gonzalez C, et al. Lipomatous polyposis of the colon. Histopathology 2001;38:81–3.
4. Baum S, Athanasoulis CA, Waltman AC, et al. Angiodysplasia of the right colon: a cause of gastrointestinal bleeding. AJR Am J Roentgenol 1977;129:789–94.
5. Gaal J, Stratakis CA, Carney JA, et al. SDHB immunohistochemistry: a useful tool in the diagnosis of Carney-Stratakis and Carney triad gastrointestinal stromal tumors. Mod Pathol 2011;24:147–51.
6. Gill AJ, Chou A, Vilain R, et al. Immunohistochemistry for SDHB divides gastrointestinal stromal tumors (GISTs) into 2 distinct types. Am J Surg Pathol 2010;34:636–44.
7. Miettinen M, Wang ZF, Sarlomo-Rikala M, et al. Succinate dehydrogenase-deficient GISTs: a clinicopathologic, immunohistochemical, and molecular genetic study of 66 gastric GISTs with predilection to young age. Am J Surg Pathol 2011;35:1712–21.
8. Doyle LA, Nelson D, Heinrich MC, et al. Loss of succinate dehydrogenase subunit B (SDHB) expression is limited to a distinctive subset of gastric wild-type gastrointestinal stromal tumours: a comprehensive genotype-phenotype correlation study. Histopathology 2012;61:801–9.
9. Wagner AJ, Remillard SP, Zhang YX, et al. Loss of expression of SDHA predicts SDHA mutations in gastrointestinal stromal tumors. Mod Pathol 2013; 26:289–94.
10. Agaram NP, Wong GC, Guo T, et al. Novel V600E BRAF mutations in imatinib-naive and imatinib-resistant gastrointestinal stromal tumors. Genes Chromosomes Cancer 2008;47:853–9.
11. Agaimy A, Terracciano LM, Dirnhofer S, et al. V600E BRAF mutations are alternative early molecular events in a subset of KIT/PDGFRA wild-type gastrointestinal stromal tumours. J Clin Pathol 2009;62:613–6.
12. Hostein I, Faur N, Primois C, et al. BRAF mutation status in gastrointestinal stromal tumors. Am J Clin Pathol 2010;133:141–8.
13. Daniels M, Lurkin I, Pauli R, et al. Spectrum of KIT/PDGFRA/BRAF mutations and Phosphatidylinositol-3-Kinase pathway gene alterations in gastrointestinal stromal tumors (GIST). Cancer Lett 2011;312:43–54.
14. Vallaeys JH, Cuvelier CA, Bekaert L, et al. Combined leiomyomatosis of the small intestine and colon. Arch Pathol Lab Med 1992;116:281–3.
15. Fernandes JP, Mascarenhas MJ, Costa CD, et al. Diffuse leiomyomatosis of the esophagus: a case report and review of the literature. Am J Dig Dis 1975;20:684–90.
16. Miettinen M, Sarlomo-Rikala M, Sobin LH, et al. Esophageal stromal tumors: a clinicopathologic, immunohistochemical, and molecular genetic study of 17 cases and comparison with esophageal leiomyomas and leiomyosarcomas. Am J Surg Pathol 2000;24:211–22.
17. Miettinen M, Sarlomo-Rikala M, Sobin LH. Mesenchymal tumors of muscularis mucosae of colon and rectum are benign leiomyomas that should be separated from gastrointestinal stromal tumors—a clinicopathologic and immunohistochemical study of eighty-eight cases. Mod Pathol 2001;14:950–6.
18. Miettinen M, Furlong M, Sarlomo-Rikala M, et al. Gastrointestinal stromal tumors, intramural leiomyomas, and leiomyosarcomas in the rectum and anus: a clinicopathologic, immunohistochemical, and molecular genetic study of 144 cases. Am J Surg Pathol 2001;25:1121–33.
19. Miettinen M, Sobin LH, Sarlomo-Rikala M. Immunohistochemical spectrum of GISTs at different sites and their differential diagnosis with a reference to CD117 (KIT). Mod Pathol 2000;13:1134–42.
20. Espinosa I, Lee CH, Kim MK, et al. A novel monoclonal antibody against DOG1 is a sensitive and specific marker for gastrointestinal stromal tumors. Am J Surg Pathol 2008;32:210–8.
21. Miettinen M, Sarlomo-Rikala M, Sobin LH, et al. Gastrointestinal stromal tumors and leiomyosarcomas in the colon: a clinicopathologic, immunohistochemical, and molecular genetic study of 44 cases. Am J Surg Pathol 2000;24:1339–52.
22. Iwata J, Fletcher CD. Immunohistochemical detection of cytokeratin and epithelial membrane antigen in leiomyosarcoma: a systematic study of 100 cases. Pathol Int 2000;50:7–14.
23. Miettinen M. Immunoreactivity for cytokeratin and epithelial membrane antigen in leiomyosarcoma. Arch Pathol Lab Med 1988;112:637–40.

24. Hornick JL, Fletcher CD. PEComa: what do we know so far? Histopathology 2006;48:75–82.

25. Shi H, Cao D, Wei L, et al. Inflammatory angiomyolipomas of the liver: a clinicopathologic and immunohistochemical analysis of 5 cases. Ann Diagn Pathol 2010;14:240–6.

26. Hornick JL, Fletcher CD. Sclerosing PEComa: clinicopathologic analysis of a distinctive variant with a predilection for the retroperitoneum. Am J Surg Pathol 2008;32:493–501.

27. Freeman HJ, Webber DL. Perivascular epithelioid cell neoplasm of the colon. World J Gastrointest Oncol 2010;2:205–8.

28. Shi HY, Wei LX, Sun L, et al. Clinicopathologic analysis of 4 perivascular epithelioid cell tumors (PEComas) of the gastrointestinal tract. Int J Surg Pathol 2010;18:243–7.

29. Ryan P, Nguyen VH, Gholoum S, et al. Polypoid PEComa in the rectum of a 15-year-old girl: case report and review of PEComa in the gastrointestinal tract. Am J Surg Pathol 2009;33:475–82.

30. Folpe AL, Mentzel T, Lehr HA, et al. Perivascular epithelioid cell neoplasms of soft tissue and gynecologic origin: a clinicopathologic study of 26 cases and review of the literature. Am J Surg Pathol 2005;29:1558–75.

31. Pan CC, Chung MY, Ng KF, et al. Constant allelic alteration on chromosome 16p (TSC2 gene) in perivascular epithelioid cell tumour (PEComa): genetic evidence for the relationship of PEComa with angiomyolipoma. J Pathol 2008;214:387–93.

32. Wagner AJ, Malinowska-Kolodziej I, Morgan JA, et al. Clinical activity of mTOR inhibition with sirolimus in malignant perivascular epithelioid cell tumors: targeting the pathogenic activation of mTORC1 in tumors. J Clin Oncol 2010;28:835–40.

33. Argani P, Aulmann S, Illei PB, et al. A distinctive subset of PEComas harbors TFE3 gene fusions. Am J Surg Pathol 2010;34:1395–406.

34. Liegl B, Hornick JL, Fletcher CD. Primary cutaneous PEComa: distinctive clear cell lesions of skin. Am J Surg Pathol 2008;32:608–14.

35. Fletcher CDM, Bridge JA, Hogendoorn PCW, et al, editors. WHO Classification of Tumours of Soft Tissue and Bone. IARC: Lyon; 2013.

36. Appelman HD, Helwig EB. Glomus tumors of the stomach. Cancer 1969;23:203–13.

37. Miettinen M, Paal E, Lasota J, et al. Gastrointestinal glomus tumors: a clinicopathologic, immunohistochemical, and molecular genetic study of 32 cases. Am J Surg Pathol 2002;26:301–11.

38. Geraghty JM, Everitt NJ, Blundell JW. Glomus tumour of the small bowel. Histopathology 1991; 19:287–9.

39. Hamilton CW, Shelburne JD, Bossen EH, et al. A glomus tumor of the jejunum masquerading as a carcinoid tumor. Hum Pathol 1982;13:859–61.

40. Barua R. Glomus tumor of the colon. First reported case. Dis Colon Rectum 1988;31:138–40.

41. Folpe AL, Fanburg-Smith JC, Miettinen M, et al. Atypical and malignant glomus tumors: analysis of 52 cases, with a proposal for the reclassification of glomus tumors. Am J Surg Pathol 2001;25:1–12.

42. Rege TA, Wagner AJ, Corless CL, et al. "Pediatric-type" gastrointestinal stromal tumors in adults: distinctive histology predicts genotype and clinical behavior. Am J Surg Pathol 2011;35:495–504.

43. West RB, Corless CL, Chen X, et al. The novel marker, DOG1, is expressed ubiquitously in gastrointestinal stromal tumors irrespective of KIT or PDGFRA mutation status. Am J Pathol 2004;165: 107–13.

44. Vanek J. Gastric submucosal granuloma with eosinophilic infiltration. Am J Pathol 1949;25: 397–411.

45. Schildhaus HU, Buttner R, Binot E, et al. Inflammatory fibroid polyps are true neoplasms with PDGFRA mutations. Pathologe 2009;30(Suppl 2): 117–20.

46. Daum O, Hes O, Vanecek T, et al. Vanek's tumor (inflammatory fibroid polyp). Report of 18 cases and comparison with three cases of original Vanek's series. Ann Diagn Pathol 2003;7:337–47.

47. Makhlouf HR, Sobin LH. Inflammatory myofibroblastic tumors (inflammatory pseudotumors) of the gastrointestinal tract: how closely are they related to inflammatory fibroid polyps? Hum Pathol 2002;33:307–15.

48. Ozolek JA, Sasatomi E, Swalsky PA, et al. Inflammatory fibroid polyps of the gastrointestinal tract: clinical, pathologic, and molecular characteristics. Appl Immunohistochem Mol Morphol 2004;12: 59–66.

49. Pantanowitz L, Antonioli DA, Pinkus GS, et al. Inflammatory fibroid polyps of the gastrointestinal tract: evidence for a dendritic cell origin. Am J Surg Pathol 2004;28:107–14.

50. Lasota J, Wang ZF, Sobin LH, et al. Gain-of-function PDGFRA mutations, earlier reported in gastrointestinal stromal tumors, are common in small intestinal inflammatory fibroid polyps. A study of 60 cases. Mod Pathol 2009;22:1049–56.

51. Schildhaus HU, Cavlar T, Binot E, et al. Inflammatory fibroid polyps harbour mutations in the platelet-derived growth factor receptor alpha (PDGFRA) gene. J Pathol 2008;216:176–82.

52. Huss S, Wardelmann E, Goltz D, et al. Activating PDGFRA mutations in inflammatory fibroid polyps occur in exons 12, 14 and 18 and are associated with tumour localization. Histopathology 2012;61: 59–68.

53. Gleason BC, Hornick JL. Inflammatory myofibroblastic tumours: where are we now? J Clin Pathol 2008;61:428–37.

54. Cook JR, Dehner LP, Collins MH, et al. Anaplastic lymphoma kinase (ALK) expression in the inflammatory myofibroblastic tumor: a comparative immunohistochemical study. Am J Surg Pathol 2001;25:1364–71.

55. Coffin CM, Hornick JL, Fletcher CD. Inflammatory myofibroblastic tumor: comparison of clinicopathologic, histologic, and immunohistochemical features including ALK expression in atypical and aggressive cases. Am J Surg Pathol 2007;31:509–20.

56. Takahashi Y, Shimizu S, Ishida T, et al. Plexiform angiomyxoid myofibroblastic tumor of the stomach. Am J Surg Pathol 2007;31:724–8.

57. Miettinen M, Makhlouf HR, Sobin LH, et al. Plexiform fibromyxoma: a distinctive benign gastric antral neoplasm not to be confused with a myxoid GIST. Am J Surg Pathol 2009;33:1624–32.

58. Takahashi Y, Suzuki M, Fukusato T. Plexiform angiomyxoid myofibroblastic tumor of the stomach. World J Gastroenterol 2010;16:2835–40.

59. Yoshida A, Klimstra DS, Antonescu CR. Plexiform angiomyxoid tumor of the stomach. Am J Surg Pathol 2008;32:1910–2.

60. Suster S, Sorace D, Moran CA. Gastrointestinal stromal tumors with prominent myxoid matrix. Clinicopathologic, immunohistochemical, and ultrastructural study of nine cases of a distinctive morphologic variant of myogenic stromal tumor. Am J Surg Pathol 1995;19:59–70.

61. Hornick JL, Fletcher CD. Soft tissue perineurioma: clinicopathologic analysis of 81 cases including those with atypical histologic features. Am J Surg Pathol 2005;29:845–58.

62. Bhattacharya B, Dilworth HP, Iacobuzio-Donahue C, et al. Nuclear beta-catenin expression distinguishes deep fibromatosis from other benign and malignant fibroblastic and myofibroblastic lesions. Am J Surg Pathol 2005;29:653–9.

63. Marino-Enriquez A, Wang WL, Roy A, et al. Epithelioid inflammatory myofibroblastic sarcoma: an aggressive intra-abdominal variant of inflammatory myofibroblastic tumor with nuclear membrane or perinuclear ALK. Am J Surg Pathol 2011;35:135–44.

64. Coffin CM, Watterson J, Priest JR, et al. Extrapulmonary inflammatory myofibroblastic tumor (inflammatory pseudotumor). A clinicopathologic and immunohistochemical study of 84 cases. Am J Surg Pathol 1995;19:859–72.

65. Yamamoto H, Oda Y, Saito T, et al. p53 Mutation and MDM2 amplification in inflammatory myofibroblastic tumours. Histopathology 2003;42:431–9.

66. Griffin CA, Hawkins AL, Dvorak C, et al. Recurrent involvement of 2p23 in inflammatory myofibroblastic tumors. Cancer Res 1999;59:2776–80.

67. Alaggio R, Cecchetto G, Bisogno G, et al. Inflammatory myofibroblastic tumors in childhood: a report from the Italian Cooperative Group studies. Cancer 2010;116:216–26.

68. Miettinen M, Shekitka KM, Sobin LH. Schwannomas in the colon and rectum: a clinicopathologic and immunohistochemical study of 20 cases. Am J Surg Pathol 2001;25:846–55.

69. Prevot S, Bienvenu L, Vaillant JC, et al. Benign schwannoma of the digestive tract: a clinicopathologic and immunohistochemical study of five cases, including a case of esophageal tumor. Am J Surg Pathol 1999;23:431–6.

70. Daimaru Y, Kido H, Hashimoto H, et al. Benign schwannoma of the gastrointestinal tract: a clinicopathologic and immunohistochemical study. Hum Pathol 1988;19:257–64.

71. Voltaggio L, Murray R, Lasota J, et al. Gastric schwannoma: a clinicopathologic study of 51 cases and critical review of the literature. Hum Pathol 2012;43:650–9.

72. Miettinen M, Sobin LH, Lasota J. Gastrointestinal stromal tumors of the stomach: a clinicopathologic, immunohistochemical, and molecular genetic study of 1765 cases with long-term follow-up. Am J Surg Pathol 2005;29:52–68.

73. Miettinen M, Lasota J. Gastrointestinal stromal tumors: pathology and prognosis at different sites. Semin Diagn Pathol 2006;23:70–83.

74. Hornick JL, Fletcher CD. Intestinal perineuriomas: clinicopathologic definition of a new anatomic subset in a series of 10 cases. Am J Surg Pathol 2005;29:859–65.

75. Groisman GM, Polak-Charcon S. Fibroblastic polyp of the colon and colonic perineurioma: 2 names for a single entity? Am J Surg Pathol 2008;32:1088–94.

76. Eslami-Varzaneh F, Washington K, Robert ME, et al. Benign fibroblastic polyps of the colon: a histologic, immunohistochemical, and ultrastructural study. Am J Surg Pathol 2004;28:374–8.

77. Groisman GM, Polak-Charcon S, Appelman HD. Fibroblastic polyp of the colon: clinicopathological analysis of 10 cases with emphasis on its common association with serrated crypts. Histopathology 2006;48:431–7.

78. Agaimy A, Stoehr R, Vieth M, et al. Benign serrated colorectal fibroblastic polyps/intramucosal perineuriomas are true mixed epithelial-stromal polyps (hybrid hyperplastic polyp/mucosal perineurioma) with frequent BRAF mutations. Am J Surg Pathol 2010;34:1663–71.

79. Gibson JA, Hornick JL. Mucosal Schwann cell "hamartoma": clinicopathologic study of 26 neural colorectal polyps distinct from neurofibromas and mucosal neuromas. Am J Surg Pathol 2009;33:781–7.

80. Shekitka KM, Sobin LH. Ganglioneuromas of the gastrointestinal tract. Relation to Von Recklinghausen

disease and other multiple tumor syndromes. Am J Surg Pathol 1994;18:250–7.

81. Fuller CE, Williams GT. Gastrointestinal manifestations of type 1 neurofibromatosis (von Recklinghausen's disease). Histopathology 1991;19:1–11.

82. Davis GB, Berk RN. Intestinal neurofibromas in von Recklinghausen's disease. Am J Gastroenterol 1973;60:410–4.

83. Lee NC, Norton JA. Multiple endocrine neoplasia type 2B–genetic basis and clinical expression. Surg Oncol 2000;9:111–8.

84. Lewin MR, Dilworth HP, Abu Alfa AK, et al. Mucosal benign epithelioid nerve sheath tumors. Am J Surg Pathol 2005;29:1310–5.

85. Kosemehmetoglu K, Folpe AL. Clear cell sarcoma of tendons and aponeuroses, and osteoclast-rich tumour of the gastrointestinal tract with features resembling clear cell sarcoma of soft parts: a review and update. J Clin Pathol 2010;63:416–23.

86. Antonescu CR, Nafa K, Segal NH, et al. EWS-CREB1: a recurrent variant fusion in clear cell sarcoma–association with gastrointestinal location and absence of melanocytic differentiation. Clin Cancer Res 2006;12:5356–62.

87. Stockman DL, Miettinen M, Suster S, et al. Malignant gastrointestinal neuroectodermal tumor: clinicopathologic, immunohistochemical, ultrastructural, and molecular analysis of 16 cases with a reappraisal of clear cell sarcoma-like tumors of the gastrointestinal tract. Am J Surg Pathol 2012; 36:857–68.

88. Zambrano E, Reyes-Mugica M, Franchi A, et al. An osteoclast-rich tumor of the gastrointestinal tract with features resembling clear cell sarcoma of soft parts: reports of 6 cases of a GIST simulator. Int J Surg Pathol 2003;11:75–81.

89. Hiraga H, Nojima T, Abe S, et al. Establishment of a new continuous clear cell sarcoma cell line: morphological and cytogenetic characterization and detection of chimaeric EWS/ATF-1 transcripts. Virchows Arch 1997;431:45–51.

90. Stenman G, Kindblom LG, Angervall L. Reciprocal translocation t(12;22)(q13]3) in clear-cell sarcoma of tendons and aponeuroses. Genes Chromosomes Cancer 1992;4:122–7.

91. Hisaoka M, Ishida T, Kuo TT, et al. Clear cell sarcoma of soft tissue: a clinicopathologic, immunohistochemical, and molecular analysis of 33 cases. Am J Surg Pathol 2008;32:452–60.

92. Meis-Kindblom JM. Clear cell sarcoma of tendons and aponeuroses: a historical perspective and tribute to the man behind the entity. Adv Anat Pathol 2006;13:286–92.

93. Shia J, Chen W, Tang LH, et al. Extranodal follicular dendritic cell sarcoma: clinical, pathologic, and histogenetic characteristics of an underrecognized disease entity. Virchows Arch 2006; 449:148–58.

94. Han JH, Kim SH, Noh SH, et al. Follicular dendritic cell sarcoma presenting as a submucosal tumor of the stomach. Arch Pathol Lab Med 2000;124: 1693–6.

95. Chan JK, Fletcher CD, Nayler SJ, et al. Follicular dendritic cell sarcoma. Clinicopathologic analysis of 17 cases suggesting a malignant potential higher than currently recognized. Cancer 1997; 79:294–313.

96. Perez-Ordonez B, Erlandson RA, Rosai J. Follicular dendritic cell tumor: report of 13 additional cases of a distinctive entity. Am J Surg Pathol 1996;20: 944–55.

97. Chang KC, Jin YT, Chen FF, et al. Follicular dendritic cell sarcoma of the colon mimicking stromal tumour. Histopathology 2001;38:25–9.

98. Grogg KL, Lae ME, Kurtin PJ, et al. Clusterin expression distinguishes follicular dendritic cell tumors from other dendritic cell neoplasms: report of a novel follicular dendritic cell marker and clinicopathologic data on 12 additional follicular dendritic cell tumors and 6 additional interdigitating dendritic cell tumors. Am J Surg Pathol 2004;28: 988–98.

99. Yu H, Gibson JA, Pinkus GS, et al. Podoplanin (D2-40) is a novel marker for follicular dendritic cell tumors. Am J Clin Pathol 2007;128:776–82.

100. Shen SC, Wu CC, Ng KF, et al. Follicular dendritic cell sarcoma mimicking giant cell carcinoma of the pancreas. Pathol Int 2006;56:466–70.

101. Miettinen M, Dow N, Lasota J, et al. A distinctive novel epitheliomesenchymal biphasic tumor of the stomach in young adults ("gastroblastoma"): a series of 3 cases. Am J Surg Pathol 2009;33: 1370–7.

102. Shin DH, Lee JH, Kang HJ, et al. Novel epitheliomesenchymal biphasic stomach tumour (gastroblastoma) in a 9-year-old: morphological, ultrastructural and immunohistochemical findings. J Clin Pathol 2010;63:270–4.

103. Wey EA, Britton AJ, Sferra JJ, et al. Gastroblastoma in a 28-year-old man with nodal metastasis: proof of the malignant potential. Arch Pathol Lab Med 2012;136:961–4.

104. Poizat F, de Chaisemartin C, Bories E, et al. A distinctive epitheliomesenchymal biphasic tumor in the duodenum: the first case of duodenoblastoma? Virchows Arch 2012;461:379–83.

105. Makhlouf HR, Ahrens W, Agarwal B, et al. Synovial sarcoma of the stomach: a clinicopathologic, immunohistochemical, and molecular genetic study of 10 cases. Am J Surg Pathol 2008;32: 275–81.

106. Terry J, Saito T, Subramanian S, et al. TLE1 as a diagnostic immunohistochemical marker for synovial sarcoma emerging from gene expression profiling studies. Am J Surg Pathol 2007; 31:240–6.

107. Foo WC, Cruise MW, Wick MR, et al. Immunohistochemical staining for TLE1 distinguishes synovial sarcoma from histologic mimics. Am J Clin Pathol 2011;135:839–44.

108. Hornick JL, Fletcher CD. Myoepithelial tumors of soft tissue: a clinicopathologic and immunohistochemical study of 101 cases with evaluation of prognostic parameters. Am J Surg Pathol 2003; 27(9):1183–96.

Barrett Esophagus
Evolving Concepts in Diagnosis and Neoplastic Progression

Mikhail Lisovsky, MD, PhD[a], Amitabh Srivastava, MD[b],*

KEYWORDS

- Esophagus • Barrett's esophagus • Metaplasia • Dysplasia • Adenocarcinoma • Cancer
- Prognosis

ABSTRACT

Surgical pathologists need to answer 2 questions when evaluating biopsies from the distal esophagus or gastroesophageal junction in patients with a history of gastroesophageal reflux disease: Are the findings consistent with Barrett esophagus? and Is there any evidence of dysplasia? Pathologists should be well informed about the controversy around the definition of Barrett esophagus and the common pitfalls that lead to a false-positive diagnosis of Barrett esophagus or Barrett esophagus–associated dysplasia. A concise description of distinct morphologic types of dysplasia in Barrett esophagus and a summary of recent data on the natural history of BE are provided in this review.

Abbreviations: Barrett's Esophagus	
BE	Barrett's Esophagus
CIM	Carditis with Intestinal Metaplasia
CLE	"Columnar lined esophagus"
EAC	Esophageal adenocarcinoma
GEJ	Gastroesophageal junction
GERD	Gastroesophageal Reflux Disease
HGD	High-grade dysplasia
IM	Intestinal metaplasia
LGD	Low-grade dysplasia
SCJ	Squamocolumnar junction (also known as the Z-line)

OVERVIEW

Barrett esophagus (BE) arises as a complication of chronic gastroesophageal reflux disease (GERD) and is a precursor of esophageal adenocarcinoma (EAC). The incidence of EAC has increased dramatically in the United States, by more than 463% in white men and 335% in white women,[1] but may have hit a plateau.[2] The incidence of BE is also rising and this represents a true increase because it persists even after adjusting for the number of endoscopies performed in the population.[3] Once a diagnosis of BE is established, these patients undergo periodic surveillance for early detection of dysplasia and cancer. In recent years, the requirement for identifying goblet cells to establish a diagnosis of BE has been challenged and there is renewed interest in the biologic significance of non–goblet columnar epithelium lining the distal esophagus. Large population-based studies have shed light on the natural history of BE and associated neoplasia. New morphologic subtypes of dysplasia have been defined and advances in endoscopic management have greatly reduced the need for esophagectomy for treating dysplasia and early cancer in BE. The aim of this review is to summarize the state of current understanding of BE and BE-related neoplasia.

Disclosures: None.
[a] Department of Pathology, Dartmouth Hitchcock Medical Center, One Medical Center Drive, Lebanon, NH 03756, USA; [b] Department of Pathology, Brigham and Women's Hospital, 75 Francis Street, Boston, MA 02115, USA
* Corresponding author.
E-mail address: ASrivastava@partners.org

Surgical Pathology 6 (2013) 475–496
http://dx.doi.org/10.1016/j.path.2013.05.002
1875-9181/13/$ – see front matter © 2013 Elsevier Inc. All rights reserved.

Pathologic Key Features
BARRETT'S ESOPHAGUS

1. Goblet cells in distal esophagus biopsies are required in making a diagnosis of BE

2. Epithelial atypia in the presence of marked inflammation or ulcer is diagnosed as indefinite for dysplasia

3. Abrupt transition in morphology and loss of surface maturation are characteristic of dysplasia

4. Pencillate, hyperchromatic, and stratified nuclei with inconspicuous nucleoli that extend from crypt base to surface epithelium are features of low-grade dysplasia (LGD)

5. High-grade dysplasia (HGD) shows crowded, back-to-back crypts with round nuclei, loss of polarity, marked nuclear pleomorphism, prominent nucleoli, and atypical mitoses

6. Cystically dilated glands with intraluminal necrosis, confluent glands, single-cell infiltration into lamina propria, and invasion of muscularis mucosae are diagnostic for intramucosal adenocarcinoma

7. Foveolar-type dysplasia shows abundant pale cytoplasmic mucin resembling gastric foveolar epithelium

8. Epithelial atypia at crypt base out of proportion with the degree of inflammation, is possibly true dysplasia confined to crypt base; diagnoses as indefinite for dysplasia and recommend close surveillance

9. Serrated dysplasia resembles traditional serrated adenoma of colorectum

THE CONTROVERSY REGARDING DEFINITION OF BARRETT ESOPHAGUS

The American Gastroenterological Association defines BE as "a change in the distal esophageal epithelium of any length that can be recognized as columnar type mucosa at endoscopy and is confirmed to have intestinal metaplasia by biopsy of the tubular esophagus."[4] There is consensus regarding the presence of columnar epithelium in the distal esophagus as a prerequisite for a diagnosis of BE. The need to demonstrate intestinal metaplasia (IM), however, to establish a diagnosis of BE is a matter of considerable debate. The British Society of Gastroenterology considers BE "a segment of columnar metaplasia of any length that must be visible endoscopically above the oesophago-gastric junction and confirmed or corroborated histologically" and does not require demonstration of IM for a diagnosis of BE.[5] The term, *columnar-lined esophagus (CLE)*, is used as a synonym for BE. Similarly, in Japan, a diagnosis of BE does not require demonstration of goblet cells.[6]

The requirement for goblet cells as a prerequisite for a diagnosis of BE is controversial for several reasons. Goblet cells are unevenly distributed in the metaplastic segment and vary in number between patients. Failure to detect goblet cells due to sampling error can lead to a false-negative

diagnosis and deprive patients of endoscopic surveillance. The likelihood of finding goblet cells in esophageal biopsies is a function of BE segment length, the number of biopsies obtained, and the number of endoscopies performed over a period of time.[7,8] Gatenby and colleagues,[8] in a study from the United Kingdom, showed that 54.8% and 90.8% of patients negative for IM at index endoscopy were positive for IM after 5 and 10 years of follow-up, respectively. Moreover, the expression of intestinal markers, such as CDX2, Hepar-1, villin, and DAS-1, in non–goblet columnar epithelium in BE has been used to support the contention that the non–goblet epithelium is already intestinalized at a molecular level and should be part of the definition of BE.[9] DNA ploidy abnormalities occur in non–goblet cell and goblet cell columnar epithelium, suggesting that the risk of neoplastic transformation may be similar in both types of mucosa.[10] There are some data to suggest that this may be true. Two longitudinal studies have shown no difference in risk of dysplasia and EAC in patients with and without IM at index endoscopy, but both have limitations.[8,11] No central review of endoscopic and pathologic findings was performed in one[8] and the criteria used to diagnose IM were different from standard practice in the other.[11] In the latter study, the presence of a brush border or a periodic acid–Schiff/Alcian blue stain was also accepted as IM even in the absence of goblet cells.[11] The absence of goblet cells in background mucosa in more than 70% of small (less than 2 cm) EACs, in some studies, also challenges the view that cancers invariably arise in mucosa with goblet cells.[12]

In contrast to the studies discussed previously, a population-based study of 8522 BE patients from Northern Ireland found the risk of cancer 0.38% per year in patients with IM and only 0.07% in those without IM.[13] In another recent study of 214 systematically biopsied patients, prevalent EAC or dysplasia was detected in 26% of patients, all of whom showed IM in the background mucosa.[14] The reported discrepancies in risk of EAC in patients with and without IM may, in part, be related to lack of standardization in biopsy protocols. An evaluation of 401 gastroenterologists participating in the AspECT trial in the United Kingdom found that 90% of them did not take adequate biopsies for histologic diagnosis.[15] There may be a small increase in risk of EAC in patients with non–goblet columnar epithelium in the esophagus but until the magnitude of risk is clearly defined, routine endoscopic surveillance cannot be recommended for these patients.[16] Moreover, non–goblet columnar mucosa is present in up to 25% of GERD patients undergoing endoscopic examination.[17] Changing the definition of BE and enrolling these patients in a surveillance program would be a significant burden on health care resources with uncertain benefit at the present time.

MACROSCOPIC FEATURES OF BARRETT ESOPHAGUS

The gastroesophageal junction (GEJ) is defined, on endoscopy, as the proximal limit of the gastric rugal folds. The squamocolumnar junction (SCJ), also known as the Z-line, is the transition between the gray-white squamous mucosa of the esophagus and the salmon-red columnar epithelium lining the stomach. In normal individuals, the GEJ and SCJ lie at the same level but in patients with BE the SCJ (neo-SCJ) is proximal to the GEJ (**Fig. 1**). It is from this columnar segment, between the GEJ and the neo-SCJ, that biopsies must be obtained to document IM and establish a diagnosis of BE. Patients with columnar epithelium lining the distal esophagus are often classified into ultrashort segment (less than 1 cm), short segment (1–3 cm), and long segment (greater than 3 cm) BE. Dysplasia in BE is usually flat and invisible by conventional endoscopy, which necessitates systematic 4-quadrant biopsies at defined intervals (known as the Seattle protocol).[18] Less frequently, dysplasia may present as an endoscopically visible lesion or nodule and the likelihood of synchronous and metachronous carcinoma is higher in these cases.[18]

MICROSCOPIC FEATURES OF BARRETT ESOPHAGUS

The diagnosis of BE is straightforward when IM is detected in biopsies obtained from the distal esophagus. Often, however, endoscopists are uncertain about the exact location of the SCJ (in relation to the GEJ) and biopsy a markedly irregular Z-line or even the GEJ and ask a pathologist to rule out the possibility of BE. In such cases, the differential diagnosis is between BE and IM involving the proximal stomach.

DISTINCTION OF BARRETT ESOPHAGUS FROM CARDITIS WITH INTESTINAL METAPLASIA

Inflammation and IM around the GEJ is etiologically related to either GERD or chronic gastritis. Distinction of BE from CIM is important because endoscopic surveillance is recommended only for patients with BE. In a prospective study, CIM was more prevalent among African Americans and showed a significantly lower prevalence of dysplasia compared with short-segment BE (1.3% vs 11.3%). HGD or cancer was detected only in BE patients on follow-up.[19] The distinction of BE from CIM remains, however, problematic. There are some morphologic features that help distinguish BE from CIM.[20] The presence of esophageal glands/ducts, squamous epithelium overlying metaplastic crypts, multilayered epithelium, and hybrid glands is typically seen in BE but not CIM (**Fig. 2**). The presence of esophageal glands/ducts is definitive evidence for BE and also for columnar-lined esophagus without IM (**Fig. 3**). The initial suggestions of a typical CK7/CK20 staining pattern characteristic of BE were not validated in subsequent studies.[21–23] Other markers, such as MUC-1, MUC-6, Das1, CDX2, Hepar-1, and CD10, also lack adequate sensitivity and/or specificity for routine clinical use.[24,25] Progression of CIM to macroscopically evident BE was reported in 25% of patients on follow-up in a recent study suggesting a possible link between the 2 conditions, at least in some patients.[26]

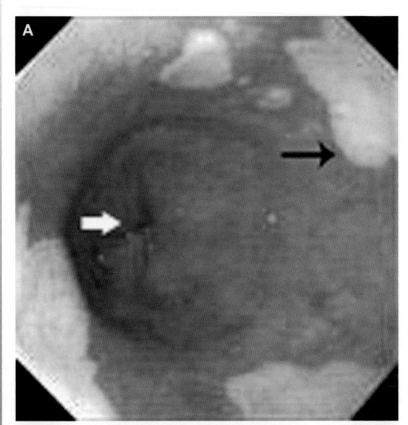

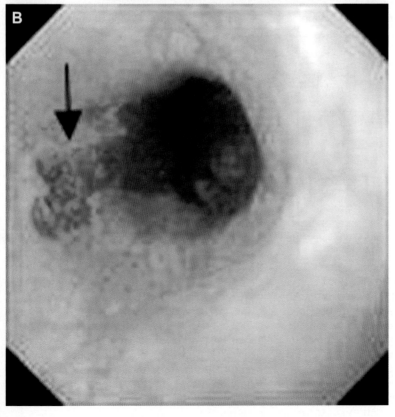

Fig. 1. Endoscopic appearance of BE. (*A*) The SCJ (*black arrow*) is proximal to the GE junction (*white arrow*) and a salmon-red columnar mucosa lines the distal esophagus. Note residual squamous islands within the columnar segment. (*B*) A discrete tongue of columnar mucosa (*arrow*) may extend into the esophagus in some patients.

Fig. 2. Presence of (*A*; H&E stain, ×100–200) esophageal mucous glands (*arrowheads*) or (*B*; H&E stain, ×100–200) esophageal gland ducts (*arrow*) is definite evidence for the esophageal location of the biopsy and BE can be diagnosed with certainty if IM is present. Hybrid glands, in which cardia-type glands at the base merge with intestinalized crypts in the upper half (*C*; H&E stain, ×100–200).

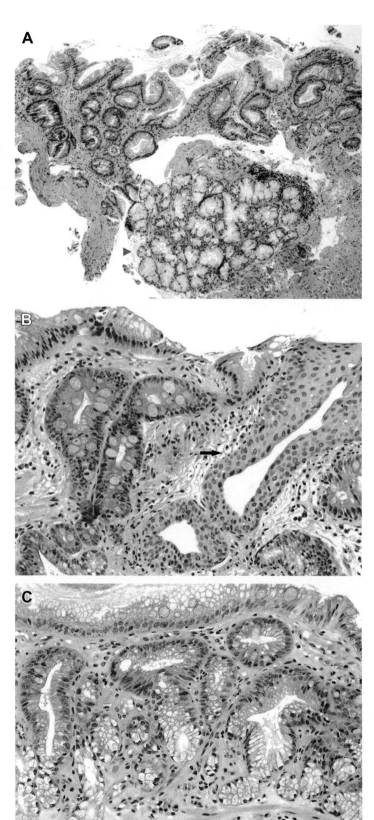

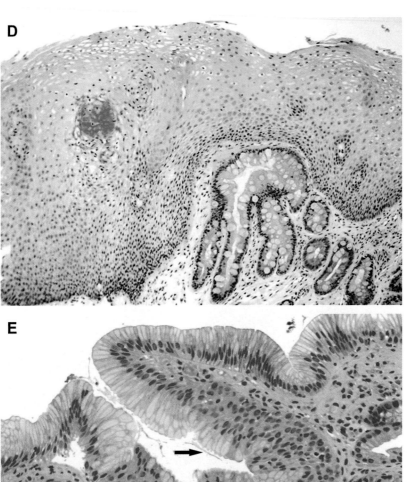

Fig. 2. Squamous mucosa overlying metaplastic crypts (*D*; H&E stain, ×100), and multilayered epithelium (*arrow*) (*E*; H&E stain, ×200) with mixed squamous and columnar features, favor a diagnosis of BE over IM of the proximal stomach in GEJ biopsies.

Fig. 3. Submucosal esophageal gland/duct confirms esophageal location but the mucosa shows no goblet cells in this columnar-lined esophagus (H&E stain, ×20).

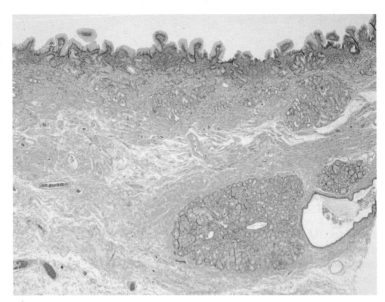

Fig. 4. (*A*; H&E stain, ×100) IM in BE occurs in a background of cardia-type mucosa. Misinterpretation of pseudogoblet cells (*arrow*) as IM can lead to a false-positive diagnosis of BE. (*B*; H&E stain, ×100) The nuclei of the intestinalized crypts are larger, more hyperchromatic, and stratified compared with the small, basal nuclei of the mucous glands (*arrow*). This baseline atypia in BE may be erroneously interpreted as dysplasia.

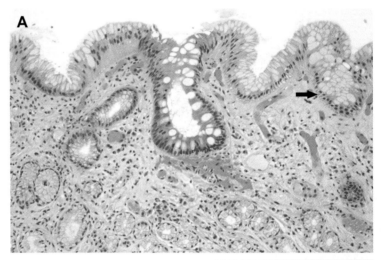

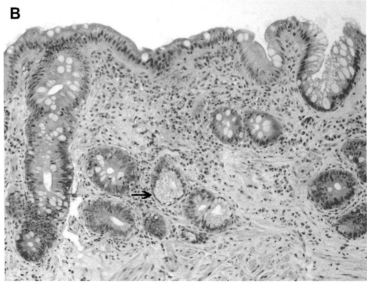

FEATURES OF NONDYSPLASTIC BARRETT ESOPHAGUS

Morphologic detection of dysplasia remains the gold standard for identification of high-risk patients most likely to benefit from close surveillance. Surveillance biopsies in patients with BE are categorized as negative for dysplasia, indefinite for dysplasia, LGD, HGD, and intramucosal adenocarcinoma.

A false-positive diagnosis of BE can be rendered when pseudogoblet cells are mistaken for IM (**Fig. 4**A) and dysplasia can be overdiagnosed if pathologists are unaware that there is a certain level of baseline or metaplastic atypia in BE. Intestinalization of crypts occurs in a background of cardia-type or oxyntocardia-type mucosa (see **Fig. 4**A). The juxtaposition of bland appearing mucous glands with small, pale, basally anchored nuclei (see **Fig. 4**B) next to intestinalized crypts with enlarged, often pencillate and hyperchromatic nuclei with some stratification can easily be misinterpreted as dysplasia. This pitfall can be avoided by paying attention to surface maturation, which consists of gradual disappearance of basal cytologic atypia and nuclear stratification toward the luminal surface. The presence of surface maturation argues strongly against a diagnosis of dysplasia,[27] except in rare instances of basal crypt dysplasia (discussed later). Another unique feature of BE is the presence of a double muscularis mucosae that can pose challenges in staging of early EAC.[28]

BARRETT ESOPHAGUS INDEFINITE FOR DYSPLASIA

The indefinite for dysplasia category is used as an interim diagnosis for cases when a definite diagnosis of dysplasia cannot be rendered due to technical issues, such as denuded surface epithelium, significant cautery artifact, or poor biopsy orientation with tangential sectioning, or in post-treatment biopsies, where metaplastic crypts may be present underneath squamous mucosa and cannot be evaluated for surface maturation. Most often, however, this diagnosis is used in the setting of significant active inflammation or ulcer with marked epithelial atypia where regenerative changes cannot be confidently distinguished from dysplasia (**Figs. 5** and **6**). Prominent regeneration can also show loss of surface maturation, nuclear enlargement, hyperchromasia, and increased mitoses. Nuclear crowding is less common, however, and the chromatin pattern remains vesicular, typically showing small nucleoli. Gradual resolution of atypia toward the periphery of the inflamed focus in contrast to abrupt transition in dysplasia is also a useful morphologic clue to the correct diagnosis.[29]

BARRETT ESOPHAGUS WITH DYSPLASIA

The biology of BE is unique in that it straddles the boundaries between metaplasia and neoplasia. The metaplastic columnar mucosa can show clonal abnormalities involving the entire BE segment despite absence of morphologic dysplasia.[30] Molecular changes, such as up-regulation of claudin-18, represent mucosal adaptation to reflux,[31,32] whereas others, such as CDKN2 A (p16) and TP53 aberrations, and DNA ploidy abnormalities, confer an increased predisposition to EAC[32,33] Thus, a subset of nondysplastic BE is already a hyperproliferative, neoplastic condition at the molecular level rather than a nonclonal metaplastic process.[34]

True morphologic dysplasia, of any grade, has 2 main characteristics at low-power examination: loss of surface maturation and abrupt transition from background nondysplastic epithelium to dysplasia (**Fig. 7**). The latter often manifests as an abrupt decrease or disappearance of goblet cells, loss of cellular mucin, higher nuclear/cytoplasmic ratio, and acquisition of additional cytologic abnormalities described under LGD and HGD below.

LGD shows a tubular architecture and the lining epithelium shows enlarged, pencillate, hyperchromatic, and overlapping nuclei with stratification (**Fig. 8**). The chromatin is uniformly hyperchromatic with inconspicuous nucleoli. By definition, these changes extend uniformly from the base of the crypt and involve the surface epithelium.[27,29,35]

HGD may show severe architectural or cytologic abnormalities but most often the 2 are present together (**Fig. 9**). Crowded back-to-back crypts with minimal intervening stroma and villiform change are the usual architectural features of HGD.[35] Cytologic abnormalities include round nuclei with loss of polarity, nuclear pleomorphism, prominent nucleoli, and increased crypt and surface mitoses, including atypical forms.

Intramucosal adenocarcinoma shows a tubular or cribriform architecture with cystically dilated

Fig. 5. Reactive atypia adjacent to mucosal ulceration shows cytoplasmic hypereosinophilia and large nuclei with vesicular chromatin and prominent nucleoli but there is minimal overlapping and stratification (H&E stain, ×100).

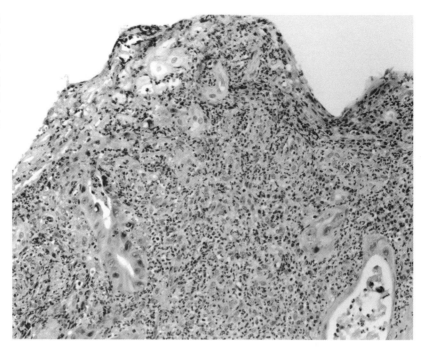

Fig. 6. The crypt surrounded by ulcer shows nuclear hyperchromasia, overlapping, and stratification as well as luminal mitosis (*arrow*). Dysplasia cannot be excluded with certainty and a diagnosis of indefinite for dysplasia is appropriate in such cases (H&E stain, ×200).

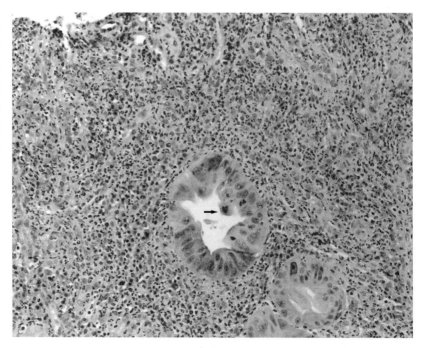

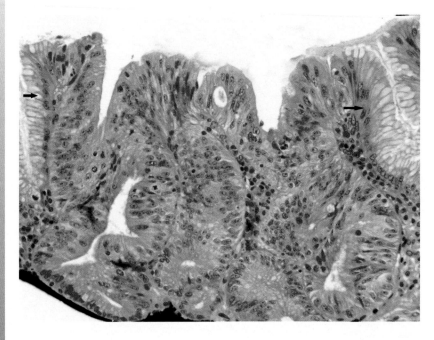

Fig. 7. Lack of surface maturation and abrupt change from surrounding mucosa are hallmarks of true dysplasia. The interface with nondysplastic epithelium (*arrows*) is sharp and the dysplastic focus shows mucin depletion and nuclear stratification that extends to the surface epithelium (H&E stain, ×200).

glands and intraluminal necrosis, intraluminal papillae or bridges, confluent and fused glandular pattern, or sheets of tumor cells devoid of gland formation, single-cell infiltration into the lamina propria, or neoplastic glands infiltrating the muscularis mucosae (**Fig. 10**).

DISTINCTIVE DYSPLASIA TYPES

The dysplasia classification (discussed previously) is based largely on cases of intestinal-type (adenomatous) dysplasia that resembles colorectal adenomas. Other distinct morphologic subtypes of dysplasia have been described recently in BE patients.

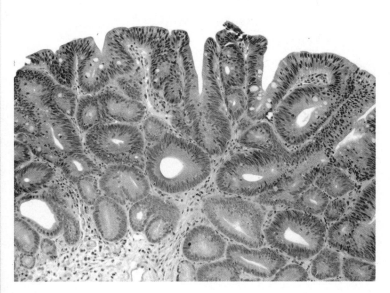

Fig. 8. Conventional LGD resembles colorectal adenomas. Elongated pencil-shaped, hyperchromatic nuclei with stratification and inconspicuous nucleoli uniformly involve the crypt base and surface epithelium (H&E stain, ×100).

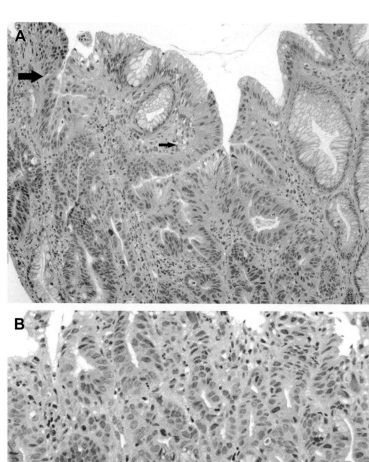

Fig. 9. (*A*; H&E stain, ×200) Conventional HGD shows greater nuclear pleomorphism, round nuclei with vesicular chromatin, and prominent nucleoli. The changes involve the surface epithelium (*arrows*). (*B*; H&E stain, ×200) Contrast nuclear features in a focus of residual LGD with elongated nuclei perpendicular to the basement membrane (*arrow*) as it transitions to HGD with round nuclei that have lost the perpendicular orientation. This loss of polarity is an important feature of HGD.

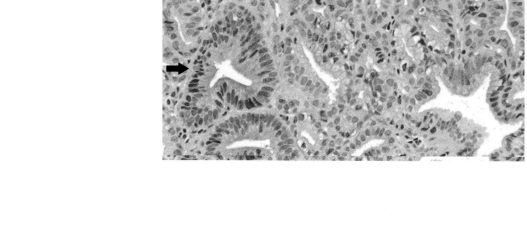

Foveolar dysplasia, which is well described in the stomach,[36] has been reported in up to 46% of dysplastic BE patients in some series,[37] but the true prevalence remains uncertain. Cases reported in literature as nonadenomatous and gastric dysplasia in BE are, most likely, part of the same spectrum.[38,39] The distinctive feature of foveolar dysplasia is the presence of abundant, pale cytoplasm resembling gastric foveolar-type epithelium (**Fig. 11**). This is in contrast to the mucin-depleted appearance typically seen in adenomatous dysplasia. The neoplastic cells stain positively with MUC5AC and are negative for MUC2. There is no validated grading scheme yet for foveolar-type dysplasia. Tubular or villiform architecture with or without significant glandular crowding may be present. The nuclei may be small and round and form a monolayer (see **Fig. 11C**) or may be pencillate and stratified, as in conventional adenomatous dysplasia (see **Fig. 11A**). There is

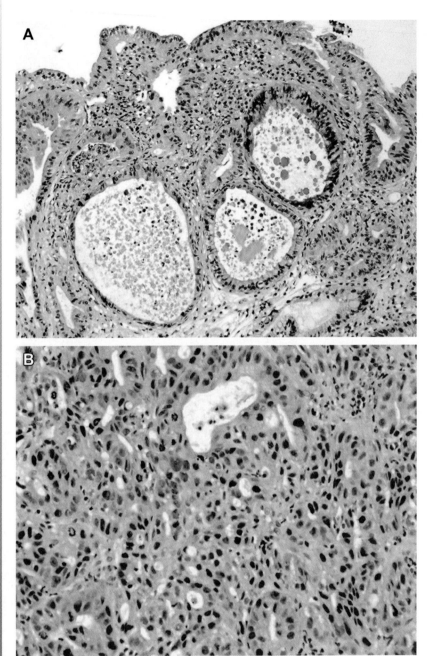

Fig.   10. Intramucosal adenocarcinoma is characterized by presence of cystically dilated crypts with (*A*; H&E stain, ×200) intraluminal necrosis, (*B*; H&E stain, ×200) confluent gland pattern

some evidence that foveolar dysplasia is more likely to arise in a goblet cell–depleted background (see **Fig. 11D**)[37,40] and carcinomas arising in this setting more often show a gastric phenotype.[41] The high prevalence of DNA abnormalities on flow cytometry and greater prevalence reported in series evaluating dysplasia adjacent to carcinoma suggest that foveolar dysplasia is a biologically high-grade lesion.[37–41]

Crypt dysplasia is a term proposed for cases of atypia in the crypt base that is beyond the acceptable range of baseline atypia in BE but still with

Fig. 10. (*C*; H&E stain, ×400) single-cell infiltration into the lamina propria, or (*D*; H&E stain, ×40) invasion through the muscularis mucosa. (*D*) BE patients often have a double muscularis mucosae as in this EMR specimen. The original compact muscularis mucosa is at the bottom of the field (*double arrows*) whereas the new one is at the top (*single arrow*). Submucosal invasion is diagnosed when the tumor breaks through the bottom compact layer.

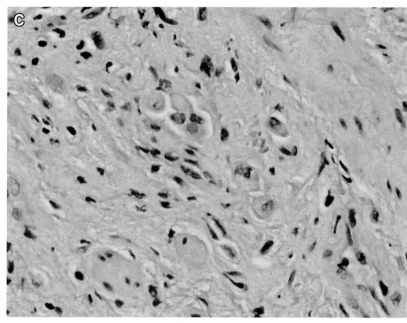

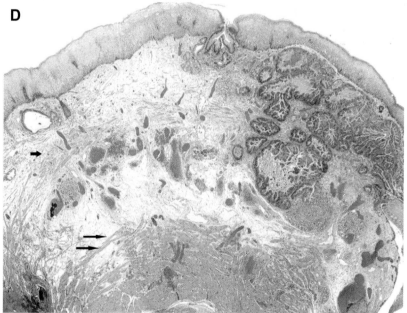

evidence of surface maturation precluding a definite diagnosis of conventional dysplasia (**Fig. 12**).[42] These foci showed overexpression of p53, *loss of heterozygosity* at 17p (*TP53*), and aneuploidy, suggesting that this may be early dysplasia confined to the crypt base. The diagnosis, however, is only moderately reproducible ($\kappa = 0.46$) among experts in the field[35] and such cases are currently diagnosed as indefinite for dysplasia to ensure proper surveillance. Serial sectioning is imperative to rule out surface involvement before rendering a diagnosis in these cases.

Serrated dysplasia in BE is rare, seldom occurs in pure form, and resembles traditional serrated adenoma of the colorectum (**Fig. 13**). Luminal serration is evident at low power and the neoplastic cells show dense eosinophilic cytoplasm with hyperchromatic and pencillate nuclei with stratification. In a small study, published in abstract form, 3 of 6 patients with serrated

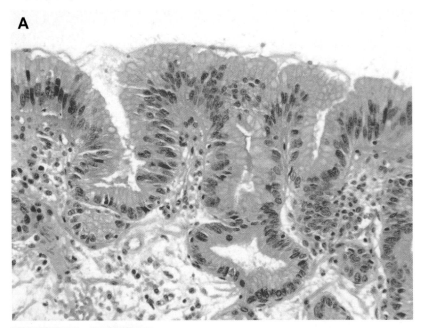

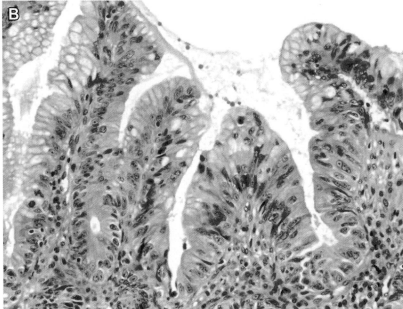

Fig. 11. In contrast to the mucin-depleted appearance in conventional dysplasia (see **Figs. 8** and **9**), foveolar dysplasia is characterized by abundant, pale cytoplasmic mucin that resembles gastric foveolar epithelium and stains positively for MUC5AC on immunohistochemistry. The nuclear features may be low grade (*A*; H&E stain, ×200) or high grade (*B*; H&E stain, ×200), and some cases show a monolayer with minimal or no stratification.

dysplasia at index examination progressed to EA on follow-up.[40]

PROBLEMS WITH DYSPLASIA DIAGNOSIS

The diagnosis of dysplasia in BE is limited by considerable interobserver variability among pathologists.[27,35,43,44] A diagnosis of negative for dysplasia or HGD is more reproducible (κ = 0.58–0.65) than LGD (κ = 0.32), and the agreement is poor for an indefinite for dysplasia diagnosis (κ = 0.17).[27] Differentiating HGD from intramucosal adenocarcinoma is also poorly reproducible in some studies[44] and may be

Fig. 11. (*C*; H&E stain, ×200), which has also been described as nonadenomatous or gastric dysplasia. Foveolar dysplasia often occurs in a goblet cell–depleted background (*D*; H&E stain, ×200) as in this case arising in a background of oxyntocardia-type mucosa (*arrow*).

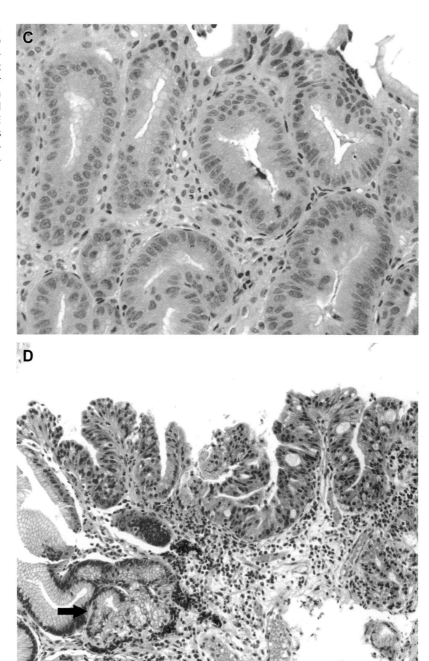

clinically important if the decision for endoscopic versus surgical management is based on this distinction.

ANCILLARY TEST FOR DYSPLASIA DIAGNOSIS

Ancillary immunohistochemical markers reported in literature are not sensitive or specific for routine diagnostic practice. Immunostaining for p53 has been studied extensively and *TP53* mutations have been reported in up to one-third of patients with nondysplastic BE.[45,46] Immunohistochemical results and gene mutation status, however, may be discordant in up to 30% of cases.[47] Regenerative BE epithelium may be positive for p53, leading to a false-positive diagnosis whereas truncating

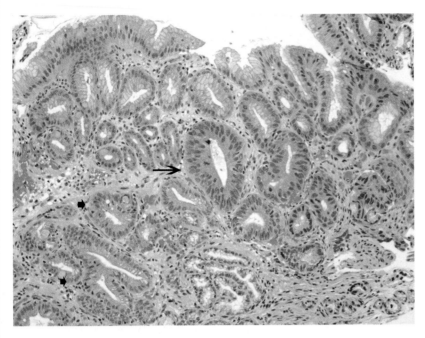

Fig. 12. Surface maturation is present but the crypts in the center (*long arrow*) stand out due to nuclear enlargement, hyperchromasia, luminal mitoses and some loss of polarity from the baseline atypia in surrounding nondysplastic crypts (*small arrows*). Note lack of significant inflammation in the biopsy. This pattern has been described as basal crypt dysplasia. If surface involvement is not seen on serial sections, these cases are best classified as indefinite for dysplasia at the present time (H&E stain, ×100).

TP53 mutations that lead to complete loss of immunoreactivity may yield a false-negative diagnosis of dysplasia. LGD cases positive for p53 are reported to have a higher risk of neoplastic progression.[48–50] It is difficult to interpret the findings of these studies because distinction of LGD from HGD can be problematic and it is possible that the p53-positive LGD cases are misclassified HGD. Moreover, LGD patients are already placed under close surveillance and results of p53 immunostaining offer no additional clinical benefit. AMACR immunoreactivity is generally reported only in dysplasia and adenocarcinoma but the reported sensitivities are not high enough to be clinically useful.[51–53] A biomarker panel consisting of *loss of heterozygosity* at 17p and 9p, aneuploidy, and tetraploidy has been shown to be a strong predictor of subsequent risk of EAC.[54,55] The methods used in these studies, however, are tedious and not suited for routine practice.

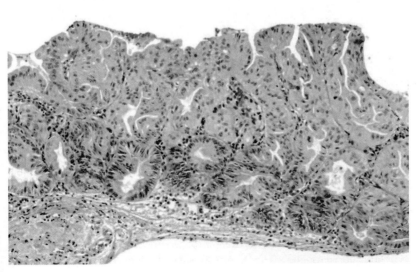

Fig. 13. Serrated dysplasia is rare in BE, occurs concurrently with conventional dysplasia, and resembles traditional serrated adenomas of the colorectum with crypt serration, intense cytoplasmic eosinophilia and nuclear stratification (H&E stain, ×100).

Differential Diagnosis
BARRETT'S ESOPHAGUS

ΔΔ

1. BE versus carditis with IM (CIM)

    a. Esophageal gland/ducts, multilayered epithelium, hybrid glands, and squamous mucosa overlying intestinalized crypts favor BE.

    b. CIM is more likely if gastric antral or body biopsies show IM in the setting of *Helicobacter pylori* gastritis or autoimmune gastritis.

2. Reactive atypia versus true dysplasia

    a. Uniform, vesicular chromatin pattern with small nucleoli are present in reactive atypia; there is a gradual transition in morphology as they move away from focus of inflammation.

    b. An abrupt transition to foci with altered morphology and involvement of surface epithelium favors dysplasia.

    c. Nuclear crowding and overlapping are more pronounced in dysplasia.

    d. Use indefinite for dysplasia as interim diagnosis when reactive versus dysplasia distinction is not possible.

3. LGD versus HGD

    a. Pencillate, hyperchromatic, stratified nuclei, oriented perpendicular to the basement membrane, are present in LGD.

    b. Marked crypt crowding with back-to-back glands and villiform architecture should raise concern for HGD.

    c. Round nuclei with loss of polarity, prominent nucleoli, and marked nuclear pleomorphism and atypical mitoses favor HGD.

4. HGD versus intramucosal adenocarcinoma

    a. There is a sharply defined basement membrane wrapping crypt epithelium in HGD.

    b. Cribriform architecture, intraluminal tufting and bridging, cystically dilated crypts with necrosis, and breach of basement membrane with confluent glandular pattern or single-cell invasion are diagnostic of intramucosal carcinoma.

NATURAL HISTORY OF BARRETT ESOPHAGUS

A consistent theme that emerges from recent population-based studies is that overall mortality is not increased in patients with BE[56] and prior literature overestimated the risk of cancer in BE. The incidence of EAC is significantly increased in BE compared with the general population but only a minority of BE patients develop cancer. The estimated annual incidence for EAC was approximately 0.5% to 0.6%[57,58] but the recent estimates are closer to 0.3% per year[13,56,59,60] and some are as low as 0.12% per year.[59] A recent multicenter BE study of 1204 patients from the United States also reported an incidence of 0.27% per year.[60] Length of BE and hiatal hernia, mucosal nodularity or ulcer, and presence of LGD at index endoscopy are risk factors associated with progression to HGD and EAC.[61]

The natural history of LGD is difficult to determine because of high interobserver variability in diagnosis. Consensus of LGD among expert gastrointestinal pathologists was reported associated with a higher risk of progression to HGD or cancer[62] but has not been confirmed in more recent studies.[60] Extent of LGD, which may contribute to diagnostic consensus, has also been reported to confer a high risk of progression to cancer.[63] LGD is estimated, in some studies, to have a 6 times higher risk for progression to EAC compared with nondysplastic BE.[61] LGD is also reported to regress in a significant proportion of patients[61] and this may, in part, be due to over-diagnosis of LGD. In one study, 85% of LGD diagnoses were downstaged to nondysplastic BE and the incidence rate for neoplastic progression was 13.4% per year for consensus LGD diagnosis and only 0.49% for patients downstaged to nondysplastic BE.[64] The current recommendation is that a diagnosis of LGD should be confirmed by a second gastrointestinal pathologist and patients be kept under surveillance at 6-month to 12-month intervals.[4]

Current estimates of HGD progressing to EA seem to be between 5.6% and 6.6% per year,[65] with a reported range of 6% to 19%.[18] It must be emphasized that these risk estimates are for patients with no endoscopic abnormalities, such as nodules or ulcers. Prior studies that reported a 60% rate of progression to EAC at 5 years are likely to have overestimated the risk.[55] HGD in biopsies obtained from areas of endoscopic abnormalities has a greater likelihood of concurrent adenocarcinoma, and endoscopic mucosal resection (EMR) of such areas leads to upgrading the diagnosis to EAC in approximately 40% of cases.[66] Similarly, in esophagectomies performed for HGD on biopsy, concurrent EAC is detected more often in those with a grossly visible abnormality.[67] Surveillance is no longer considered a viable strategy for management of patients with HGD unless significant comorbidities prevent endoscopic or surgical therapy.

MANAGEMENT OF BARRETT ESOPHAGUS–ASSOCIATED NEOPLASIA

A detailed discussion of management of dysplasia and early cancer in patients with BE is beyond the scope of this review and has been extensively reviewed elsewhere.[68] Dysplasia can be eliminated by EMR, ablation, or esophagectomy. Endoscopic therapy for HGD and early EAC is more cost effective than esophagectomy, particularly in patients at high intraoperative risk.[69] Of the various forms of mucosal ablation, radiofrequency ablation is currently the most widely used modality. Most patients (70%–80%) with HGD are successfully treated with a combination of EMR and mucosal ablation.[4] Visible lesions are removed by EMR and if no submucosal invasion is identified the remaining columnar segment is ablated. The AIM Dysplasia Trial showed complete eradication of HGD by radiofrequency ablation in 81% patients at 1-year follow-up, and the 2-year and 3-year outcomes confirmed durability of response.[70,71] After successful ablation of columnar epithelium, the esophageal lining epithelium reverts to its normal squamous phenotype. Buried metaplasia or dysplasia is infrequent in patients undergoing radiofrequency ablation[71] but may be present anywhere along the prior columnar segment (**Fig. 14**)

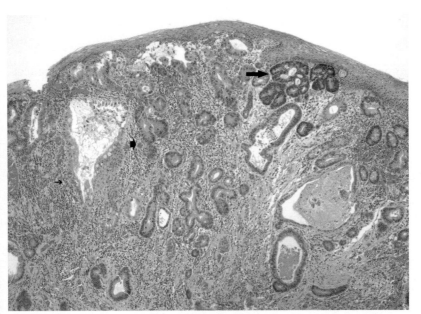

Fig. 14. Postradiofrequency ablation EMR specimen with metaplastic (*small arrow*) and dysplastic (*smal, thick arrow*) crypts, and adenocarcinoma (*long thick arrow*) buried underneath squamous mucosa (H&E stain, ×40).

Pitfalls
BARRETT'S ESOPHAGUS

1. For false-positive diagnosis of BE
   a. Mistaking pseudogoblet cells for IM
   b. Misdiagnosing IM of proximal stomach in a GE junction biopsy as BE (which leads to lifelong endoscopic surveillance)
2. For false-positive diagnosis of dysplasia in BE
   a. Reactive atypia in the setting of significant inflammation or ulcer mistaken for dysplasia
   b. Enlarged nuclei in intestinalized crypts next to bland cardia-type mucous glands misdiagnosed as dysplasia (look for surface maturation)
   c. Diagnosis of dysplasia, in particular LGD, not highly reproducible; should be confirmed by a GI pathologist before implementing appropriate surveillance strategy
   d. HGD in a mucosal biopsy from an area of nodularity more likely associated with carcinoma on EMR or esophagectomy

and is the reason for continued surveillance of these patients.

REFERENCES

1. Brown LM, Devesa SS, Chow WH. Incidence of adenocarcinoma of the esophagus among white Americans by sex, stage, and age. J Natl Cancer Inst 2008;100:1184–7.
2. Pohl H, Sirovich B, Welch HG. Esophageal adenocarcinoma incidence: are we reaching the peak? Cancer Epidemiol Biomarkers Prev 2010;19: 1468–70.
3. Prach AT, MacDonald TA, Hopwood DA, et al. Increasing incidence of Barrett's oesophagus: education, enthusiasm, or epidemiology? Lancet 1997; 350:933.
4. Wang KK, Sampliner RE, Practice Parameters Committee of the American College of Gastroenterology. Updated guidelines 2008 for the diagnosis, surveillance and therapy of Barrett's esophagus. Am J Gastroenterol 2008;103:788–97.
5. Playford RJ. New British Society of Gastroenterology (BSG) guidelines for the diagnosis and management of Barrett's oesophagus. Gut 2006; 55:442.
6. Ogiya K, Kawano T, Ito E, et al. Lower esophageal palisade vessels and the definition of Barrett's esophagus. Dis Esophagus 2008;21:645–9.
7. Harrison R, Perry I, Haddadin W, et al. Detection of intestinal metaplasia in Barrett's esophagus: an observational comparator study suggests the need for a minimum of eight biopsies. Am J Gastroenterol 2007;102:1154–61.
8. Gatenby PA, Ramus JR, Caygill CP, et al. Relevance of the detection of intestinal metaplasia in non-dysplastic columnar-lined oesophagus. Scand J Gastroenterol 2008;43:524–30.
9. Hahn HP, Blount PL, Ayub K, et al. Intestinal differentiation in metaplastic, nongoblet columnar epithelium in the esophagus. Am J Surg Pathol 2009;33: 1006–15.
10. Liu W, Hahn H, Odze RD, et al. Metaplastic esophageal columnar epithelium without goblet cells shows DNA content abnormalities similar to goblet cell-containing epithelium. Am J Gastroenterol 2009;104:816–24.
11. Kelty CJ, Gough MD, Van Wyk Q, et al. Barrett's oesophagus: intestinal metaplasia is not essential for cancer risk. Scand J Gastroenterol 2007;42: 1271–4.
12. Takubo K, Aida J, Naomoto Y, et al. Cardiac rather than intestinal-type background in endoscopic resection specimens of minute Barrett adenocarcinoma. Hum Pathol 2009;40:65–74.
13. Bhat S, Coleman HG, Yousef F, et al. Risk of malignant progression in Barrett's esophagus patients: results from a large population-based study. J Natl Cancer Inst 2011;103:1049–57.
14. Chandrasoma P, Wijetunge S, Demeester S, et al. Columnar-lined esophagus without intestinal metaplasia has no proven risk of adenocarcinoma. Am J Surg Pathol 2012;36:1–7.
15. Das D, Ishaq S, Harrison R, et al. Management of Barrett's esophagus in the UK: overtreated and underbiopsied but improved by the introduction of a national randomized trial. Am J Gastroenterol 2008;103:1079–89.

16. Spechler SJ, Sharma P, Souza RF, et al. American Gastroenterological Association medical position statement on the management of Barrett's esophagus. Gastroenterology 2011;140:1084–91.

17. Balasubramanian G, Singh M, Gupta N, et al. Prevalence and predictors of columnar lined esophagus in gastroesophageal reflux disease (GERD) patients undergoing upper endoscopy. Am J Gastroenterol 2012;107:1655–61.

18. Bennett C, Vakil N, Bergman J, et al. Consensus statements for management of Barrett's dysplasia and early-stage esophageal adenocarcinoma, based on a Delphi process. Gastroenterology 2012;143:336–46.

19. Sharma P, Weston AP, Morales T, et al. Relative risk of dysplasia for patients with intestinal metaplasia in the distal oesophagus and in the gastric cardia. Gut 2000;46:9–13.

20. Srivastava A, Odze RD, Lauwers GY, et al. Morphologic features are useful in distinguishing Barrett esophagus from carditis with intestinal metaplasia. Am J Surg Pathol 2007;31:1733–41.

21. Ormsby AH, Goldblum JR, Rice TW, et al. Cytokeratin subsets can reliably distinguish Barrett's esophagus from intestinal metaplasia of the stomach. Hum Pathol 1999;30:288–94.

22. Mohammed IA, Streutker CJ, Riddell RH. Utilization of cytokeratins 7 and 20 does not differentiate between Barrett's esophagus and gastric cardiac intestinal metaplasia. Mod Pathol 2002;15:611–6.

23. Glickman JN, Wang H, Das KM, et al. Phenotype of Barrett's esophagus and intestinal metaplasia of the distal esophagus and gastroesophageal junction: an immunohistochemical study of cytokeratins 7 and 20, Das-1 and 45 MI. Am J Surg Pathol 2001; 25:87–94.

24. Gulmann C, Shaqaqi OA, Grace A, et al. Cytokeratin 7/20 and MUC1, 2, 5AC, and 6 expression patterns in Barrett's esophagus and intestinal metaplasia of the stomach: intestinal metaplasia of the cardia is related to Barrett's esophagus. Appl Immunohistochem Mol Morphol 2004;12:142–7.

25. Odze RD. Unraveling the mystery of the gastroesophageal junction: a pathologist's perspective. Am J Gastroenterol 2005;100:1853–67.

26. Leodolter A, Nocon M, Vieth M, et al. Progression of specialized intestinal metaplasia at the cardia to macroscopically evident Barrett's esophagus: an entity of concern in the ProGERD study. Scand J Gastroenterol 2012;47:1429–35.

27. Montgomery E, Goldblum JR, Greenson JK, et al. Dysplasia as a predictive marker for invasive carcinoma in Barrett esophagus: a follow-up study based on 138 cases from a diagnostic variability study. Hum Pathol 2001;32:379–88.

28. Abraham SC, Krasinskas AM, Correa AM, et al. Duplication of the muscularis mucosae in Barrett esophagus: an underrecognized feature and its implication for staging of adenocarcinoma. Am J Surg Pathol 2007;31:1719–25.

29. Odze RD. Diagnosis and grading of dysplasia in Barrett's oesophagus. J Clin Pathol 2006;59: 1029–38.

30. Reid BJ, Li X, Galipeau PC, et al. Barrett's oesophagus and oesophageal adenocarcinoma: time for a new synthesis. Nat Rev Cancer 2010;10:87–101.

31. Jovov B, Van Itallie CM, Shaheen NJ, et al. Claudin-18: a dominant tight junction protein in Barrett's esophagus and likely contributor to its acid resistance. Am J Physiol Gastrointest Liver Physiol 2007;293:G1106–13.

32. Reid BJ. Early events during neoplastic progression in Barrett's esophagus. Cancer Biomark 2011;9:307–24.

33. Wong DJ, Paulson TG, Prevo LJ, et al. p16(INK4a) lesions are common, early abnormalities that undergo clonal expansion in Barrett's metaplastic epithelium. Cancer Res 2001;61:8284–9.

34. Paulson TG, Reid BJ. Focus on Barrett's esophagus and esophageal adenocarcinoma. Cancer Cell 2004;6:11–6.

35. Coco DP, Goldblum JR, Hornick JL, et al. Interobserver variability in the diagnosis of crypt dysplasia in barrett esophagus. Am J Surg Pathol 2011;35: 45–54.

36. Park do Y, Srivastava A, Kim GH, et al. Adenomatous and foveolar gastric dysplasia: distinct patterns of mucin expression and background intestinal metaplasia. Am J Surg Pathol 2008;32:524–33.

37. Brown IS, Whiteman DC, Lauwers GY. Foveolar type dysplasia in Barrett esophagus. Mod Pathol 2010;23:834–43.

38. Mahajan D, Bennett AE, Liu X, et al. Grading of gastric foveolar-type dysplasia in Barrett's esophagus. Mod Pathol 2010;23:1–11.

39. Rucker-Schmidt RL, Sanchez CA, Blount PL, et al. Nonadenomatous dysplasia in barrett esophagus: a clinical, pathologic, and DNA content flow cytometric study. Am J Surg Pathol 2009;33:886–93.

40. Srivastava A, Sanchez CA, Cowan DS, et al. Foveolar and serrated dysplasia are rare high-risk lesions in Barrett's esophagus: a prospective outcome analysis of 214 patients. Mod Pathol 2010;23a.

41. Khor TS, Alfaro EE, Ooi EM, et al. Divergent expression of MUC5AC, MUC6, MUC2, CD10, and CDX-2 in dysplasia and intramucosal adenocarcinomas with intestinal and foveolar morphology: is this evidence of distinct gastric and intestinal pathways to carcinogenesis in Barrett Esophagus? Am J Surg Pathol 2012;36:331–42.

42. Lomo LC, Blount PL, Sanchez CA, et al. Crypt dysplasia with surface maturation: a clinical, pathologic, and molecular study of a Barrett's esophagus cohort. Am J Surg Pathol 2006;30:423–35.

43. Reid BJ, Haggitt RC, Rubin CE, et al. Observer variation in the diagnosis of dysplasia in Barrett's esophagus. Hum Pathol 1988;19:166–78.

44. Downs-Kelly E, Mendelin JE, Bennett AE, et al. Poor interobserver agreement in the distinction of high-grade dysplasia and adenocarcinoma in pretreatment Barrett's esophagus biopsies. Am J Gastroenterol 2008;103:2333–40.

45. Jenkins GJ, Doak SH, Griffiths AP, et al. Early p53 mutations in nondysplastic Barrett's tissue detected by the restriction site mutation (RSM) methodology. Br J Cancer 2003;88:1271–6.

46. Campomenosi P, Conio M, Bogliolo M, et al. p53 is frequently mutated in Barrett's metaplasia of the intestinal type. Cancer Epidemiol Biomarkers Prev 1996;5:559–65.

47. Hamelin R, Flejou JF, Muzeau F, et al. TP53 gene mutations and p53 protein immunoreactivity in malignant and premalignant Barrett's esophagus. Gastroenterology 1994;107:1012–8.

48. Skacel M, Petras RE, Rybicki LA, et al. p53 expression in low grade dysplasia in Barrett's esophagus: correlation with interobserver agreement and disease progression. Am J Gastroenterol 2002;97:2508–13.

49. Sikkema M, Kerkhof M, Steyerberg EW, et al. Aneuploidy and overexpression of Ki67 and p53 as markers for neoplastic progression in Barrett's esophagus: a case-control study. Am J Gastroenterol 2009;104:2673–80.

50. Weston AP, Banerjee SK, Sharma P, et al. p53 protein overexpression in low grade dysplasia (LGD) in Barrett's esophagus: immunohistochemical marker predictive of progression. Am J Gastroenterol 2001;96:1355–62.

51. Lisovsky M, Falkowski O, Bhuiya T. Expression of alpha-methylacyl-coenzyme a racemase in dysplastic Barrett's epithelium. Hum Pathol 2006;37:1601–6.

52. Scheil-Bertram S, Lorenz D, Ell C, et al. Expression of alpha-methylacyl coenzyme a racemase in the dysplasia carcinoma sequence associated with Barrett's esophagus. Mod Pathol 2008;21:961–7.

53. Sonwalkar SA, Rotimi O, Scott N, et al. A study of indefinite for dysplasia in Barrett's oesophagus: reproducibility of diagnosis, clinical outcomes and predicting progression with AMACR (alpha-methylacyl-CoA-racemase). Histopathology 2010;56:900–7.

54. Galipeau PC, Li X, Blount PL, et al. NSAIDs modulate CDKN2A, TP53, and DNA content risk for progression to esophageal adenocarcinoma. PLoS Med 2007;4:342–53.

55. Reid BJ, Levine DS, Longton G, et al. Predictors of progression to cancer in Barrett's esophagus: baseline histology and flow cytometry identify low- and high-risk patient subsets. Am J Gastroenterol 2000;95:1669–76.

56. Schouten LJ, Steevens J, Huysentruyt CJ, et al. Total cancer incidence and overall mortality are not increased among patients with Barrett's esophagus. Clin Gastroenterol Hepatol 2011;9:754–61.

57. Shaheen NJ, Crosby MA, Bozymski EM, et al. Is there publication bias in the reporting of cancer risk in Barrett's esophagus? Gastroenterology 2000;119:333–8.

58. Wani S, Puli SR, Shaheen NJ, et al. Esophageal adenocarcinoma in Barrett's esophagus after endoscopic ablative therapy: a meta-analysis and systematic review. Am J Gastroenterol 2009;104:502–13.

59. Hvid-Jensen F, Pedersen L, Drewes AM, et al. Incidence of adenocarcinoma among patients with Barrett's esophagus. N Engl J Med 2011;365:1375–83.

60. Wani S, Falk GW, Post J, et al. Risk factors for progression of low-grade dysplasia in patients with Barrett's esophagus. Gastroenterology 2011;141:1179–86 1186.e1.

61. Rugge M, Zaninotto G, Parente P, et al. Barrett's esophagus and adenocarcinoma risk: the experience of the North-Eastern Italian Registry (EBRA). Ann Surg 2012;256:788–94.

62. Skacel M, Petras RE, Gramlich TL, et al. The diagnosis of low-grade dysplasia in Barrett's esophagus and its implications for disease progression. Am J Gastroenterol 2000;95:3383–7.

63. Srivastava A, Hornick JL, Li X, et al. Extent of low-grade dysplasia is a risk factor for the development of esophageal adenocarcinoma in Barrett's esophagus. Am J Gastroenterol 2007;102:483–93.

64. Curvers WL, ten Kate FJ, Krishnadath KK, et al. Low-grade dysplasia in Barrett's esophagus: overdiagnosed and underestimated. Am J Gastroenterol 2010;105:1523–30.

65. Rastogi A, Puli S, El-Serag HB, et al. Incidence of esophageal adenocarcinoma in patients with Barrett's esophagus and high-grade dysplasia: a meta-analysis. Gastrointest Endosc 2008;67:394–8.

66. Mino-Kenudson M, Brugge WR, Puricelli WP, et al. Management of superficial Barrett's epithelium-related neoplasms by endoscopic mucosal resection: clinicopathologic analysis of 27 cases. Am J Surg Pathol 2005;29:680–6.

67. Tharavej C, Hagen JA, Peters JH, et al. Predictive factors of coexisting cancer in Barrett's high-grade dysplasia. Surg Endosc 2006;20:439–43.

68. Odze RD, Lauwers GY. Histopathology of Barrett's esophagus after ablation and endoscopic mucosal resection therapy. Endoscopy 2008;40:1008–15.

69. Pohl H, Sonnenberg A, Strobel S, et al. Endoscopic versus surgical therapy for early cancer in Barrett's esophagus: a decision analysis. Gastrointest Endosc 2009;70:623–31.

70. Shaheen NJ, Sharma P, Overholt BF, et al. Radiofrequency ablation in Barrett's esophagus with dysplasia. N Engl J Med 2009;360: 2277–88.

71. Shaheen NJ, Overholt BF, Sampliner RE, et al. Durability of radiofrequency ablation in Barrett's esophagus with dysplasia. Gastroenterology 2011;141: 460–8.

IgG4-related Disorders of the Gastrointestinal Tract

Madelyn Lew, MD, Vikram Deshpande, MD*

KEYWORDS

- Autoimmune pancreatitis • IgG4-related disease • IgG4-related sclerosing cholangitis • IgG4

ABSTRACT

IgG4-related disease, a newly established multisystemic disease can affect virtually every organ. Histologically, it is characterized by the presence of a dense lymphoplasmacytic infiltrate, storiform-type fibrosis, and obliterative phlebitis. The disease shows elevated serum and tissue IgG4. The pancreas and hepatobiliary tract are involved far more commonly than the tubular gut. This review summarizes the clinical and pathologic features of the gastrointestinal manifestations of IgG4-related disease and discusses the wide spectrum of diseases that this entity may mimic.

OVERVIEW

Immunoglobulin G4 (IgG4)-related disease is by no means a new disease—it has been either misclassified or dismissed by pathologists as a nonspecific inflammatory infiltrate (**Box 1**).[1–3] Among the various manifestations of the disease, autoimmune pancreatitis (IgG4-related pancreatitis) was the first to be recognized as a unique clinicopathologic entity.[4] Before its recognition, it was often mistaken clinically for pancreatic malignancy and histologically misdiagnosed as chronic pancreatitis. Similarly, IgG4-related sclerosing cholangitis was erroneously classified as primary sclerosing cholangitis. Autoimmune pancreatitis and IgG4-related sclerosing cholangitis, like all the other manifestations of this disease, are responsive to immunosuppressive therapy, whereas the majority of cases of chronic pancreatitis and primary sclerosing cholangitis are not, and therein lies the clinical relevance of this entity.[5] For reasons that are currently unknown, the tubular gut is seldom affected by IgG4-related disease.

Elevated numbers of IgG4+ plasma cells in tissue constitute a key diagnostic feature of IgG4-related disease.[1,6] Elevated numbers of IgG4+ plasma cells, however, are also identified in a variety of other diseases, including inflammatory bowel disease.[3] Although inflammatory bowel disease does not belong to the IgG4-related disease spectrum, the identification of IgG4+ plasma cells within the colon and ileal pouch may have diagnostic and/or prognostic relevance.

This article provides readers an in-depth discussion on the hepatic and pancreatic manifestations of IgG4-related disease, with particular emphasis on its mimics. This review also sheds light on the diseases of the gastrointestinal tract that are associated with elevated numbers of IgG4+ plasma cells but do not belong to the IgG4-related disease spectrum.

AN INTRODUCTION TO IGG4-RELATED DISEASE

This disease can involve virtually every organ and tissue type (although glandular organs are

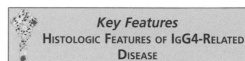

Key Features
HISTOLOGIC FEATURES OF IGG4-RELATED DISEASE

1. Dense lymphoplasmacytic infiltrate

2. Storiform-type fibrosis

3. Obliterative phlebitis

4. Elevated numbers of IgG4+ plasma cells

5. Elevated ratio of IgG4 to IgG-positive plasma cells

Department of Pathology, Massachusetts General Hospital, 55 Fruit street, Boston, MA 02114, USA
* Corresponding author.
E-mail address: vikramdirdeshpande@gmail.com

Surgical Pathology 6 (2013) 497–521
http://dx.doi.org/10.1016/j.path.2013.05.004
1875-9181/13/$ – see front matter © 2013 Elsevier Inc. All rights reserved.

most commonly affected)[1,7] and is characterized by[1,7]

1. Presence of tumefactive lesions that often mimic malignancy
2. Involvement of multiple organs, either synchronously or metachronously
3. Presence of elevated serum IgG4
4. Characteristic histologic appearance
5. Elevated numbers of IgG4+ plasma cells as well as elevated IgG4 to IgG ratio

Histology is the gold standard; hence, the onus for an accurate diagnosis lies squarely with the surgical pathologist.[6] The disease is remarkably analogous to sarcoidosis, a condition that involves virtually every organ, and shows a uniform histologic appearance—the presence of non-necrotizing epithelioid cell granulomas.

THE HISTOLOGIC DIAGNOSIS OF IGG4-RELATED DISEASE

The disease is characterized by 3 histologic features[6]:

1. A dense lymphoplasmacytic infiltrate (**Figs. 1** and **2**)
2. Dense fibrosis, invariably arranged in a storiform pattern (see **Figs. 1** and **2**)
3. Obliterative phlebitis (**Figs. 2** and **3**)

In most instances, a definitive diagnosis of IgG4-related disease requires at least 2 of these 3 histologic features. Storiform pattern of fibrosis is a characteristic feature of IgG4-related disease. This pattern is somewhat analogous to that seen in mesenchymal tumors, such as dermatofibrosarcoma protuberans. In contrast to these neoplastic lesions, however, the spindle cell population (and these cells may appear prominent in some examples of this disease) lacks nuclear atypia or mitotic activity. Obliterative phlebitis, the least common of the 3 histologic features, is nonetheless a unique feature of this disease. Medium-sized veins are involved, and the lumen is obliterated by a lymphoplasmacytic infiltrate.

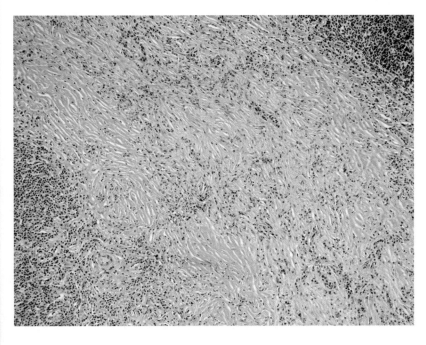

Fig. 1. Type 1 autoimmune pancreatitis. This high-power image shows a dense lymphoplasmacytic infiltrate embedded within a collagenous background.

Fig. 2. Obliterative phlebitis (*arrow*) in type 1 autoimmune pancreatitis.

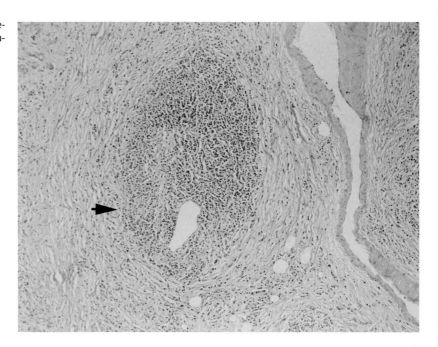

Vessels obliterated by fibrosis but devoid of inflammatory cells are not necessarily characteristic of IgG4-related disease, because this histologic appearance is seen in other conditions (see **Fig. 3**). Medium-sized arterial channels are also involved (**Fig. 4**). The arteritis respects the structure of the vessel, however, unlike destructive vasculitides, such as polyarteritis nodosa: necrotizing vasculitis with fibrin deposition is not a feature of IgG4-related disease.

A categorical diagnosis of IgG4-related disease requires both the presence of a characteristic morphologic appearance and elevated numbers of IgG4+ plasma cells (**Table 1**): an IgG4 to IgG ratio of greater than 40% provides additional support to the diagnosis.

Fig. 3. The lumen of this vein is totally obliterated. It lacks, however, the characteristic intraluminal lymphoplasmacytic infiltrate, hence does not constitute obliterative phlebitis.

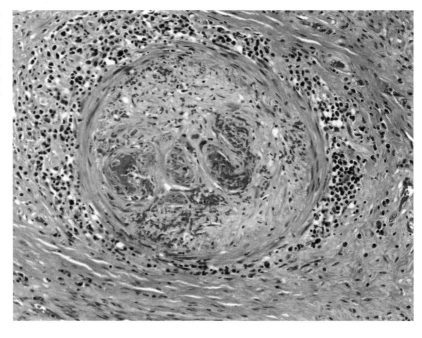

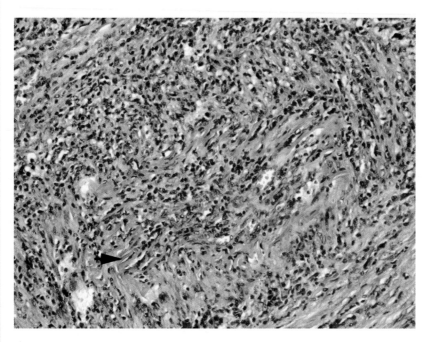

Fig. 4. Obliterative arteritis in type 1 autoimmune pancreatitis. The obliterated lumen is outlined by the internal elastic lamina (*arrow*); the media and lumen of the arterial wall are replaced by inflammation.

CLINICAL FEATURES THAT ASSIST IN THE DIAGNOSIS OF IGG4-RELATED DISEASE

There are 4 cardinal features help a clinical team (and this includes a pathologist) distinguish IgG4-related disease from its mimics[1,7–10]:

1. Elevated serum IgG4
2. Radiologic appearance
3. Other organ involvement
4. Response to immunosuppressive therapy

Elevated Serum IgG4

The frequency of serum IgG4 elevation varies in published series from 44% to 100%.[11] An elevated serum IgG4, although characteristic of IgG4-related disease, is unfortunately also seen in a variety of other etiologies, including neoplastic diseases. Nonetheless, elevation of serum IgG4 is highly suggestive of IgG4-related disease, particularly in patients with characteristic organ involvement, such as a tumefactive orbital lesion. An elevation greater than 2-fold the upper limit of normal (normal 140 mg/dL) has a specificity of greater than 90% for IgG4-related disease and is rarely observed in other conditions. A normal serum IgG4 does not exclude the diagnosis.

Radiologic Appearance

On imaging, autoimmune pancreatitis, the pancreatic manifestation of IgG4-related disease, shows a characteristic appearance. Similarly, imaging may help distinguish IgG4-related sclerosing cholangitis from cholangiocarcinoma. At other sites, however, the appearance is generally nonspecific.

Other Organ Involvement

IgG4-related disease is a multisystemic disease with either synchronous or more often metachronous involvement. Tumefactive enlargement of a second organ, particularly one that is commonly affected by this condition, argues in favor of a diagnosis of IgG4-related disease. For example, it is not uncommon to elucidate a history of chronic sialadenitis in patients with autoimmune pancreatitis.[12] The histologic evaluation of the gland demonstrates classic features of IgG4-related sialadenitis (IgG4-related disease of the salivary gland). Similarly, IgG4-related sclerosing cholangitis is frequently associated with autoimmune pancreatitis.

Table 1
Suggested IgG4 cutpoint for the diagnosis of IgG4-related disease of the gastrointestinal tract

Organ	Number of IgG4+ Cells
Pancreas (surgical specimen)	>50
Pancreas (biopsy)	>10
Bile duct (surgical specimen)	>50
Bile duct (biopsy)	>10
Liver (surgical specimen)	>50
Liver (biopsy)	>10

Response to Immunosuppressive Therapy

IgG4-related disease shows a swift response to immunosuppressive therapy, with a dramatic decrease in size of the mass as well as normalization of pancreatic and bile duct strictures.[1,9,13,14] The absence of a swift response to steroids should prompt reevaluation of the diagnosis, specifically to rule out a malignant process. A therapeutic trial with steroids may also help unravel an otherwise knotty diagnostic problem. A pancreatic adenocarcinoma may show, however, a partial response to steroid therapy; hence, a trial should be monitored closely, with a low threshold to rebiopsy.

THERAPY

As discussed previously, a swift and often dramatic response to steroids is the norm, although relapses are common.[14] To minimize relapses, maintenance therapy with steroids is often used, particularly in cases with pancreatic involvement. Rituximab, an anti-CD20 antibody, is equally efficacious and avoids the many complications associated with long-term steroid usage.[15] Immunosuppressive therapy is generally associated with a decline in serum IgG4.

PANCREAS

Overview

IgG4-related disease was initially recognized in the pancreas, and autoimmune pancreatitis is its

best-characterized manifestation. Autoimmune pancreatitis is not a homogenous entity and 2 unique subtypes are recognized—type 1 (previously known as lymphoplasmacytic sclerosing pancreatitis or lobulocentric pancreatitis) and type 2 (also known as idiopathic duct-centric chronic pancreatitis or ductocentric pancreatitis).[16–18] Type 1 autoimmune pancreatitis bears all the histologic hallmarks of IgG4-related disease, whereas the histologic features of type 2 disease show little resemblance to this entity. Although there is considerable overlap in the clinical and radiologic features, the histologic features and the outcome of these forms of pancreatitis are distinctive. Clinically, autoimmune pancreatitis mimics pancreatic carcinoma, and familiarization with the morphology and immunohistochemical features is key to the prevention of unnecessary procedures.

Clinical Features

Typical patients are middle aged or elderly, but there is a wide age range.[16,19,20] Type 1 variant is generally limited to elderly men, whereas the majority of patients with type 2 disease are middle aged (**Table 2**). The age group affected by type 1 autoimmune pancreatitis (7th decade) coincides with the demographic affected by pancreatic ductal adenocarcinoma. There is also significant overlap in clinical presentation between type 1 autoimmune pancreatitis and pancreatic adenocarcinoma—both cohorts present with painless obstructive jaundice and a pancreatic mass. This makes the distinction of type 1 autoimmune pancreatitis from pancreatic adenocarcinoma particularly challenging. Studies have demonstrated that autoimmune pancreatitis is responsible for up to one-third of benign pancreatic diseases treated unintentionally by pancreaticoduodenectomies.

The type 2 variant of autoimmune pancreatitis may also present with obstructive jaundice and a pancreatic mass on imaging. Individuals with this variant, however, are equally likely to have abdominal pain and in general show overlapping features with other forms of chronic pancreatitis, such as alcohol-related pancreatitis.

Radiologic Features

On CT and ultrasound, the affected area appears hypodense or hypoechoic, respectively. A hypoattenuating rim may be seen surrounding the pancreas (halo sign). Endoscopic retrograde cholangiopancreatography and magnetic resonance cholangiopancreatography show irregular narrowing of the pancreatic duct.

Table 2
Differences between type 1 and type 2 autoimmune pancreatitis

	Type 1 AIP	Type 2 AIP
Age	Elderly, 7th decades	Middle age, 5th decade
Gender	Predominantly male	M = F
Presentation	Jaundice (75%), acute pancreatitis (15%)	Acute pancreatitis (~33%) Jaundice (~50%)
Systemic disease	Yes	No
Elevated serum IgG4	80%	Uncommon
Inflammatory bowel disease	No association	16%–30% of Cases have inflammatory bowel disease
Histopathology	Periductal inflammation with 1 or more of the following features: 1. Storiform fibrosis 2. Obliterative phlebitis	Periductal inflammation with 1 or more of the following features: 1. Ductal/lobular abscesses 2. Ductal ulceration with neutrophils
Long-term outcome	Frequent relapses	No relapses

Abbreviations: AIP, autoimmune pancreatitis; M, male; F, female.
   Adapted from Shinagare S, Shinagare AB, Deshpande V. Autoimmune pancreatitis: a guide for the histopathologist [review]. Semin Diagn Pathol 2012;29(4):198. Elsevier. http://dx.doi.org/10.1053/j.semdp.2012.07.007; with permission.

Gross Features

A firm to hard ill-defined pancreatic lesion is the most common gross appearance. A less common form of presentation is a discrete pancreatic mass. Regardless, the pancreas is diffusely fibrotic and the main pancreatic duct is typically narrow with multiple strictures. Unlike pancreatic malignancy, an upstream dilatation of the pancreatic duct is distinctly uncommon. A stricture may involve the intrapancreatic portion of the bile duct as well, an event generally associated with marked proximal dilatation of this duct.

Microscopic Features

Type 1 autoimmune pancreatitis

As with other organs involved by IgG4-related disease, the histologic triad of autoimmune pancreatitis includes a dense lymphoplasmacytic infiltrate, storiform fibrosis (**Figs. 5** and **6**), and obliterative phlebitis.[16,19,20] The disease is

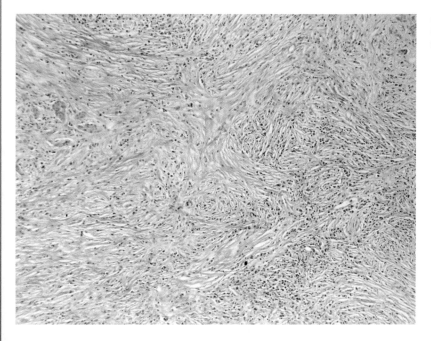

Fig. 5. Type 1 autoimmune pancreatitis with storiform-type fibrosis.

Fig. 6. This high-power view shows a dense lymphoplasmacytic infiltrate with fibrosis organized in a storiform pattern, a feature characteristic of IgG4-related disease.

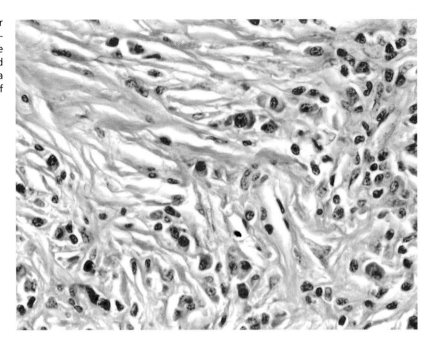

accompanied by progressive destruction of the pancreatic parenchyma. The lymphoplasmacytic infiltrate and fibrosis may extend into the peripancreatic soft tissue—an appearance that mimics idiopathic retroperitoneal fibrosis. The inflammatory infiltrate comprises lymphocytes, plasma cells, and a generous sprinkling of eosinophils. Storiform fibrosis is best appreciated in the interlobular septa. A dense collar of inflammation is often seen around pancreatic ducts (**Fig. 7**). A circumscribed aggregate of lymphocytes adjacent to an artery is suspicious for obliterative phlebitis. Inflamed venous channels (phlebitis) lacking obliteration is common in other forms of chronic pancreatitis, as well as adjacent to pancreatic

Fig. 7. Type 1 autoimmune pancreatitis. The lymphoplasmacytic infiltrate aggregates around ductal structures. The ductal epithelium itself, however, shows little evidence of damage.

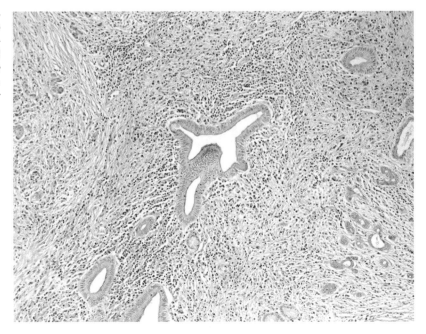

malignancy, and should be considered a non-specific histologic appearance.

Type 1 autoimmune pancreatitis is invariably associated with a diffuse and marked increase in IgG4+ plasma cells. A recent international consensus effort suggests a cutoff concentration of greater than 50 IgG4+ plasma cells per high-power field (HPF) on resection specimens (**Fig. 8**).[6] It is not uncommon, however, to find occasional clusters of IgG4+ plasma cells approaching this cutpoint in peritumoral inflammatory infiltrates as well as other forms of chronic pancreatitis (including type 2 autoimmune pancreatitis) (**Fig. 9**). In contrast to the hot spots of IgG4+ plasma cells found in these diseases, the infiltrate in type 1 disease diffusely involves the pancreatic parenchyma. Some additional caveats also deserve mention. A lower number of IgG4+ plasma cells are often acceptable on pancreatic biopsies—greater than 10 IgG4+ plasma cells per HPF.[21] Furthermore, patients with long-standing autoimmune pancreatitis as well as those on immunosuppressive therapy may show a lower number of plasma cells. In these instances, an elevated ratio of IgG4+/IgG+ plasma cells (greater than 40%) may assist in distinguishing IgG4-related disease from its mimics.

Diagnostic algorithm for type 1 autoimmune pancreatitis

Histopathology constitutes only 1 component of a larger algorithm used to diagnose autoimmune pancreatitis. This statement applies chiefly to needle biopsy samples: on a pancreatic resection specimen, histopathology remains the de facto gold standard. Pancreatic involvement is often patchy; hence, biopsies may be nonrepresentative or, more commonly, lack the complete spectrum of histologic features (**Fig. 10**). Furthermore, immunohistochemical stains for IgG4 and IgG on needle biopsies tend to show a more intense background stain. Several clinical diagnostic algorithms have been suggested, all of which rely on a combination of clinical, radiologic, and pathologic features: serology (increased serum IgG4 or auto-antibodies), histology, response to steroid therapy, and involvement of other organs.[10]

Type 2 autoimmune pancreatitis

Both forms of autoimmune pancreatitis are immune mediated and are associated with a dense lymphoplasmacytic infiltrate; however, histologically the 2 diseases are dissimilar.

The histologic hallmarks of the type 2 variant are a dense periductal lymphoplasmacytic infiltrate and a neutrophilic form of ductal injury (granulocytic epithelial lesions) (**Figs. 11–13**).[16,19,20,22] Typically, neutrophilic microabscesses are identified within the lumen of the duct, and often the overall appearance resembles that seen in inflammatory bowel disease. Among patients with type 2 autoimmune pancreatitis, 15% to 30% are associated with inflammatory bowel disease, most commonly ulcerative colitis. Neutrophils are also identified within the lobules. The ductal injury may be severe enough to result in complete loss of ductal structures (see **Fig. 13**). In contrast to type 1 autoimmune pancreatitis, storiform fibrosis

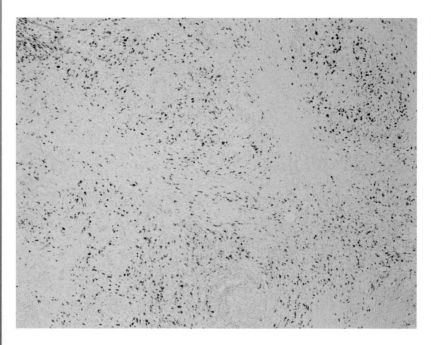

Fig. 8. Type 1 autoimmune pancreatitis with a diffuse infiltration of IgG4+ plasma cells (IgG4 immunoperoxidase stain).

Fig. 9. Type 2 autoimmune pancreatitis with a sparse IgG4 plasma cell infiltrate. The infiltrate is often confined to the periductal region (IgG4 immunoperoxidase stain).

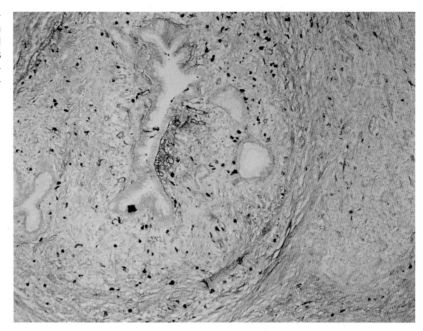

and obliterative phlebitis are seldom seen. The interlobular tissue in type 1 autoimmune pancreatitis is expanded by an inflamed and cellular stromal reaction; in contrast, the interlobular stroma in type 2 disease is acellular and fibrotic and lacks a dense lymphoplasmacytic infiltrate (see **Figs. 1** and **11**). Periductal epithelioid cell granulomas are occasionally seen (**Fig. 14**).

Type 2 disease also lacks a dense population of IgG4+ plasma cells. In a minority of cases, however, aggregates of IgG4+ plasma cells may be identified.

Diagnostic algorithm for type 2 autoimmune pancreatitis

Many of the diagnostic criteria that help with the diagnosis of type 1 disease are absent in the type 2 variant. Serum IgG4 levels are seldom elevated, the disease is confined to the pancreas, and this cohort lacks the presence of other organ involvement. The radiologic features are often nonspecific. As a result, the diagnosis of type 2 disease rests principally on a biopsy. Biopsy samples that show a periductal lymphoplasmacytic infiltrate with intraductal neutrophils are virtually diagnostic for type 2 autoimmune pancreatitis. Rarely, however, periductal lymphoplasmacytic infiltrates containing neutrophils may be seen adjacent to a pancreatic ductal adenocarcinoma. The diagnosis of autoimmune pancreatitis generally requires an exhaustive effort to exclude malignancy.

Differential Diagnosis

The clinical distinction of autoimmune pancreatitis from pancreatic carcinoma is difficult, particularly if classic clinical and radiologic features are not observed. On a core biopsy, a well-differentiated adenocarcinoma with a brisk intratumoral lymphoplasmacytic infiltrate may mimic autoimmune pancreatitis. Even well-differentiated adenocarcinomas, however, show variation in nuclear size and architectural features, such as the presence of perineural infiltration. The differential diagnosis also includes other forms of pancreatitis, such as hereditary pancreatitis and alcohol-related pancreatitis.

Prognosis and Outcome

Although both form of the disease show a high response to immunosuppressive therapy, relapses are frequently seen, particularly in the pancreas and biliary tree.

Potential long-term sequelae include pancreatic duct stones and malignancy, although both are uncommon.

HEPATOBILIARY SYSTEM

Overview

Clinically, 2 forms of the disease are recognized in the hepatobiliary system. The more common manifestation of the disease, diffuse involvement of the biliary tract, mimics primary sclerosing cholangitis.[5] This variant is often associated with a

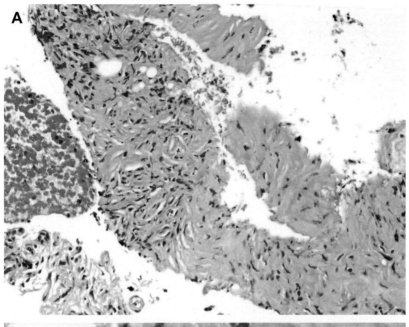

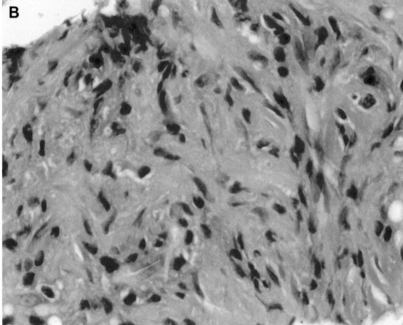

Fig. 10. (*A*) Tru-Cut biopsy from a pancreatic mass. The biopsy is dominated by collagen with fibroblasts. Storiform pattern of fibrosis is present, albeit subtle. An immunohistochemical stain showed greater than 10 IgG4+ plasma cells per HPF. The biopsy findings supported the clinical impression of type 1 autoimmune pancreatitis. (*B*) A high-powered view of a core biopsy from a patient with type 1 autoimmune pancreatitis. The fibroblasts are prominent. Scattered embedded lymphocytes are present.

peribiliary tumefactive lesion.[23,24] The second form of the disease is a solitary tumefactive lesion that mimics an intrahepatic cholangiocarcinoma.[25]

IgG4-related sclerosing cholangitis

Clinical features Affected individuals are greater than 50 years of age, and a great majority of patients are men.[5] It is currently thought that greater

than 90% of these patients have type 1 autoimmune pancreatitis.[23] It is likely, however, that this number underestimates the true extent of isolated IgG4-related sclerosing cholangitis and, with wider recognition of this entity, this number is likely to rise.

An elderly man with either a concurrent or prior history of autoimmune pancreatitis presenting with obstructive jaundice and sclerosing cholangitis is

Fig. 11. Low-power image of type 2 autoimmune pancreatitis. The inflammation is for the most part confined to an area around the duct. The adjacent pancreas shows extensive atrophy but lacks storiform type fibrosis.

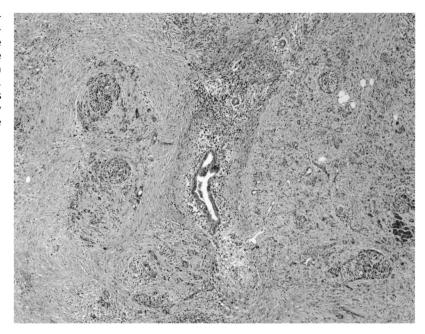

almost certain to have IgG4-related sclerosing cholangitis. In individuals who lack clinical evidence of pancreatic involvement, however, the distinction of IgG4-related disease from primary sclerosing cholangitis/extrahepatic biliary adenocarcinoma is problematic. Radiologically, there is significant overlap between these entities, with both primary sclerosing cholangitis and IgG4-related sclerosing cholangitis showing multiple narrowing and dilatation of intrahepatic and extrahepatic bile ducts (**Fig. 15**). Furthermore, patients with primary sclerosing cholangitis as well as bile duct carcinoma may show elevated serum IgG4. Approximately 10% of patients with primary sclerosing cholangitis show elevated serum levels of IgG4.[26] The association of elevated levels of serum and tissue IgG4 in patients with pancreaticobiliary malignancies is also well established.[11] Elevations above 4 times

Fig. 12. This pancreatic lobule is infiltrated by neutrophils, a finding that is highly suggestive of type 2 variant of autoimmune pancreatitis.

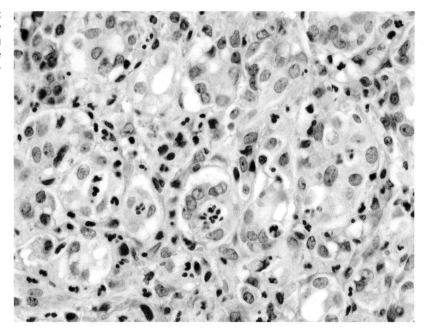

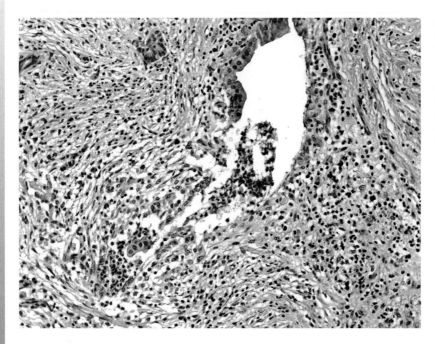

Fig. 13. Type 2 autoimmune pancreatitis. The doctor surrounded by a brisk lymphoplasmacytic infiltrate. A neutrophilic abscess identified within the lumen. Additionally, extensive denudation of the lining epithelium is also seen.

normal (normal IgG4 ≤140 mg/dL) are unlikely, however, in either of these mimics of IgG4-related sclerosing cholangitis.[27] Serum levels of IgG4, however, are not elevated in all patients with IgG4-related sclerosing cholangitis, and surgical excision may be the only alternative to exclude malignancy.

Gross features The disease typically affects large extrahepatic and intrahepatic bile ducts. The gallbladder may also be involved (discussed later). The ducts are markedly thickened and show a pipe stem fibrosis-like appearance. Unlike primary sclerosing cholangitis, the mucosal surfaces are

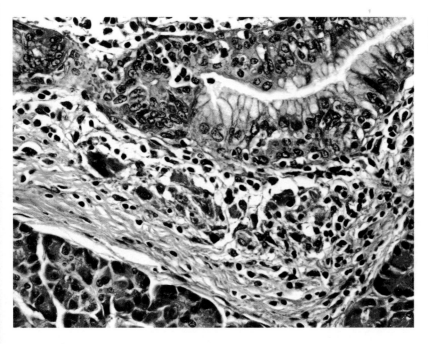

Fig. 14. Type 2 autoimmune pancreatitis with a periductal granuloma.

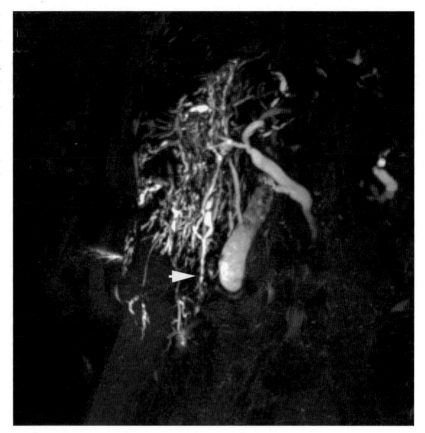

Fig. 15. Magnetic resonance cholangiogram show narrowing and dilatation of the biliary tree. The differential diagnosis includes IgG4-related sclerosing cholangitis and primary sclerosing cholangitis. A biopsy confirmed a diagnosis of IgG4-related sclerosing cholangitis. *Arrow* highlights the characteristic beaded appearance of sclerosing cholangitis.

uninvolved, and ulceration, if present, is related to an indwelling stent. A fleshy to fibrotic soft tissue mass may be seen adjacent to the bile duct.[24] The peripheral regions of the liver may show small gray white nodules, representing microscopic inflammatory pseudotumor-like lesions.[28]

Microscopic features

Large Bile Ducts The large bile ducts show a dense transmural lymphoplasmacytic infiltrate, generally associated with an eosinophil cell infiltrate (**Fig. 16**).[24,29] Occasionally, eosinophils may be sufficiently prominent to raise the possibility of eosinophilic cholangitis. The inflammatory infiltrate is associated with storiform-type fibrosis. This characteristic pattern may not be appreciable, however, on a needle biopsy. Obliterative phlebitis is often only seen in the outer half of the bile duct wall. The peribiliary glands are also involved by this fibroinflammatory process. These glands, as well as the surface epithelium, lack cellular atypia.

On immunohistochemistry, the transmural infiltrate is rich in IgG4+ plasma cells and, as in the pancreas, these cells are seen to diffusely infiltrate the duct wall. On a resection specimen, greater than 100 IgG4+ plasma cells are effortlessly found. As in other forms of IgG4-related disease, an IgG4 to IgG ratio of greater than 40% often helps distinguish IgG4-related sclerosing cholangitis from other mimics of the disease.

Differential Diagnosis

Primary sclerosing cholangitis The distinction of primary sclerosing cholangitis from IgG4-related cholangitis is straightforward when a segment of the bile duct is available for histologic study (**Table 3**).[24,29] The periluminal inflammatory infiltrate of primary sclerosing cholangitis is distinctly different from the transmural inflammation seen in IgG4-related sclerosing cholangitis. Moreover, storiform-type fibrosis and obliterative phlebitis are absent in primary sclerosing cholangitis. Unfortunately, these changes are rarely as obvious on a bile duct biopsy, and an unqualified diagnosis of IgG4-related sclerosing cholangitis is seldom possible on these small tissue samples.

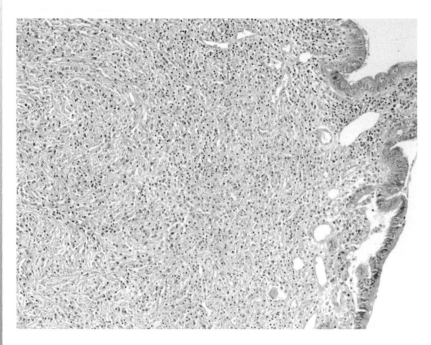

Fig. 16. A low-power photomicrograph shows the intrapancreatic portion of the common bile duct with transmural inflammation. The presence of this dense lymphoplasmacytic infiltrate in the outer layer of the common bile duct distinguishes IgG4-related sclerosing cholangitis from primary sclerosing cholangitis.

An immunohistochemical stain for IgG4 may not be a panacea—elevated numbers of IgG4+ plasma cells are seen in both primary sclerosing cholangitis and bile duct carcinoma. In a series of 98 resected cases of primary sclerosing cholangitis, 23% were found to have greater than 10 IgG4+ plasma cells per HPF, whereas another study revealed 5% of cases with greater than 100 IgG4+ cells per HPF (**Figs. 17** and **18**).[30,31] Nonetheless, the mean numbers of IgG4+ plasma cells in IgG4-related sclerosing cholangitis far exceeds those seen in primary sclerosing cholangitis, and counts in excess of 50 are uncommon in the latter disease.[32] Patients with elevated numbers of IgG4+ plasma cells may occupy a unique clinicopathologic niche. Patients with primary sclerosing cholangitis and elevated serum IgG4 seem to show a more aggressive clinical course.[26]

Bile duct carcinoma As in the pancreas, the most egregious error lies in misinterpreting a distal bile duct carcinoma for IgG4-related sclerosing

Table 3
Comparison of clinical and histologic features of primary sclerosing cholangitis and IgG4-related sclerosing cholangitis

	Primary Sclerosing Cholangitis	IgG4- Related Sclerosing Cholangitis
Mean age	62	39
Gender	M>F	M ≫ F
Clinical presentation	Abnormal LFT, asymptomatic	Obstructive jaundice
Serum IgG4	Normal or mildly elevated*	Elevated - moderate to marked (>4x normal)
Histopathological features *Large ducts*	• Inflammation involving inner half of bile duct • Erosion/ulceration	• Transmural inflammation • Storiform fibrosis • Obliterative phlebitis
Histopathologic features *Small ducts*	Sparse inflammation	Portal inflammatory nodules*
Tissue IgG4+ plasma cells	Present around large bile ducts	Present around both large ducts and in portal tracts

* Uncommon on a random biopsy of the liver.
Abbreviation: LFT, liver function test.

Fig. 17. Primary sclerosing cholangitis. A large bile duct shows extensive denudation of epithelium. Adjacent to the lumen a dense lymphoplasmacytic infiltrate is present. This infiltrate showed 25 IgG4+ plasma cells per HPF (see Fig. 18).

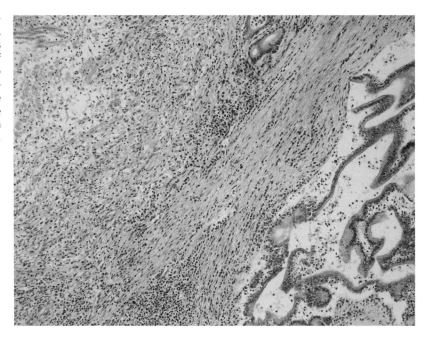

cholangitis.[33] The clinical presentation of the 2 diseases is similar; both present with localized bile duct stricture. The distinction is obvious if overt malignancy is identified on a biopsy. Unfortunately, in some cases, the histologic features of malignancy are less obvious; instead, a peritumoral infiltrate rich in IgG4+ plasma cells could raise the specter of IgG4-related sclerosing cholangitis. In one study, a cutoff of greater than 10 IgG4+ plasma cells per HPF showed a moderate sensitivity and high specificity for distinguishing IgG4-related sclerosing cholangitis from malignancy—52% and 96%, respectively.[34] As in the pancreas, however, the optimal approach is to avoid committing to a diagnosis based solely on the presence of elevated numbers of IgG4+ plasma cells. Unfortunately, a full gamut of morphologic changes is seldom seen on a biopsy sample, and it may thus

Fig. 18. Infiltrate adjacent to lumen showing 25 IgG4+ plasma cells per HPF.

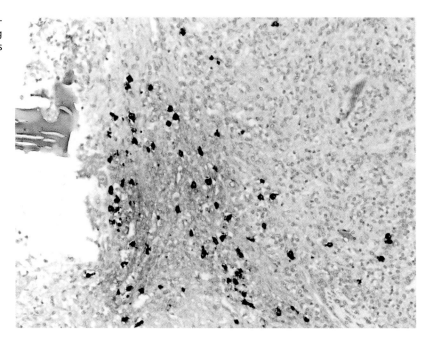

prove virtually impossible to exclude a bile duct carcinoma.

Other forms of cholangitis Two recently described diseases may also mimic IgG4-related sclerosing cholangitis. The first of these is follicular cholangitis, a lesion somewhat reminiscent of follicular cholecystitis in that numerous lymphoid follicles are seen surrounding the hilar and perihilar ducts.[35] Although lymphoid follicles and germinal centers may be seen in other forms of IgG4-related disease, such as IgG4-related sialadenitis, they are seldom as prominent in the hepatobiliary manifestations of this disease. Like IgG4-related sclerosing cholangitis, individuals with follicular cholangitis show with bile duct strictures. Histologically, however, this disease lacks storiform-type fibrosis and obliterative phlebitis, and although elevated numbers of IgG4+ plasma cells may be seen, their distribution is patchy and the IgG4 to IgG ratio is less than 40%.

Another histologically unique form of cholangitis is the so-called sclerosing cholangitis with granulocytic epithelial lesions.[36] This disease also shows neutrophil-rich infiltrates and bile duct damage, an appearance that resembles granulocytic epithelial lesions of type 2 autoimmune pancreatitis. Although only a few cases have been described and the clinical significance of this disease has not been fully explored, it is likely that this represents another steroid responsive form of cholangitis.[36]

Small Duct Lesions The changes on a nonfocal needle biopsy are seldom diagnostic for IgG4-related sclerosing cholangitis. This situation is somewhat analogous to needle biopsies from patients with primary sclerosing cholangitis: although several histologic changes are appreciable, they are seldom of themselves diagnostic. A core liver biopsy from patients with IgG4-related sclerosing cholangitis may show a variety of changes, including sclerosis of the portal tract, lobular and portal inflammatory infiltrates, bile ductular reaction, and canalicular cholestasis. Nonetheless, 2 features, if present, suggest IgG4-related sclerosing cholangitis[28]:

1. Presence of portal-based fibroinflammatory lesions
2. Elevated numbers of IgG4+ plasma cells

These portal-based inflammatory nodules show histologic features that are typical for IgG4-related disease: a dense lymphoplasmacytic infiltrate with eosinophils and elevated numbers of IgG4+ plasma cells (**Figs. 19–23**). Needle biopsies from

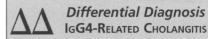

Differential Diagnosis
IgG4-RELATED CHOLANGITIS

1. Extrahepatic bile duct carcinoma
2. Intrahepatic cholangiocarcinoma
3. Hepatic inflammatory pseudotumor
4. Primary sclerosing cholangitis
5. Other forms of sclerosing cholangitis

patients with primary sclerosing cholangitis typically show only a sparse portal lymphoplasmacytic infiltrate and seldom show greater than 10 IgG4+ plasma cells per HPF (unlike the periductal inflammatory infiltrates around large ducts that may show a hot spot of IgG4+ cells). The onionskin–like fibrosis around ducts, often touted as a unique feature of primary sclerosing cholangitis, is also seen in IgG4-related sclerosing cholangitis.

Hepatic Inflammatory Pseudotumor of Liver

Overview Hepatic inflammatory pseudotumors of the liver, like pseudotumors at other sites, are characterized histologically by a proliferation of fibroblasts, myofibroblasts, and inflammatory cells (**Fig. 24**).[24,25] This term refers to a heterogeneous group of entities, and only a third of these cases belong to the IgG4-related disease spectrum. IgG4-related hepatic pseudotumors are typically seen in elderly men and the lesion is located in the hilum of the liver.

Microscopic Features Histologically, these lesions show characteristic features of IgG4-related disease, including obliterative phlebitis and elevated numbers of IgG4+ plasma cells. Inflammatory tumefactive lesions of the liver that lack these histologic features, and that instead show xanthogranulomatous inflammation and giant cell formation, do not belong to the IgG4-related disease spectrum. The differential diagnosis of IgG4-related hepatic pseudotumor also includes inflammatory myofibroblastic tumor.

IgG4+ Cells in Autoimmune Hepatitis
IgG4+ plasma cells are identified in a variety of inflammatory diseases, including some in the gastrointestinal tract, such as autoimmune hepatitis and ulcerative colitis (discussed later). There is little evidence to suggest that either entity is a member of the IgG4-related disease family. Nonetheless, a substantial number of patients with

Fig. 19. IgG4-related sclerosing cholangitis. The image shows a subcapsular fibroinflammatory nodule.

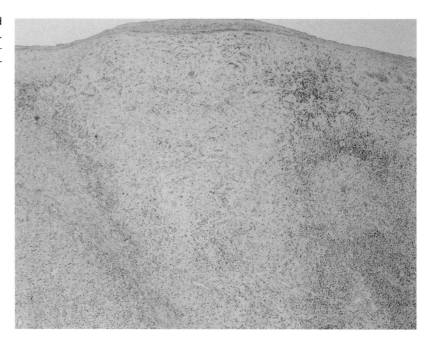

these diseases show elevated numbers of IgG4+ plasma cells. In one study, 1 in 3 liver biopsies from patients with autoimmune pancreatitis shows elevated numbers of IgG4+ plasma cells (defined as >5/HPF).[37] In comparison with patients who lacked elevated numbers of IgG4+ plasma cells, these cases seemed to show a sustained response to steroids and did not relapse on maintenance steroids, suggesting that the presence of IgG4+ plasma cells may be a surrogate marker of response to therapy.[37]

There is some debate as to whether a pure form of IgG4-related liver disease without bile duct involvement exists.[38] Histologically, this variant of IgG4-related disease, labeled IgG4-related hepatopathy, mimics autoimmune hepatitis, and shows

Fig. 20. On higher power, the infiltrate is composed of lymphocytes, plasma cells, and scattered eosinophils in an edematous background. On an immunoperoxidase stain, virtually all the plasma cells were positive for IgG4 (image not shown).

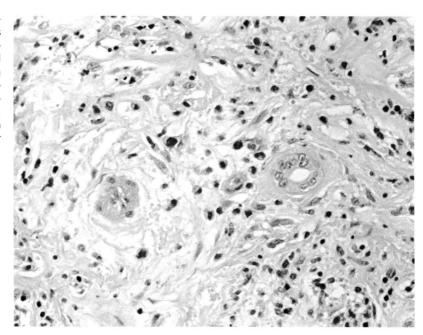

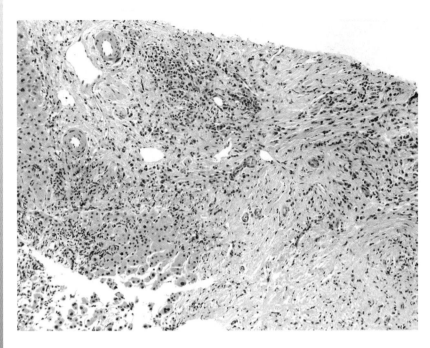

Fig. 21. A needle biopsy from an elderly man with obstructive jaundice. A fibroinflammatory nodule is seen within this portal tract. Lymphocytes, plasma cells, and scattered eosinophils are present.

elevated serum and tissue levels of IgG4+ plasma cells.

Gallbladder

Overview Although it is common to see gallbladder involvement in type 1 autoimmune pancreatitis, clinically symptomatic gallbladder disease has not been reported. Nonetheless, the gallbladder, if available for histologic review, is another tool in the diagnostic armamentarium. Remarkably, little is known about the prevalence of gallbladder involvement in nonpancreatic forms of IgG4-related disease.

Gross Features The gallbladder may be appreciably thickened and fibrotic, although a discrete mass is generally not observed.

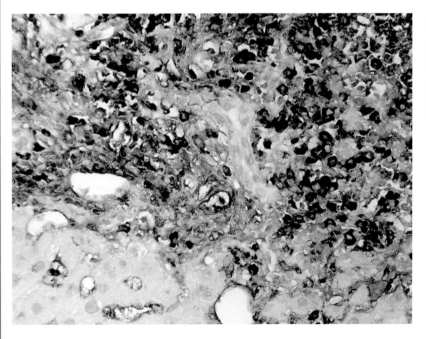

Fig. 22. A majority of the plasma cells in the nodule in **Fig. 21** were positive for IgG4. This individual subsequently developed radiologic evidence of autoimmune pancreatitis.

Fig.   23. IgG4-related sclerosing cholangitis. This photomicrograph shows a large portal tract infiltrated by a dense lymphoplasmacytic infiltrate. Focal interface hepatitis is also present. Note the acellular collar around the bile duct.

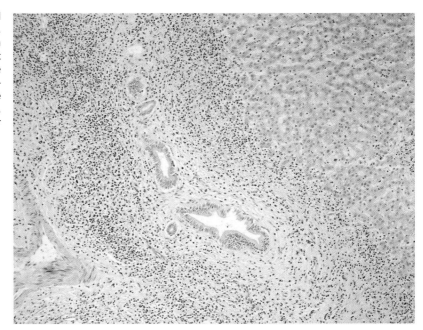

Microscopic Features Gallbladders resected in the course of a Whipple procedure often show a dense mucosal-based lymphoplasmacytic infiltrate (the so-called lymphoplasmacytic cholecystitis), and this infiltrate is a consequence of biliary obstruction, commonly by tumor or inflammatory disease. In contrast, the lymphoplasmacytic infiltrate in patients with type 1 autoimmune pancreatitis extends through the muscularis propria and into subserosal tissue and occasionally forms circumscribed nodules (**Figs. 25** and **26**).[39] Obliterative phlebitis is frequently identified within subserosal tissue. A marked increase in IgG4+ plasma cells is found both in the mucosal compartment and in the subserosal infiltrate.

Fig.   24. IgG4-related inflammatory pseudotumor of the liver. On immunohistochemistry, this solitary hepatic lesion showed large numbers of IgG4+ plasma cells.

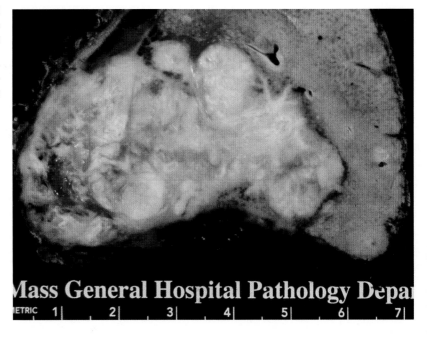

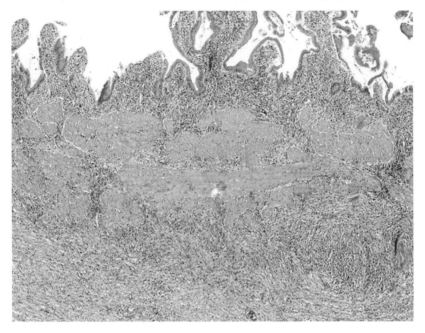

Fig. 25. IgG4-related cholecystitis. This patient also had type 1 autoimmune pancreatitis. The transmural inflammatory infiltrate, as well as a robust serosal inflammatory infiltrate, is typical of IgG4-related cholecystitis, distinguishing it from other forms of lymphoplasmacytic cholecystitis.

Differential Diagnosis Key features that distinguish IgG4-related cholecystitis from other inflammatory diseases of the gallbladder (including lymphoplasmacytic cholecystitis) are the presence of subserosal/transmural inflammation, obliterative phlebitis, and increased numbers of IgG4+ plasma cells.[39] As with other forms of the disease, it is prudent to require both a characteristic morphologic appearance as well as elevated numbers of IgG4+ plasma cells.

TUBULAR GUT

It is remarkable that although the liver and the pancreas are frequently targeted by IgG4-related disease, the tubular gut is seldom involved.

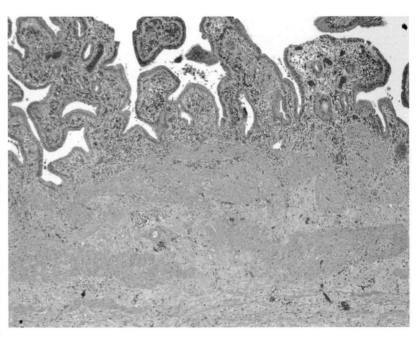

Fig. 26. Lymphoplasmacytic cholecystitis secondary to bile duct obstruction by a pancreatic adenocarcinoma. The inflammation is confined to the mucosa, without involvement of the muscularis propria or subserosa layer.

Fig. 27. IgG4-related gastropathy. The lymphoplasmacytic infiltrate is predominantly located in the basal half of the mucosa.

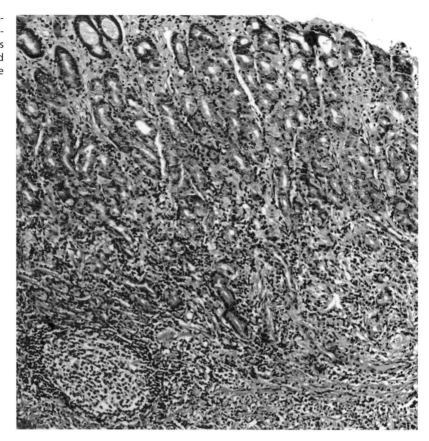

Fig. 28. IgG4-related gastropathy. The lymphoplasmacytic infiltrate involves the muscularis mucosae and the basal glands.

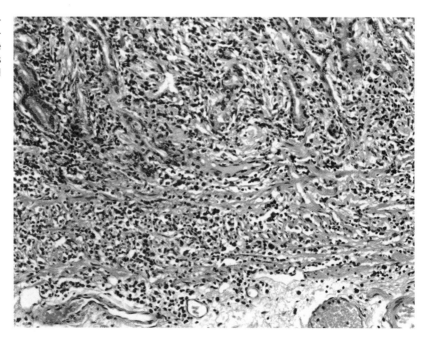

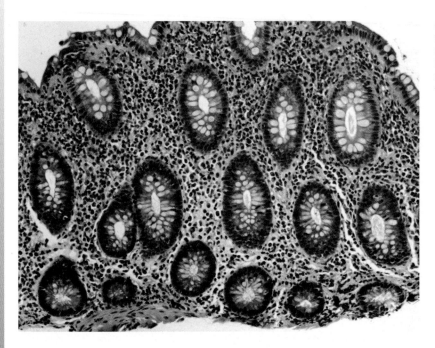

Fig. 29. Colonic biopsies showing expansion of mononuclear cells in the lamina propria without significant crypt architectural distortion.

Nonetheless, there are now a substantial number of reports that convincingly document involvement of the tubular gut.[40]

Stomach

Overview

IgG4-related gastropathy is a well-characterized entity. The endoscopic features of IgG4-related gastropathy are nonspecific, although chronic gastric ulceration has been reported.[41]

Microscopic features

Histologically, both the corpus and antral mucosa show a diffuse transmucosal lymphoplasmacytic infiltrate, a pattern that may mimic *Helicobacter pylori* gastritis.[42] Unlike active *Helicobacter pylori* gastritis, however, neutrophils are uncommon.

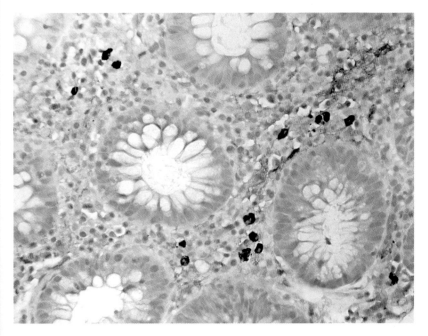

Fig. 30. The colonic biopsy from **Fig. 29**, taken within weeks of the initial presentation of the disease, shows elevated numbers of IgG4+ plasma cells.

A deep mucosal lymphoplasmacytic infiltrate is also more typical of IgG4-related gastropathy (**Figs. 27** and **28**). In addition, IgG4+ plasma cells are absent in *Helicobacter pylori* gastritis, although they are easily found in IgG4-related gastropathy. IgG4-related gastropathy may also resemble autoimmune gastritis; however, unlike in autoimmune gastritis, the antrum is not spared.

Ampulla

The ampulla seems commonly involved in autoimmune pancreatitis, although this involvement is clinically inapparent. Endoscopically, the duodenal papilla may appear swollen.[43] A blind biopsy from the ampulla may assist in distinguishing pancreatic ductal adenocarcinoma from autoimmune pancreatitis: using a cutoff of greater than 10 IgG4+ plasma cells, the sensitivity and specificity in one study was 52% and specificity 91%, respectively.[34] Although other studies report a higher specificity and sensitivity, it is unwise to base a diagnosis of autoimmune pancreatitis solely on the presence of elevated numbers of IgG4+ cells. Type 2 autoimmune pancreatitis is not an IgG4-related disease; hence, elevated numbers of IgG4+ plasma cells may not be found.

DISEASE ENTITIES THAT DO NOT BELONG TO THE IGG4-RELATED DISEASE SPECTRUM BUT ARE ASSOCIATED WITH ELEVATED NUMBERS OF IGG4+ PLASMA CELLS

Overview

Several other entities are associated with elevated numbers of IgG4+ plasma cells, foremost among which are rheumatologic diseases, such as Wegener granulomatosis and rheumatoid arthritis. Within the gastrointestinal tract, IgG4+ plasma cells are consistently detected in autoimmune gastritis and inflammatory bowel disease, and in each of these instances their presence seems (at least based on the limited evidence available to date) to have diagnostic and/or prognostic value.

Stomach

In the stomach, IgG4+ plasma cells (>10/HPF) are identified in autoimmune gastritis, although they are absent in other forms of chronic atrophic gastritis as well as *Helicobacter pylori* gastritis. In one study, increased IgG4+ plasma cells were present in 37% of patients with autoimmune gastritis and pernicious anemia, whereas patients who lack pernicious anemia were negative for IgG4.[44] Although the etiopathogenic and therapeutic implications of this serendipitous association are unclear, this finding may have clinical relevance.

Inflammatory bowel disease

Similarly, elevated numbers of IgG4+ plasma cells are identified in inflammatory bowel disease (**Figs. 29** and **30**). The authors' experience suggests that patients with ulcerative colitis show higher numbers of IgG4+ plasma cells than those with Crohn colitis—19 (38%) ulcerative colitis patients had IgG4 counts greater than 10 per HPF compared with 2 (5%) patients with Crohn disease. Colonic biopsies from patients with lymphocytic/collagenous colitis are virtually devoid of IgG4+ plasma cells—mean 1 per HPF.[45] Thus, elevated numbers of IgG4+ plasma cells (>10/HPF) may assist in the distinction of ulcerative colitis from Crohn disease.

IgG4+ plasma cells are also seen in individuals with pouchitis, a finding that seems to have predictive value—patients with greater than 10 IgG4+ plasma cells in biopsies from the pouch had higher pouch inflammatory scores as measured by endoscopic evaluation.[46,47] Furthermore, these individuals did not respond to conventional agents used for the treatment pouchitis and patients with chronic antibiotic refractory pouchitis also show elevated serum IgG4 levels.[46,47] These studies have not been validated, and the diagnostic and predictive significance of IgG4+ plasma cells in these inflammatory diseases of the gut awaits further studies.

REFERENCES

1. Stone JH, Zen Y, Deshpande V. IgG4-related disease. N Engl J Med 2012;366(6):539–51.
2. Deshpande V. IgG4-related disease. Introduction. Semin Diagn Pathol 2012;29(4):175–6.
3. Deshpande V. The pathology of IgG4-related disease: critical issues and challenges. Semin Diagn Pathol 2012;29(4):191–6.
4. Finkelberg DL, Sahani D, Deshpande V, et al. Autoimmune pancreatitis. N Engl J Med 2006;355(25):2670–6.
5. Ghazale A, Chari ST, Zhang L, et al. Immunoglobulin G4-associated cholangitis: clinical profile and response to therapy. Gastroenterology 2008;134(3):706–15.
6. Deshpande V, Zen Y, Chan JK, et al. Consensus statement on the pathology of IgG4-related disease. Mod Pathol 2012;25(9):1181–92.
7. Stone JH. IgG4-related disease: nomenclature, clinical features, and treatment. Semin Diagn Pathol 2012;29(4):177–90.
8. Khosroshahi A, Stone JH. A clinical overview of IgG4-related systemic disease. Curr Opin Rheumatol 2011;23(1):57–66.

9. Khosroshahi A, Stone JH. Treatment approaches to IgG4-related systemic disease. Curr Opin Rheumatol 2011;23(1):67–71.

10. Chari ST. Diagnosis of autoimmune pancreatitis using its five cardinal features: introducing the Mayo Clinic's HISORt criteria. J Gastroenterol 2007; 42(Suppl 18):39–41.

11. Sah RP, Chari ST. Serologic issues in IgG4-related systemic disease and autoimmune pancreatitis. Curr Opin Rheumatol 2011;23(1):108–13.

12. Geyer JT, Ferry JA, Harris NL, et al. Chronic sclerosing sialadenitis (Kuttner tumor) is an IgG4-associated disease. Am J Surg Pathol 2010;34(2):202–10.

13. Sugumar A. Diagnosis and management of autoimmune pancreatitis. Gastroenterol Clin North Am 2012;41(1):9–22.

14. Kamisawa T, Shimosegawa T, Okazaki K, et al. Standard steroid treatment for autoimmune pancreatitis. Gut 2009;58(11):1504–7.

15. Khosroshahi A, Bloch DB, Deshpande V, et al. Rituximab therapy leads to rapid decline of serum IgG4 levels and prompt clinical improvement in IgG4-related systemic disease. Arthritis Rheum 2010; 62(6):1755–62.

16. Deshpande V, Gupta R, Sainani N, et al. Subclassification of autoimmune pancreatitis: a histologic classification with clinical significance. Am J Surg Pathol 2011;35(1):26–35.

17. Sah RP, Chari ST, Pannala R, et al. Differences in clinical profile and relapse rate of type 1 versus type 2 autoimmune pancreatitis. Gastroenterology 2010;139(1):140–8 [quiz: e12–3].

18. Notohara K, Burgart LJ, Yadav D, et al. Idiopathic chronic pancreatitis with periductal lymphoplasmacytic infiltration: clinicopathologic features of 35 cases. Am J Surg Pathol 2003;27(8):1119–27.

19. Shinagare S, Shinagare AB, Deshpande V. Autoimmune pancreatitis: a guide for the histopathologist. Semin Diagn Pathol 2012;29(4):197–204.

20. Zhang L, Chari S, Smyrk TC, et al. Autoimmune pancreatitis (AIP) type 1 and type 2: an international consensus study on histopathologic diagnostic criteria. Pancreas 2011;40(8):1172–9.

21. Shimosegawa T, Chari ST, Frulloni L, et al. International consensus diagnostic criteria for autoimmune pancreatitis: guidelines of the International Association of Pancreatology. Pancreas 2011; 40(3):352–8.

22. Zamboni G, Luttges J, Capelli P, et al. Histopathological features of diagnostic and clinical relevance in autoimmune pancreatitis: a study on 53 resection specimens and 9 biopsy specimens. Virchows Arch 2004;445(6):552–63.

23. Zen Y, Nakanuma Y, Portmann B. Immunoglobulin G4-related sclerosing cholangitis: pathologic features and histologic mimics. Semin Diagn Pathol 2012;29(4):205–11.

24. Zen Y, Harada K, Sasaki M, et al. IgG4-related sclerosing cholangitis with and without hepatic inflammatory pseudotumor, and sclerosing pancreatitis-associated sclerosing cholangitis: do they belong to a spectrum of sclerosing pancreatitis? Am J Surg Pathol 2004;28(9):1193–203.

25. Zen Y, Fujii T, Sato Y, et al. Pathological classification of hepatic inflammatory pseudotumor with respect to IgG4-related disease. Mod Pathol 2007;20(8): 884–94.

26. Mendes FD, Jorgensen R, Keach J, et al. Elevated serum IgG4 concentration in patients with primary sclerosing cholangitis. Am J Gastroenterol 2006; 101(9):2070–5.

27. Oseini AM, Chaiteerakij R, Shire AM, et al. Utility of serum immunoglobulin G4 in distinguishing immunoglobulin G4-associated cholangitis from cholangiocarcinoma. Hepatology 2011;54(3):940–8.

28. Deshpande V, Sainani NI, Chung RT, et al. IgG4-associated cholangitis: a comparative histological and immunophenotypic study with primary sclerosing cholangitis on liver biopsy material. Mod Pathol 2009;22(10):1287–95.

29. Zen Y, Nakanuma Y. IgG4 Cholangiopathy. Int J Hepatol 2012;2012:472376.

30. Zen Y, Quaglia A, Portmann B. Immunoglobulin G4-positive plasma cell infiltration in explanted livers for primary sclerosing cholangitis. Histopathology 2011;58(3):414–22.

31. Zhang L, Lewis JT, Abraham SC, et al. IgG4+ plasma cell infiltrates in liver explants with primary sclerosing cholangitis. Am J Surg Pathol 2010; 34(1):88–94.

32. Kimura Y, Harada K, Nakanuma Y. Pathologic significance of immunoglobulin G4-positive plasma cells in extrahepatic cholangiocarcinoma. Hum Pathol 2012;43(12):2149–56.

33. Gardner TB, Levy MJ, Takahashi N, et al. Misdiagnosis of autoimmune pancreatitis: a caution to clinicians. Am J Gastroenterol 2009;104(7):1620–3.

34. Kawakami H, Zen Y, Kuwatani M, et al. IgG4-related sclerosing cholangitis and autoimmune pancreatitis: histological assessment of biopsies from Vater's ampulla and the bile duct. J Gastroenterol Hepatol 2010;25(10):1648–55.

35. Zen Y, Ishikawa A, Ogiso S, et al. Follicular cholangitis and pancreatitis—clinicopathological features and differential diagnosis of an under-recognized entity. Histopathology 2012;60(2):261–9.

36. Zen Y, Grammatikopoulos T, Heneghan MA, et al. Sclerosing cholangitis with granulocytic epithelial lesion: a benign form of sclerosing cholangiopathy. Am J Surg Pathol 2012;36(10):1555–61.

37. Umemura T, Zen Y, Hamano H, et al. Clinical significance of immunoglobulin G4-associated autoimmune hepatitis. J Gastroenterol 2011;46(Suppl 1): 48–55.

38. Umemura T, Zen Y, Nakanuma Y, et al. Another cause of autoimmune hepatitis. Hepatology 2010; 52(1):389–90.
39. Wang WL, Farris AB, Lauwers GY, et al. Autoimmune pancreatitis-related cholecystitis: a morphologically and immunologically distinctive form of lymphoplasmacytic sclerosing cholecystitis. Histopathology 2009;54(7):829–36.
40. Wong DD, Pillai SR, Kumarasinghe MP, et al. IgG4-related sclerosing disease of the small bowel presenting as necrotizing mesenteric arteritis and a solitary jejunal ulcer. Am J Surg Pathol 2012;36(6):929–34.
41. Bateman AC, Sommerlad M, Underwood TJ. Chronic gastric ulceration: a novel manifestation of IgG4-related disease? J Clin Pathol 2012;65(6):569–70.
42. Uehara T, Hamano H, Kawa S, et al. Chronic gastritis in the setting of autoimmune pancreatitis. Am J Surg Pathol 2010;34(9):1241–9.
43. Kubota K, Kato S, Akiyama T, et al. Differentiating sclerosing cholangitis caused by autoimmune pancreatitis and primary sclerosing cholangitis according to endoscopic duodenal papillary features. Gastrointest Endosc 2008;68(6):1204–8.
44. Bedeir AS, Lash RH, Lash JG, et al. Significant increase in IgG4+ plasma cells in gastric biopsy specimens from patients with pernicious anaemia. J Clin Pathol 2010;63(11):999–1001.
45. Virk R, Shinagare, S, Yajnik V, Stone JH, Deshpande V. Tissue IgG4+ plasma cells in inflammatory bowel disease: A study of 88 treatment-naïve biopsies of inflammatory bowel disease. Modern Pathology (in press).
46. Navaneethan U, Bennett AE, Venkatesh PG, et al. Tissue infiltration of IgG4+ plasma cells in symptomatic patients with ileal pouch-anal anastomosis. J Crohns Colitis 2011;5(6):570–6.
47. Navaneethan U, Venkatesh PG, Kapoor S, et al. Elevated serum IgG4 is associated with chronic antibiotic-refractory pouchitis. J Gastrointest Surg 2011;15(9):1556–61.

Diarrheal Illness in the Pediatric Population
A Review of Neonatal Enteropathies and Childhood Idiopathic Inflammatory Bowel Disease

Eric U. Yee, MD, Jeffrey D. Goldsmith, MD*

KEYWORDS

- Microvillous inclusion disease • Tufting enteropathy • Autoimmune enteropathy
- Hypobetalipoproteinemias • Enteroendocrine cell dysgenesis • Chronic granulomatous disease
- Immunodeficiencies

ABSTRACT

In the clinical context of pediatric diarrheal illness, the interpretation of endoscopic mucosal biopsies varies significantly from that of adults. This review outlines these differences by first describing a host of diarrheal illnesses that are nearly exclusive to the pediatric age group. The final portion of this article describes salient pathologic differences between adult and pediatric idiopathic inflammatory bowel disease. The goal of this review is to provide a brief description of each disease process and focus on practical aspects of diagnosis that are applicable for pathologists working in general practice settings.

the associated crucial clinical management decisions in the pediatric age group, it is important for pathologists to recognize the histologic and clinical differences in the work-up of pediatric diarrheal illness compared with that of adults. The first section of this review discusses entities that have characteristic histologic findings that occur almost exclusively in neonates and infants (**Box 1**); the second portion of this article highlights key differences in inflammatory bowel disease (IBD) in children compared with adults.

OVERVIEW

Diarrhea, defined as an excess of 200 g per day of stool in those over age 3 years and more than 10 g/kg per day in infants, is a common indication for endoscopic biopsy in the pediatric population. With continued advances in anesthesia and endoscopy, the frequency of endoscopic biopsy continues to increase.[1] Despite this, pathologists' exposure to these samples is limited in most practice settings. Given the morbidity and potential mortality associated with protracted diarrhea and

MICROVILLOUS INCLUSION DISEASE

OVERVIEW

MVID, also referred to as microvillous atrophy, is the most common noninfectious cause of severe protracted watery diarrhea during the first week of life.[2] Most patients present during the neonatal period, but some have a later onset and symptoms may not commence until the 60th day of life. The diarrhea is of secretory type, has a watery consistency, and tends to persist at a high rate (up to 500 mL/kg/d).[3] The disease is life threatening and urgent total parenteral nutrition and hydration support are needed.[2] Sustained parenteral nutritional supplementation and intestinal transplant

Funding Sources: None.
Conflicts of Interest: None.
Department of Pathology, Harvard Medical School, Beth Israel Deaconess Medical Center, Children's Hospital Boston, 330 Brookline Avenue, Boston, MA 02215, USA
* Corresponding author.
E-mail address: jgoldsmi@bidmc.harvard.edu

Surgical Pathology 6 (2013) 523–543
http://dx.doi.org/10.1016/j.path.2013.05.006

Abbreviations: Diarrheal illness in the pediatric population	
ABL	Abetalipoproteinemia
AEA	Antienterocyte autoantibodies
APECED	Autoimmune polyendocrinopathy-candidiasis-ectodermal dystrophy
APOB	Apolipoprotein B
CD	Crohn's disease
CGD	Chronic granulomatous disease
CRD	Chylomicron retention disease
CVID	Common variable immunodeficiency
ECD	Enteroendocrine cell dysgenesis
FHBL	Familial hypobetalipoproteinemia
IBD	Inflammatory bowel disease
IPEX	Immune dysfunction, polyendocrinopathy, enteropathy, and X-linked inheritance
LDL	Low-density lipoprotein
MTP	Microsomal triglyceride transfer protein
MVID	Microvillous inclusion disease
NEUROG3	Neurogenin-3 gene
TE	Tufting enteropathy
UC	Ulcerative colitis
XLA	X-linked agammaglobulinemia

Box 1
Causes of diarrheal illness that are nearly exclusive to the pediatric population

- Microvillous inclusion disease (MVID)
- Tufting enteropathy (TE)
- Autoimmune enteropathy (AE)
- Hypobetalipoproteinemias
- Enteroendocrine cell dysgenesis (ECD)
- Chronic granulomatous disease (CGD)
- Immunodeficiencies
  - X-linked agammaglobulinemia (XLA)
  - Common variable immunodeficiency (CVID)

Key Features
MICROVILLOUS INCLUSION DISEASE

1. Villous atrophy without crypt hyperplasia.
2. Normal amount of lamina propria inflammation.
3. Periodic acid–Schiff (PAS), CD10, and carcinoembryonic antigen (CEA) stains show patchy disruption and internalization of the brush border.
4. Electron microscopy shows diagnostic microvillous inclusions.

have been reported as long-term treatment options.[3,4]

Recent studies have implicated loss-of-function mutations in *MYO5B*, a gene encoding type Vb myosin motor protein, as the main defect causing MVID. Myo5B, together with Rab8, is believed to be involved in intracellular protein trafficking, with mutations in *MYO5B* leading to disruption of enterocyte cell polarization.[5–7]

MICROSCOPIC FEATURES

Although endoscopy usually demonstrates no specific alterations, histology reveals distinctive features. In small bowel specimens, the most noticeable feature at low power is diffuse, subtotal to total villous atrophy without crypt hyperplasia; the lamina propria does not show increased inflammation.[3,8] At high power, fine cytoplasmic vacuoles may be seen along the apical surface and the brush border appears poorly developed or indiscernable.[8,9] Cytoplasmic vacuoles are most commonly seen along the upper crypts but occasionally are found in the lower villus and deeper crypt areas as well (**Fig. 1**A, B).[3]

Although definitive diagnosis relies on demonstration of intracytoplasmic microvillous inclusions by electron microscopy,[10,11] typical features identified on hematoxylin-eosin (H&E) stain and corroborative evidence by special stains strongly support the diagnosis of MVID.[12] These adjunctive stains include PAS histochemistry, CD10, and polyclonal CEA immunohistochemistry; all of these show patchy disruption of the normal band-like apical brush border with internalization of the brush border into the apical cytoplasm. Also, these stains tend to highlight the intracytoplasmic microvillous inclusions by showing punctuate apical cytoplasmic staining (see **Fig. 1**C–F).[8,12] Meanwhile, genetic studies for *MYO5B* mutations have

Fig. 1. MVID, small intestine. (*A*) Complete villous atrophy with a normal amount of lamina propria inflammation (H&E, ×200,). (*B*) The apical cytoplasm of the surface epithelium shows a bubbly appearance (H&E, ×400). (*C*) PAS stain shows abnormal brush border morphology with internalization of the normal PAS-positive signal. Also, punctate PAS positivity is seen within the apical cytoplasm, which corresponds to the microvillous inclusions seen ultrastructurally (PAS, ×400).

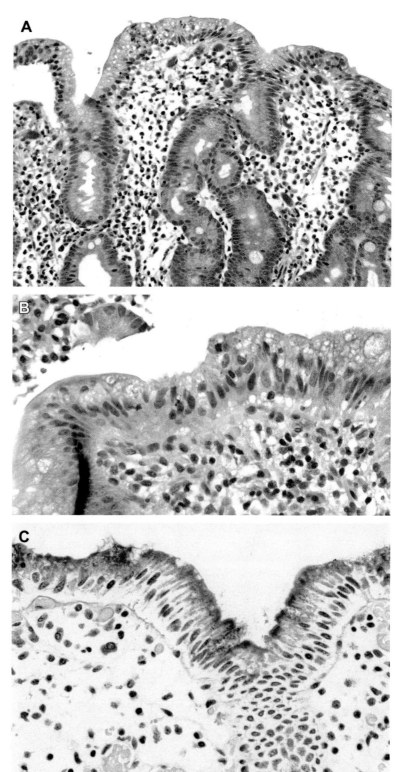

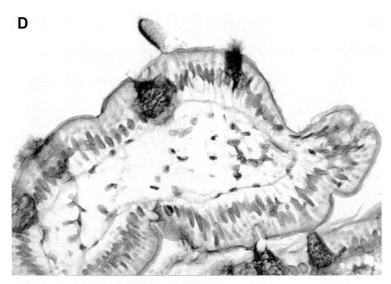

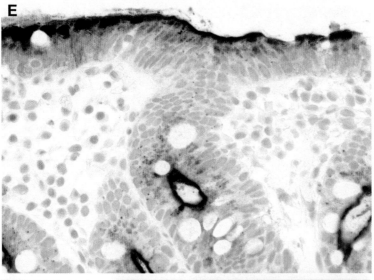

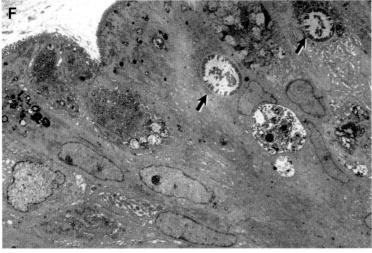

Fig. 1. (*D*, PAS, ×400) PAS on normal small intestinal epithelium for comparison with (*C*). (*E*) CD10 immunohistochemistry shows similar findings as the PAS stains with loss of normal brush border morphology and punctuate staining in the apical cytoplasm (CD10 immunohistochemistry, ×400). (*F*) Transmission electron microscopy showing the diagnostic microvillous inclusions (*arrows*).

been used clinically in at least 1 case as a diagnostic adjunct and may play a more prominent role in the future.[13]

Although the features described previously are typical for MVID, pathologists should be aware of some potential pitfalls in diagnosis. Variant forms have been reported that can present with normal-appearing villous architecture.[3,11] Although the bubbly apical cytoplasmic vacuolation is distinctive, this change may occasionally be confused with gastric foveolar metaplasia and can be subtle by H&E alone; thus, the special stains (discussed previously) should always be evaluated when MVID is in the differential diagnosis.[3,12] Lastly, clinical correlation is essential. Even negative work-up on special stains and absence of classic findings by electron microscopy on initial biopsy cannot entirely exclude MVID due to the sometimes patchy nature of typical changes.[14]

DIFFERENTIAL DIAGNOSIS

The differential diagnosis includes entities described later, notably TE and AE. TE shares histologic features with MVID in that the villous architecture is typically altered in both conditions. TE has, however, normal, or nearly normal, brush border morphology and exhibits the classic epithelial tufts of teardrop-appearing enterocytes that are a sine qua non of this disorder. AE, however, is characterized by markedly increased lamina propria inflammation with prominent, destructive neutrophilic inflammation, including neutrophilic crypt abscesses. These inflammatory infiltrates are not characteristic of MVID.

TUFTING ENTEROPATHY (INTESTINAL EPITHELIAL DYSPLASIA)

OVERVIEW

First reported in 1994 by Reifen and colleagues,[15] TE is rare condition with a prevalence estimated at 1/50,000 to 1/100,000 live births in Western Europe.[16] It seems more common among those of Arabic descent and those with consanguineous parents. Infants may present with severe, life-threatening watery diarrhea (up to 200 mL/kg body weight/d) within the first days to weeks of life that persists despite bowel rest. Clinically, TE can sometimes be associated with congenital anomalies, such as dysmorphic facial features, esophageal atresia, choanal atresia, imporforate anus, and punctate keratitis.[16–18] Treatment options include long-term parenteral nutrition, parenteral nutrition with progressive weaning, small bowel transplantation, and, in cases of

> **Key Features**
> **TUFTING ENTEROPATHY**
>
> 1. Villous atrophy and crypt hyperplasia.
>
> 2. Normal amount of lamina propria inflammation.
>
> 3. Abnormal enterocyte morphology with teardrop-shaped enterocytes, which are most prominent at abortive villous tips.

development of end-stage liver disease (cirrhosis), combined small bowel and liver transplantation.[16]

Early studies suggested an association between basement membrane abnormalities, such as alterations in $\alpha 2\beta 1$ integrin adhesion molecule distribution.[19] More recently, studies have identified mutations in EpCAM, the product of which is thought to be involved in cell-cell interactions.[20–22]

MICROSCOPIC FEATURES

No distinctive endoscopic abnormalities have been reported to date. Microscopically, small bowel biopsies demonstrate partial to total villous atrophy and crypt hyperplasia without significant expansion of the lamina propria by inflammatory cells or increase in intraepithelial lymphocytes.[11,15] Characteristic features include disorganized, closely packed surface enterocytes with apical rounding of plasma membrane that imparts a teardrop appearance to the cells (**Fig. 2**). These features are responsible for the tufted appearance, particularly when seen at the villous tips.[15] Meanwhile, crypts can show enterocyte crowding with regenerative features as well as crypt hyperplasia, mild dilation, and branching.[16] Tufts are occasionally seen in colonic biopsies as well.[19] Recently, reports of decreased or complete loss of EpCAM expression, as measured by immunohistochemistry, have been noted in subsets of TE patients.[20,23] It is unclear, however, if the immunohistochemical assay is sufficiently specific to be used as a definitive diagnostic test.

DIFFERENTIAL DIAGNOSIS

Clinically, congenital chloride diarrhea, congenital sodium diarrhea, and glucose-galactose malabsorption are in the differential diagnosis. Laboratory stool studies and electrolyte chemistries usually identify the former 2 entities whereas dietary modification can control the latter. MVID is also in the differential diagnosis given the similar age of onset. As discussed previously, supportive

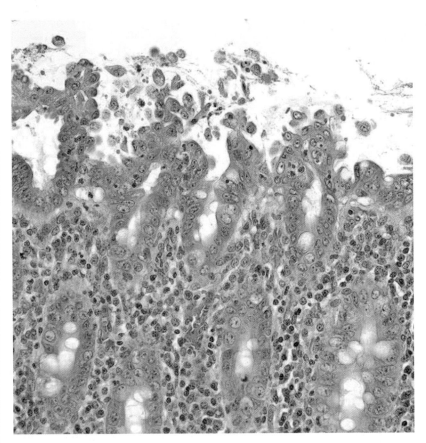

Fig. 2. TE, small intestine: marked villous atrophy is present with marked disorganization and teardrop morphology of the surface epithelium (H&E, ×400). (*Courtesy of* Ronald Jaffe, MBBCh, Children's Hospital of Pittsburgh, University of Pittsburgh Medical Center, Pittsburgh, PA.)

studies with PAS or CD10 and negative electron microscopy help rule out MVID.[16]

The characteristic tufts may be rare or absent, particularly in early life, and repeat biopsies may be needed to establish the correct diagnosis. When tufts are absent, the disease sometimes is misinterpreted as AE; this is a critical distinction, because the treatments of these 2 entities are drastically different.[16] Also, although tufts are characteristic, they are not specific or exclusive to TE. Up to 16% of small bowel biopsies in patients with celiac disease show similar tufts; however, they are not as well developed.[15] Additionally, in patients who have undergone small bowel transplantation, follow-up biopsies from the nontransplanted colon can show resolution of histologic abnormalities.[24]

AUTOIMMUNE ENTEROPATHY

OVERVIEW

AE is the most frequent cause of severe and protracted secretory diarrhea in infants, responsible for up to 25% of cases of severe neonatal diarrhea.[25] Patients are affected any time from birth to adulthood but usually tend to be male and present within the first 6 months of life.[26,27] Malabsorption leads to impaired growth, and patients can have local or systemic infections. Patients with AE can also present with or develop other autoimmune disorders, which may involve the pancreas, kidneys, liver, bone marrow, lungs, or skin.[27] Two unique syndromes can occur with AE as a component: immune dysfunction, polyendocrinopathy, enteropathy, and X-linked inheritance (IPEX) and autoimmune polyendocrinopathy–candidiasis–ectodermal dystrophy (APECED).[28] Mortality for AE is high, being fatal in up to one-third of patients.[29] Patients usually require parenteral or enteral support, depending on the severity of disease. Corticosteroids, tacrolimus, mycophenalate mofetil, infliximab, and cyclophosphamide have been used with variable success.[30–33]

Antienterocyte autoantibodies (AEAs) were originally described by Unsworth and colleagues[34] and have been used as diagnostic criteria for AE. AEAs are usually of IgG subtype but can also be IgA or IgM.[35] They do not seem to be[36] a key

Key Features
AUTOIMMUNE ENTEROPATHY

1. Villous atrophy and crypt hyperplasia are characteristic.

2. Lamina propria is markedly expanded by lymphocytes, plasma cells, and neutrophils.

3. Neutrophilic cryptitis and neutrophilic crypt abscess formation may be prominent.

4. Increased intraepithelial lymphocytes may be increased in the crypts.

5. Paucity or absence of goblet cells and/or Paneth cells may be seen.

factor, however, in pathogenesis because they can appear after the mucosa has been damaged and can become undetectable after treatment but before complete resolution of epithelial injury. Therefore, titers of AEAs do not seem to correspond to histologic severity of disease.[34,37] Furthermore, the presence of AEAs is not specific to AE because they are detected in other disorders, including idiopathic IBD.[35,38] Meanwhile, antibodies against goblet cell mucus have also been described in patients with AE.[39] These antibodies, however, are similarly nonspecific and also occur outside the setting of AE.[40,41]

MICROSCOPIC FEATURES

Histology typically demonstrates duodenal and jejunal total villous atrophy, crypt hyperplasia, marked expansion of the lamina propria by polymorphic inflammatory cells including an increase in CD3+ lymphocytes.[26,27] Neutrophilic cryptitis and neutrophilic crypt abscesses may be seen (**Fig. 3**A).[26-28] In contrast to celiac disease, which is in the differential diagnosis, there is not a prominent increase in surface intraepithelial lymphocytes, although intraepithelial lymphocytes may be increased in the deep crypts. In patients with anti–goblet cell antibodies, small intestinal biopsies can demonstrate preserved villous architecture but a paucity or absence of goblet cells, Paneth cells, and endocrine cells (see **Fig. 3**B).[27,39] Small bowel biopsies can also show foci of apoptoses within the deep crypt epithelium, which can mimic graft-versus-host disease.[27] Meanwhile, the stomach and colon can also show abnormalities. The stomach may show a pattern of atrophic gastritis, including destruction of oxyntic glands and intestinal metaplasia with expansion of the lamina propria by CD8+

and CD4+ T lymphocytes.[42] Colonic biopsies may show varying severity of colitis, rarely with architectural distortion.[43]

AE can be life threatening and needs to be considered if clinical and histologic findings are consistent, even in the absence of antienterocyte or anti–goblet cell antibodies; and particularly with a developing immune system in the neonatal and early infant period.[26] Before initiating immunomodulatory agents, work-up to exclude a concurrent immunodeficiency is warranted, because studies have demonstrated defects in T-cell function in some patients with AE.[44,45]

DIFFERENTIAL DIAGNOSIS

The principal differential diagnosis of AE includes celiac disease and Crohn disease. Both celiac disease and Crohn disease are rare in those under age 2 years, which is when AE typically presents. Celiac disease, however, tends to show a marked increase in intraepithelial lymphocytes with a paucity of intraepithelial neutrophils, whereas the inflammatory infiltrate in AE tends to be more neutrophil-rich and intraepithelial lympocytes are not a prominent component. Crohn disease is typified by its patchy nature of destructive acute and chronic inflammation, whereas AE is characteristically diffuse in nature. The presence of non-necrotizing granulomas strongly argues for a diagnosis of Crohn disease in the appropriate clinical and endocsopic context. The expansion of the

Differential Diagnosis
AUTOIMMUNE ENTEROPATHY

Differentials	Compared with Autoimmune Enteropathy
Celiac disease	Intraepithelial lymphocytosis of the surface epithelium is a prominent feature. Typically lacks exuberant neutrophilic inflammation. Celiac disease usually presents in children older than 1–2 years of age.
Crohn disease	Inflammatory changes are patchier in distribution; non-necrotizing granulomas are helpful, when present. Crohn disease is rare in children under 1 year of age.
MVID and TE	Both of these do not show increased lamina propria inflammation.

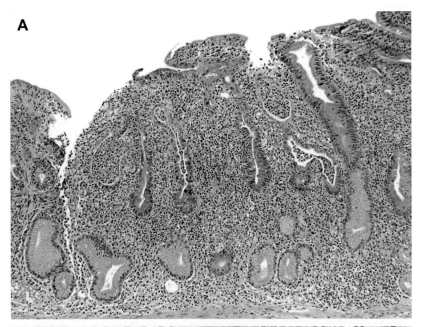

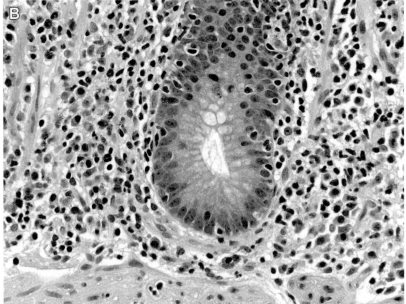

Fig. 3. AE, small intestine. (*A*) Marked villous atrophy and crypt hyperplasia with significant expansion of the lamina propria by inflammatory cells. Marked neutrophilic infiltration of the epithelium is present with neutrophilic crypt abscesses; only rare goblet cells are present (H&E, ×40). (*B*) The base of the crypts shows a lack of Paneth cells with increased intraepithelial lymphocytes (H&E, ×400).

lamina propria by inflammatory cells argues against MVID and TE, which are classically pauci-inflammatory. Other differential diagnostic possibilities include infection; cow's milk intolerance, which often shows patchy increase in lamina propria and intraepithelial eosinophils; and immunodeficiency syndromes (discussed later).[27,46]

HYPOBETALIPOPROTEINEMIAS

OVERVIEW

Hypobetalipoproteinemias encompasse a group of diseases that have a similar clinical and pathologic presentation and include abetalipoproteinemia

(ABL), a rare autosomal recessive condition; familial hypobetalipoproteinemia (FBHL) a rare autosomal dominant condition; and chylomicron retention disease (CRD), a very rare autosomal recessive condition.[47–49] These diseases manifest with malabsorption, neurologic problems, abnormal lipid profiles, and, possibly, altered red blood cell morphology.[47,50] Steatorrhea usually starts in infancy but may not become prominent until the second decade of life.[47] Without treatment, neurologic defects can become progressive and may include tremors, weakness, increased or decreased reflexes, diminished sensation, and nystagmus.[47,49,51] Fundoscopic examination may reveal retinitis pigmentosa–like retinopathy, which is characteristic of ABL and FHBL.[52] Early identification and diagnosis is prudent, because treatment can prevent neurologic complications and improve gastrointestinal symptoms. Treatment generally consists of fat-soluble vitamin replacement and a low-fat diet.[47,49,53]

Laboratory studies in patients with hypobetalipoproteinemias show distinctive fasting lipid profiles. ABL and homozygous FHBL patients show markedly decreased triglycerides and total cholesterol with absent low-density lipoprotein. Heterozygous FHBL patients tend to have only mildly decreased triglycerides and total cholesterol, with 10% to 60% normal levels of low-density lipoprotein. Patients with CRD have normal triglyceride levels, moderately decreased total cholesterol, and moderately decreased low-density lipoprotein levels with normal or only mildly decreased apolipoprotein B.[53] Peripheral blood smears can demonstrate acanthocytes, comprising up to 5% of erythrocytes in patients heterozygous for HBL and more than 50% of erythrocytes in patients with ABL.[53]

ABL is thought to be caused by mutations in the microsomal triglyceride transfer protein (MTP) gene, the product of which is involved in the transfer of lipids to apolipoprotein B.[54–56] Recent studies suggest that missense mutations may lead to diminished MTP activity whereas an array of frameshift, nonsense, and splice site mutations likely lead to nonfunctional MTP, explaining the variability in disease phenotype.[57] Meanwhile, FHBL is thought mainly caused by mutations in the *APOB* gene itself, perhaps leading to truncations in apolipoprotein B. Some forms of FHBL, however, that may not be caused by direct defects in apolipoprotein B have also been identified.[58] CRD seems to be caused by mutations in the *SARA2* gene, which leads to a defect in its product, Sar1b, a protein believed involved in intracellular trafficking of chylomicrons.[59]

ENDOSCOPIC AND MICROSCOPIC FEATURES

On endoscopic examination, patients with ABL have been described as having a diffusely gray, dirty-appearing duodenal mucosa whereas those with CRD have shown white duodenal mucosa.[47,49] Low-power microscopic examination of small bowel biopsies in patients with ABL, homozygous FHBL, and CRD demonstrate normal villous architecture without an increase in lamina propria inflammation. Higher-power magnification reveals foamy, cytoplasmic vacuolization, mainly along the apical aspect of enterocytes along the entirety of the villous length, imparting a pale appearance to the epithelial surface (**Fig. 4**A).[47,50,51,60] Although special stains are usually not needed, an oil red O stain may be performed on frozen section tissue to confirm the lipid content within enterocytes.[61]

DIFFERENTIAL DIAGNOSIS

Cytoplasmic vacuolization within enterocytes are not specific. Enterocyte vacuolization may also be seen in celiac disease, tropical sprue, and megaloblastic anemia.[47,62] Meanwhile, lipid droplets can be seen in any small bowel biopsy after a recent fatty meal; however, these changes are restricted to the villous tips (see **Fig. 4**B).[63]

ENTEROENDOCRINE CELL DYSGENESIS

OVERVIEW

Wang and colleagues[64] first described ECD as a diarrheal syndrome in humans associated with mutations in the Neurogenin-3 (*NEUROG3*) gene. *NEUROG3* is believed to play an important role in endocrine cell development in the gastrointestinal tract.[65,66] These patients present within the first weeks of life with diarrheal volumes of up to 120 mL/kg body weight per day. The diarrhea is characterized as malabsorptive, with diarrhea

---

Key Features
HYPOBETALIPOPROTEINEMIAS

1. Patients present with fat malabsorption.

2. Enterocytes contain clear cytoplasmic vacuoles that uniformly line the tips and sides of the villi.

3. Cytoplasmic vacuolization at the villous tips is associated with a fatty meal before endoscopy and should not be mistaken FHBL.

Key Features
ENTEROENDOCRINE CELL DYSGENESIS

1. H&E appears normal.

2. Immunohistochemistry for chromogranin shows decreased numbers of endocrine cells (0–4 endocrine cells/50 crypts) in both the large and small intestine.

Key Features
CHRONIC GRANULOMATOUS DISEASE

1. Pigment-laden macrophages within the lamina propria of the stomach, small intestine, and colon are present.

2. Non-necrotizing granulomas may also be seen.

3. Some cases show inflammatory changes that may resemble Crohn disease.

ceasing on stopping enteral feeds.[64] Patients are usually treated with total parenteral nutrition.[64]

MICROSCOPIC FEATURES

Microscopically, duodenal and jejunal biopsies appear normal at low power, showing normal villous architecture, enterocytes with preserved brush borders, goblet cells, Paneth cells, and no expansion of the lamina propria by inflammatory cells or intraepithelial lymphocytosis (**Fig. 5**A). Careful inspection at high power reveals absent or significantly decreased numbers of enteroendocrine cells within the small and large bowel. Meanwhile, no decrease in G cells is seen in the gastric antrum or duodenum.[67]

Immunohistochemical studies for chromogranin A demonstrate only 0 to 4 endocrine cells per 50 crypts in both small and large bowel of affected patients compared with averages of 145 and 84 endocrine cells per 50 crypts in small and large bowel specimens, respectively, from age-matched normal controls (see **Fig. 5**B, C). In addition, the intensity of chromogranin A staining appears less intense compared with controls.[67]

DIFFERENTIAL DIAGNOSIS

Other diseases associated with a decrease in enteroendocrine cells include AE and APECED. AE usually is distinguished from ECD by the accompanying inflammation, epithelial injury, and presence of AEAs. Meanwhile, if present, esophageal candidiasis helps suggest a diagnosis of APECED. Otherwise, genetic studies for *NEUROG3* or *AIRE* gene mutations may be needed to distinguish the 2 entities.[68]

CHRONIC GRANULOMATOUS DISEASE

OVERVIEW

CGD is an uncommon primary immunodeficiency that is estimated to affect up to 1 in 200,000 live births. A majority of patients are diagnosed with CGD before the age of 5, with almost 40% diagnosed within the first year of life. Affected patients are highly susceptible to serious infections by catalase-positive bacteria and fungi. Common presenting infections include pneumonia, abscesses in a variety of organs, suppurative adenitis, osteomyeltitis, cellulitis, meningitis, and sepsis.[69] Gastrointestinal manifestations include oral ulcers, granulomatous stomatitis, esophageal dysmotility, gastric outlet obstruction, small bowel obstruction, enteritis, and colitis.[69–71]

CGD is caused by a mutation in any 1 of 4 genes, which results in a defective subunit of NADPH oxidase within phagocytic cells. Most cases are X-linked, due to a mutation in the *CYBB* gene that encodes the gp91-*phox* subunit; the remainder of cases are autosomal recessive, due to defects in the *CYBA*, *NCF-1*, and *NCF-2* genes, which encode the p22-*phox*, p47-*phox*, and p67-*phox* subunits, respectively. Regardless of the subunit involved, the resulting defect prevents phagocytes from forming effective quantities of superoxide derivatives, including hydrogen peroxide, hypohalous acids, and hydroxyl radicals, which are critical for microbicidal activity.[72]

ENDOSCOPIC AND MICROSCOPIC FEATURES

Endoscopic biopsies of the stomach, small bowel, and colon are generally unremarkable except for the finding of variable numbers of brownish-yellow, PAS-positive, pigmented histiocytes present within the lamina propria, which are usually adjacent to crypts.[73] Occasionally, non-necrotizing granulomas are also seen (**Fig. 6**), and a subset of patients may present with intestinal manifestations that simulate Crohn disease, including bowel wall thickening, mural abscesses with non-necrotizing granulomas, and mucosal ulceration.[74] In some cases, however, pigmented histiocytes are not identified and only nonspecific mucosal inflammatory changes are found.[71,74,75]

Fig. 4. ABL, small intestine. (*A*) The villous architecture is normal. The enterocytes are distended, however, by optically clear, fat-containing vesicles along the entire length of the villous (H&E, ×400). (*B*) The finding in (*A*) is compared with focal fat accumulation in a patient without a lipid transport disorder who ingested a fatty meal before endoscopy. Note that this finding is only present in a portion of the villous epithelium (H&E, ×400).

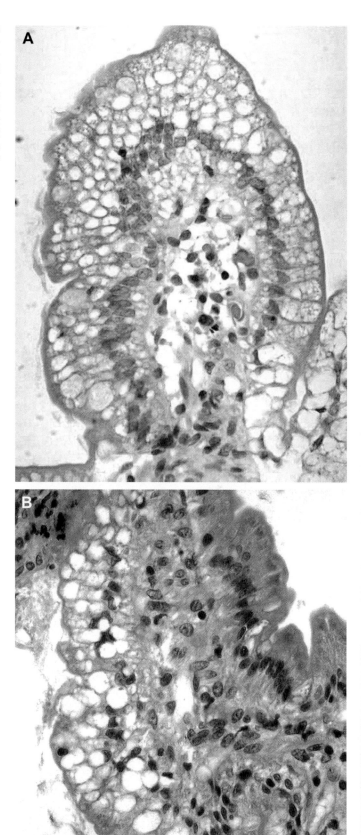

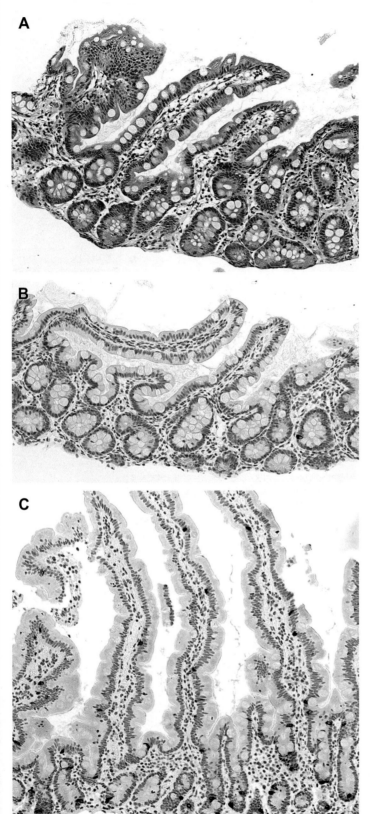

Fig. 5. ECD, small intestine. (*A*) Normal H&E histology (H&E, ×40). (*B*) Immunohistochemistry for chromogranin shows markedly reduced enterendocrine cells in this patient with ECD (chromogranin immunohistochemistry, ×40). (*C*) Normal compliment of enteroendocrine cells as shown on chromogranin immunohistochemsitry from a normal patient (chromogranin immunohistochemistry, ×40). (*Courtesy of* Galen Cortina, MD, PhD, David Geffen School of Medicine at the University of California, Los Angeles, CA.)

Fig. 6. CGD, colon. Modestly increased lamina propria inflammation with neutrophilic cryptitis, crypt abscesses, and poorly formed, non-necrotizing granulomas (H&E, ×40).

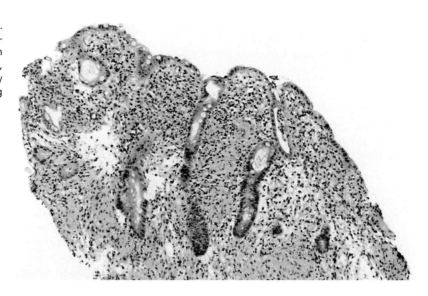

DIFFERENTIAL DIAGNOSIS

The differential diagnosis of pigment-laden histiocytes within the lamina propria in the gastrointestinal tract includes causes of melanosis and pseudomelanosis. The finding of granulomas is not specific and can be indistinguishable from those found in Crohn disease.[74] Clinical correlation assists in distinguishing Crohn disease from CGD, particularly if a patient is an infant or has a history of recurrent infections. In either case, diagnosis of CGD requires additional testing; the diagnosis is usually made by a negative or markedly reduced response to the nitroblue-tetrazolium test and/or genetic analysis to identify the disease-causing mutation.[70]

IMMUNODEFICIENCIES

OVERVIEW

Selective IgA deficiency and CVID are the most common primary immunodeficiency diseases, affecting 1 in 700 Caucasians and up to 1 in 50,000 persons in the general population respectively,[76] whereas XLA is rare and occurs in 1 of 100,000 live male births. Selective IgA deficiency and CVID are thought by some investigators to represent mild and severe forms along a spectrum of the same disease,[77] whereas XLA is known to be due to a mutation in Bruton protein kinase (Xq22).[78]

Patients are defined as having selective IgA deficiency if have they are older than 4 years, have no other explanation for having a serum IgA level less than 7 mg/dL, and have normal IgM and IgG levels. CVID is diagnosed in patients older than 2 years that have no other explanation for having hypogammaglobulinemia, have absent isohemagglutinins and/or a poor response to vaccines, and a serum IgG and IgA level 2 SDs below the mean for age.[79] The mean age at onset of symptoms is 16.9 years and up to 33% of patients affected with CVID are under age 14 years.[80] Onset of symptoms in early life seems rare, but it is still important to keep CVID in mind when examining samples from pediatric patients; since approximately half of patients are diagnosed within 5 years of symptom onset, some patients experience delays in diagnosis of 20 years or more.[80]

Most patients with selective IgA deficiency are asymptomatic.[81] Symptoms, when present, include increased susceptibility to infections, particularly of the respiratory and gastrointestinal tract; commonly reported GI infections include salmonellosis and giardiasis.[82] In addition, children above age 4 years may show an increased risk for food allergy.[83] Several autoimmune diseases have also been seen in association with IgA deficiency, including diabetes mellitus, and autoimmune thyroid disease[84,85]; up to 7.7% of patients with IgA deficiency have celiac disease.[86]

IgA deficiency in both pediatric and adult patients may evolve into CVID.[87,88] Clinical manifestations of CVID include infections, pulmonary disease, gastrointestinal illness, autoimmune disease, and malignancy.[89] A minority of patients (4.6%) may be asymptomatic at diagnosis,[80] and approximately 36% of patients younger than age 14 years have autoimmune manifestations before a diagnosis of CVID has been rendered compared with 17.4% of adults.[80]

> ### *Key Features*
> #### COMMON VARIABLE IMMUNODEFICIENCY
>
> 1. Plasma cells are absent in up to two-thirds of patients.
>
> 2. Variable villous atrophy, crypt hyperplasia, and patchy intraepithelial lymphocytosis may be seen.
>
> 3. Epithelial apoptosis may be present in the midzone of the stomach, and the deep crypts in the small intestine.
>
> 4. Superimposed infection with organisms, such as cytomegalovirus and Giardia, may be present.

Patients with XLA typically present with life-threatening infections that begin at an early age; some patients also present with diarrhea and protein-losing enteropathy. Laboratory studies show profound hypogammaglobulinemia.

MICROSCOPIC FEATURES

Duodenal biopsies in patients with XLA may show marked villous atrophy, crypt hyperplasia; a complete absence of plasma cells is often seen with an empty lamina propria and atrophic lymphoid tissue that lack germinal centers.

A variety of histologic findings have been described in patients with CVID. The most common finding throughout the GI tract is paucity or a complete absence of plasma cells in 63% to 68% of patients.[90] Small intestinal biopsies in CVID patients typically show villous atrophy, crypt hyperplasia, patchy increase in intraepithelial lymphocytes, and nodular lymphoid hyperplasia; frequently, increased number of apoptotic epithelial cells are seen in the depths of the small intestinal crypts or in the midzone of the gastric pits (**Fig. 7**).[90,91] In addition, multifocal atrophic gastritis can be seen in patients with or without associated *Helicobacter pylori* infection.[92] Because these patients are at increased risk for infection, particular effort should be made toward identifying infectious organisms, such as cytomegalovirus and giardia.

Histologic features of IgA deficiency are mild and nonspecific, with nodular lymphoid hyperplasia the most well-described feature. If IgA deficiency needs to be confirmed on biopsy materials, which is rarely necessary, immunohistochemistry for IgA show a complete lack of IgA positive plasma cells.[90,93,94]

INFLAMMATORY BOWEL DISEASE

OVERVIEW

Although many classic precepts that allow gastroenterologists and pathologists to distinguish ulcerative colitis (UC) from Crohn disease in adults apply to pediatric patients, there are many exceptions recently described in the pediatric population that are important to understand because the proper categorization of IBD patients is critical for patient management and prognosis.

From an epidemiologic perspective, only 1% of IBD patients are diagnosed within the first year of life.[95] In contrast, approximately 25% of IBD cases are diagnosed between ages 2 and 20.[96] Although IBD in pediatric and adult patients share many clinical features, presenting signs unique to children include growth retardation and delayed puberty.[97]

DISTRIBUTION AND EXTENT OF DISEASE AT INITIAL PRESENTION

At initial presentation, the distribution and extent of endoscopic involvement of both Crohn disease and UC differs between adults and children. Approximately 43% of pediatric patients who present with Crohn disease present with both ileal and colonic disease compared with only 3% of adults. Pediatric UC patients tend to exhibit more extensive colonic disease, with 82% of children demonstrating disease proximal to the splenic flexure compared with 48% of adults at initial diagnosis in one study.[36]

> ### *Key Features*
> #### IDIOPATHIC INFLAMMATORY BOWEL DISEASE IN CHILDREN
>
> 1. Relative or absolute rectal sparing and/or patchy distribution of colonic inflammatory changes at initial presentation of IBD may be seen in both UC and Crohn disease.
>
> 2. Nonspecific inflammatory changes in the upper gastrointestinal tract should not be used as a sole criterion for the diagnosis of Crohn disease because patients with UC may show similar findings.
>
> 3. Non-necrotizing granulomas that are unassociated with ruptured crypts are an important diagnostic feature of Crohn disease. They are more common in children and may be exclusively seen in upper gastrointestinal biopsies.

Fig. 7. CVID, small intestine. (*A*) Marked villous atrophy and crypt hyperplasia with a normal amount of lamina propria inflammation (H&E, ×200). (*B*) High power shows a paucity of plasma cells in the lamina propria (H&E, ×400).

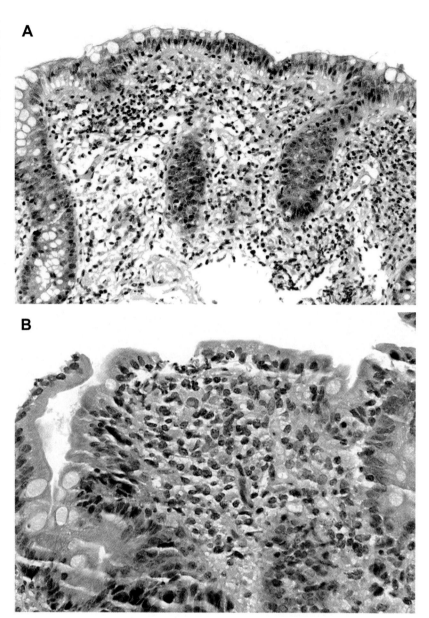

From a histologic perspective, there are important exceptions and differences in pathologic findings in pediatric IBD patients compared with adults. Classically, UC is thought of as a disease of that affects the colon in a continuous fashion, with the rectum most severely affected.[98] Recent studies have shown, however, that biopsies from pediatric patients with UC at initial presentation are more likely to show rectal sparing or patchiness of disease. Glickman and colleagues[99] observed that 15% of children (n = 73) compared with 0% of adults (n = 38) were found to have patchy disease at presentation. In the same study, 30% of children compared with 3% of adults showed rectal sparing for both histologic features of chronic mucosal injury as well as severity of acute inflammation. In another study, Washington and colleagues[100] found that 34% of pediatric patients (n = 53) were found to have normal rectal biopsies compared with 11% of adults (n = 38). Furthermore, histologic findings at initial presentation of UC tend to be less developed compared with adults (**Fig. 8**). A study by Robert and colleagues[101] used a scoring system for various features of inflammatory activity and chronicity; they found that in children under 10 years of age, histologic features tend to be less pronounced compared with adults on initial presentation of UC. Odds ratios comparing 12 children and 25 adults reached statistical significance for architectural distortion, cellularity of lamina propria plasma cells, and active inflammation. Therefore, rectal sparing and variability of acute and chronic inflammatory changes in colonic biopsies at initial presentation of IBD should not be misconstrued as evidence for Crohn disease.

UPPER GASTROINTESTINAL TRACT INVOLVEMENT

In general, Crohn disease is conceptualized as a disease that involves any segment of the GI tract whereas UC is thought to be restricted to the lower GI tract.[98,102] In the pediatric population, however, the upper GI tract can show histologic abnormalities in both Crohn disease and UC. Early case reports and a study comparing Crohn disease and UC found that up to 55% and 60% of children with Crohn disease and UC, respectively, had nonspecific inflammatory changes in the upper GI tract; 50% of the time, the mucosa was endoscopically normal.[103] A more recent follow-up study of pediatric patients confirmed these findings, demonstrating that 82% with Crohn disease (n = 81) and 71% with UC (n = 34) had

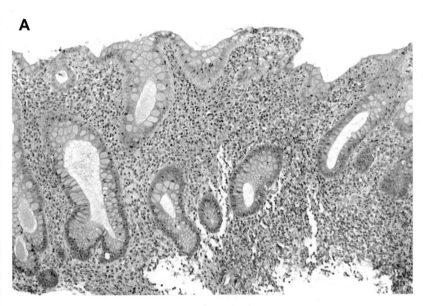

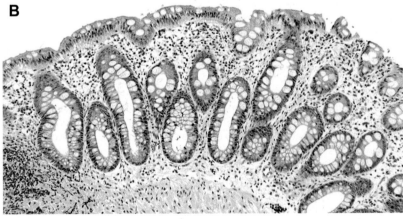

Fig. 8. Rectal sparing at initial presentation of UC in a pediatric patient. (*A*) Sigmoid colon biopsy shows chronic active colitis with markedly abnormal crypt architecture and modest amounts of neutrophilic infiltration of the surface epithelium (H&E, ×40). (*B*) The rectal biopsy shows normal crypt architecture and only rare intraepithelial neutrophils (H&E, ×40).

Fig. 9. Non-necrotizing granuloma at initial presentation of Crohn disease in a small intestinal biopsy. Note that this granuloma is in the deep aspect of the mucosa and is not associated with inflamed crypts (H&E, ×200).

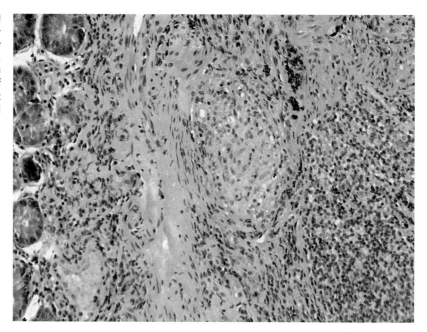

predominantly inflammatory-type histologic abnormalities in the upper GI tract.[104] Therefore the finding of histologic abnormalities in the upper GI tract should not be used as unequivocal evidence of Crohn disease in the pediatric population.

NON-NECROTIZING GRANULOMAS

The finding of non-necrotizing granulomas unassociated with crypt rupture provides important corroborating evidence that helps distinguish Crohn disease from UC (**Fig. 9**).[102] Granulomas are more frequently found in pediatric patients than in adult patients with Crohn disease, reported in up to 42% of children, which is almost twice the incidence in adults in one study.[105–107] Two separate studies showed that 11% of granulomas were exclusively found in the upper GI tract of children.[104,108] Meanwhile, De Matos and colleagues[109] found that upper GI tract and terminal ileal biopsies were essential to identifying granulomas in 42% of children (n = 117), leading to a diagnosis of Crohn disease. These findings stress the importance of complete endoscopic evaluation in pediatric patients regardless of whether upper GI symptoms are present.[110]

SUMMARY

The histologic differential diagnosis of diarrheal illness in early life differs significantly from that in adults and includes diseases, such as MVID, TE,

AE, and immunodeficiency states. Knowledge of the varying pathologic appearance of pediatric idiopathic IBD enables pathologists to more accurately separate Crohn disease from UC.

REFERENCES

1. Volonaki E, Sebire NJ, Borrelli O, et al. Gastrointestinal endoscopy and mucosal biopsy in the first year of life: indications and outcome. J Pediatr Gastroenterol Nutr 2012;55(1):62–5.
2. Ruemmele FM, Schmitz J, Goulet O. Microvillous inclusion disease (microvillous atrophy). Orphanet J Rare Dis 2006;1:22.
3. Phillips AD, Schmitz J. Familial microvillous atrophy: a clinicopathological survey of 23 cases. J Pediatr Gastroenterol Nutr 1992;14(4):380–96.
4. Croft NM, Howatson AG, Ling SC, et al. Microvillous inclusion disease: an evolving condition. J Pediatr Gastroenterol Nutr 2000;31(2):185–9.
5. Muller T, Hess MW, Schiefermeier N, et al. MYO5B mutations cause microvillus inclusion disease and disrupt epithelial cell polarity. Nat Genet 2008; 40(10):1163–5.
6. Ruemmele FM, Muller T, Schiefermeier N, et al. Loss-of-function of MYO5B is the main cause of microvillus inclusion disease: 15 novel mutations and a CaCo-2 RNAi cell model. Hum Mutat 2010; 31(5):544–51.
7. Sato T, Mushiake S, Kato Y, et al. The Rab8 GTPase regulates apical protein localization in intestinal cells. Nature 2007;448(7151):366–9.

8. Groisman GM, Amar M, Livne E. CD10: a valuable tool for the light microscopic diagnosis of microvillous inclusion disease (familial microvillous atrophy). Am J Surg Pathol 2002;26(7): 902–7.

9. Khubchandani SR, Vohra P, Chitale AR, et al. Microvillous inclusion disease—an ultrastructural diagnosis: with a review of the literature. Ultrastruct Pathol 2011;35(2):87–91.

10. Bell SW, Kerner JA Jr, Sibley RK. Microvillous inclusion disease. The importance of electron microscopy for diagnosis. Am J Surg Pathol 1991; 15(12):1157–64.

11. Sherman PM, Mitchell DJ, Cutz E. Neonatal enteropathies: defining the causes of protracted diarrhea of infancy. J Pediatr Gastroenterol Nutr 2004; 38(1):16–26.

12. Al-Daraji WI, Zelger B, Hussein MR. Microvillous inclusion disease: a clinicopathologic study of 17 cases from the UK. Ultrastruct Pathol 2010;34(6): 327–32.

13. Chen CP, Chiang MC, Wang TH, et al. Microvillus inclusion disease: prenatal ultrasound findings, molecular diagnosis and genetic counseling of congenital diarrhea. Taiwan J Obstet Gynecol 2010;49(4):487–94.

14. Mierau GW, Wills EJ, Wyatt-Ashmead J, et al. Microvillous inclusion disease: report of a case with atypical features. Ultrastruct Pathol 2001; 25(3):275–9.

15. Reifen RM, Cutz E, Griffiths AM, et al. Tufting enteropathy: a newly recognized clinicopathological entity associated with refractory diarrhea in infants. J Pediatr Gastroenterol Nutr 1994;18(3): 379–85.

16. Goulet O, Salomon J, Ruemmele F, et al. Intestinal epithelial dysplasia (tufting enteropathy). Orphanet J Rare Dis 2007;2:20.

17. Abely M, Hankard GF, Hugot JP, et al. Intractable infant diarrhea with epithelial dysplasia associated with polymalformation. J Pediatr Gastroenterol Nutr 1998;27(3):348–52.

18. Roche O, Putterman M, Salomon J, et al. Superficial punctate keratitis and conjunctival erosions associated with congenital tufting enteropathy. Am J Ophthalmol 2010;150(1):116–121.e1.

19. Patey N, Scoazec JY, Cuenod-Jabri B, et al. Distribution of cell adhesion molecules in infants with intestinal epithelial dysplasia (tufting enteropathy). Gastroenterology 1997;113(3):833–43.

20. Sivagnanam M, Mueller JL, Lee H, et al. Identification of EpCAM as the gene for congenital tufting enteropathy. Gastroenterology 2008;135(2):429–37.

21. Sivagnanam M, Schaible T, Szigeti R, et al. Further evidence for EpCAM as the gene for congenital tufting enteropathy. Am J Med Genet A 2010; 152A(1):222–4.

22. Ko JS, Seo JK, Shim JO, et al. Tufting enteropathy with EpCAM mutations in two siblings. Gut Liver 2010;4(3):407–10.

23. Salomon J, Espinosa-Parrilla Y, Goulet O, et al. A founder effect at the EPCAM locus in Congenital Tufting Enteropathy in the Arabic Gulf. Eur J Med Genet 2011;54(3):319–22.

24. Paramesh AS, Fishbein T, Tschernia A, et al. Isolated small bowel transplantation for tufting enteropathy. J Pediatr Gastroenterol Nutr 2003;36(1): 138–40.

25. Catassi C, Fabiani E, Spagnuolo MI, et al. Severe and protracted diarrhea: results of the 3-year SIGEP multicenter survey. Working Group of the Italian Society of Pediatric Gastroenterology and Hepatology (SIGEP). J Pediatr Gastroenterol Nutr 1999;29(1):63–8.

26. Hartfield D, Turner J, Huynh H, et al. The role of histopathology in diagnosing protracted diarrhea of infancy. Fetal Pediatr Pathol 2010;29(3):144–57.

27. Russo PA, Brochu P, Seidman EG, et al. Autoimmune enteropathy. Pediatr Dev Pathol 1999;2(1): 65–71.

28. Montalto M, D'Onofrio F, Santoro L, et al. Autoimmune enteropathy in children and adults. Scand J Gastroenterol 2009;44(9):1029–36.

29. Lachaux A. Autoimmune enteropathy. Arch Pediatr 1996;3(3):261–6 [in French].

30. Bousvaros A, Leichtner AM, Book L, et al. Treatment of pediatric autoimmune enteropathy with tacrolimus (FK506). Gastroenterology 1996;111(1):237–43.

31. Oliva-Hemker MM, Loeb DM, Abraham SC, et al. Remission of severe autoimmune enteropathy after treatment with high-dose cyclophosphamide. J Pediatr Gastroenterol Nutr 2003;36(5):639–43.

32. Quiros-Tejeira RE, Ament ME, Vargas JH. Induction of remission in a child with autoimmune enteropathy using mycophenolate mofetil. J Pediatr Gastroenterol Nutr 2003;36(4):482–5.

33. Elwing JE, Clouse RE. Adult-onset autoimmune enteropathy in the setting of thymoma successfully treated with infliximab. Dig Dis Sci 2005;50(5): 928–32.

34. Unsworth J, Hutchins P, Mitchell J, et al. Flat small intestinal mucosa and autoantibodies against the gut epithelium. J Pediatr Gastroenterol Nutr 1982; 1(4):503–13.

35. Mirakian R, Richardson A, Milla PJ, et al. Protracted diarrhoea of infancy: evidence in support of an autoimmune variant. Br Med J (Clin Res Ed) 1986;293(6555):1132–6.

36. Van Limbergen J, Russell RK, Drummond HE, et al. Definition of phenotypic characteristics of childhood-onset inflammatory bowel disease. Gastroenterology 2008;135(4):1114–22.

37. Walker-Smith JA, Unsworth DJ, Hutchins P, et al. Autoantibodies against gut epithelium in child

with small-intestinal enteropathy. Lancet 1982; 1(8271):566–7.

38. Martin-Villa JM, Camblor S, Costa R, et al. Gut epithelial cell autoantibodies in AIDS pathogenesis. Lancet 1993;342(8867):380.

39. Moore L, Xu X, Davidson G, et al. Autoimmune enteropathy with anti-goblet cell antibodies. Hum Pathol 1995;26(10):1162–8.

40. Hibi T, Ohara M, Kobayashi K, et al. Enzyme linked immunosorbent assay (ELISA) and immunoprecipitation studies on anti-goblet cell antibody using a mucin producing cell line in patients with inflammatory bowel disease. Gut 1994;35(2):224–30.

41. Folwaczny C, Noehl N, Tschop K, et al. Goblet cell autoantibodies in patients with inflammatory bowel disease and their first-degree relatives. Gastroenterology 1997;113(1):101–6.

42. Mitomi H, Tanabe S, Igarashi M, et al. Autoimmune enteropathy with severe atrophic gastritis and colitis in an adult: proposal of a generalized autoimmune disorder of the alimentary tract. Scand J Gastroenterol 1998;33(7):716–20.

43. Hill SM, Milla PJ, Bottazzo GF, et al. Autoimmune enteropathy and colitis: is there a generalised autoimmune gut disorder? Gut 1991;32(1):36–42.

44. Murch SH, Fertleman CR, Rodrigues C, et al. Autoimmune enteropathy with distinct mucosal features in T-cell activation deficiency: the contribution of T cells to the mucosal lesion. J Pediatr Gastroenterol Nutr 1999;28(4):393–9.

45. Seidman EG, Hollander GA. Autoimmunity with immunodeficiency: a logical paradox. J Pediatr Gastroenterol Nutr 1999;28(4):377–9.

46. Guarino A, Spagnuolo MI, Russo S, et al. Etiology and risk factors of severe and protracted diarrhea. J Pediatr Gastroenterol Nutr 1995;20(2):173–8.

47. Triantafillidis JK, Kottaras G, Sgourous S, et al. A-beta-lipoproteinemia: clinical and laboratory features, therapeutic manipulations, and follow-up study of three members of a Greek family. J Clin Gastroenterol 1998;26(3):207–11.

48. Levy E. The genetic basis of primary disorders of intestinal fat transport. Clin Invest Med 1996; 19(5):317–24.

49. Peretti N, Sassolas A, Roy CC, et al. Guidelines for the diagnosis and management of chylomicron retention disease based on a review of the literature and the experience of two centers. Orphanet J Rare Dis 2010;5:24.

50. Levy E, Roy CC, Thibault L, et al. Variable expression of familial heterozygous hypobetalipoproteinemia: transient malabsorption during infancy. J Lipid Res 1994;35(12):2170–7.

51. Mars H, Lewis LA, Robertson AL Jr, et al. Familial hypo-beta-lipoproteinemia: a genetic disorder of lipid metabolism with nervous system involvement. Am J Med 1969;46(6):886–900.

52. Chowers I, Banin E, Merin S, et al. Long-term assessment of combined vitamin A and E treatment for the prevention of retinal degeneration in abetalipoproteinaemia and hypobetalipoproteinaemia patients. Eye 2001;15(Pt 4):525–30.

53. Granot E, Deckelbaum RJ. Hypocholesterolemia in childhood. J Pediatr 1989;115(2):171–85.

54. Sharp D, Blinderman L, Combs KA, et al. Cloning and gene defects in microsomal triglyceride transfer protein associated with abetalipoproteinaemia. Nature 1993;365(6441):65–9.

55. Shoulders CC, Brett DJ, Bayliss JD, et al. Abetalipoproteinemia is caused by defects of the gene encoding the 97 kDa subunit of a microsomal triglyceride transfer protein. Hum Mol Genet 1993; 2(12):2109–16.

56. Ohashi K, Ishibashi S, Osuga J, et al. Novel mutations in the microsomal triglyceride transfer protein gene causing abetalipoproteinemia. J Lipid Res 2000;41(8):1199–204.

57. Chardon L, Sassolas A, Dingeon B, et al. Identification of two novel mutations and long-term follow-up in abetalipoproteinemia: a report of four cases. Eur J Pediatr 2009;168(8):983–9.

58. Schonfeld G, Lin X, Yue P. Familial hypobetalipoproteinemia: genetics and metabolism. Cell Mol Life Sci 2005;62(12):1372–8.

59. Jones B, Jones EL, Bonney SA, et al. Mutations in a Sar1 GTPase of COPII vesicles are associated with lipid absorption disorders. Nat Genet 2003;34(1): 29–31.

60. Boldrini R, Biselli R, Bosman C. Chylomicron retention disease—the role of ultrastructural examination in differential diagnosis. Pathol Res Pract 2001; 197(11):753–7.

61. Lewin DN, Klaus J. Small intestine. In: Weidner NC, Richard J, Suster S, et al, editors. Modern surgical pathology. 2nd edition. Philadelphia: Saunders Elsevier; 2009. p. 748–9.

62. Joshi M, Hyams J, Treem W, et al. Cytoplasmic vacuolization of enterocytes: an unusual histopathologic finding in juvenile nutritional megaloblastic anemia. Mod Pathol 1991;4(1):62–5.

63. Lewin DN. Systemic illnesses involving the GI Tract. In: Odze RD, Goldblum JR, editors. Surgical pathology of the GI tract, liver, biliary tract and pancreas. 2nd edition. Philadelphia: Saunders Elsevier; 2009. p. 107.

64. Wang J, Cortina G, Wu SV, et al. Mutant neurogenin-3 in congenital malabsorptive diarrhea. N Engl J Med 2006;355(3):270–80.

65. Lee CS, Kaestner KH. Clinical endocrinology and metabolism. Development of gut endocrine cells. Best Pract Res Clin Endocrinol Metab 2004;18(4): 453–62.

66. Schonhoff SE, Giel-Moloney M, Leiter AB. Neurogenin 3-expressing progenitor cells in the

gastrointestinal tract differentiate into both endo-crine and non-endocrine cell types. Dev Biol 2004;270(2):443–54.

67. Cortina G, Smart CN, Farmer DG, et al. Enteroendo-crine cell dysgenesis and malabsorption, a histopath-ologic and immunohistochemical characterization. Hum Pathol 2007;38(4):570–80.

68. Ohsie S, Gerney G, Gui D, et al. A paucity of colonic enteroendocrine and/or enterochromaffin cells characterizes a subset of patients with chronic unexplained diarrhea/malabsorption. Hum Pathol 2009;40(7):1006–14.

69. Winkelstein JA, Marino MC, Johnston RB Jr, et al. Chronic granulomatous disease. Report on a na-tional registry of 368 patients. Medicine (Baltimore) 2000;79(3):155–69.

70. Huang A, Abbasakoor F, Vaizey CJ. Gastrointes-tinal manifestations of chronic granulomatous dis-ease. Colorectal Dis 2006;8(8):637–44.

71. Stopyrowa J, Fyderek K, Sikorska B, et al. Chronic granulomatous disease of childhood: gastric mani-festation and response to salazosulfapyridine ther-apy. Eur J Pediatr 1989;149(1):28–30.

72. Heyworth PG, Cross AR, Curnutte JT. Chronic gran-ulomatous disease. Curr Opin Immunol 2003;15(5):578–84.

73. Dickerman JD, Colletti RB, Tampas JP. Gastric outlet obstruction in chronic granulomatous disease of childhood. Am J Dis Child 1986;140(6):567–70.

74. Ament ME, Ochs HD. Gastrointestinal manifesta-tions of chronic granulomatous disease. N Engl J Med 1973;288(8):382–7.

75. al-Tawil YS, Abramson SL, Gilger MA, et al. Steroid-responsive esophageal obstruction in a child with chronic granulomatous disease (CGD). J Pediatr Gastroenterol Nutr 1996;23(2):182–5.

76. Primary immunodeficiency diseases. Report of a WHO Scientific Group. Clin Exp Immunol 1995;99(Suppl 1):1–24.

77. Hammarstrom L, Vorechovsky I, Webster D. Selec-tive IgA deficiency (SIgAD) and common variable immunodeficiency (CVID). Clin Exp Immunol 2000;120(2):225–31.

78. Ochs HD, Ament ME, Davis SD. Giardiasis with malabsorption in X-linked agammaglobulinemia. N Engl J Med 1972;287(7):341–2.

79. Conley ME, Notarangelo LD, Etzioni A. Diagnostic criteria for primary immunodeficiencies. Repre-senting PAGID (Pan-American Group for Immunode-ficiency) and ESID (European Society for Immunodeficiencies). Clin Immunol 1999;93(3):190–7.

80. Quinti I, Soresina A, Spadaro G, et al. Long-term follow-up and outcome of a large cohort of patients with common variable immunodeficiency. J Clin Immunol 2007;27(3):308–16.

81. Latiff AH, Kerr MA. The clinical significance of immunoglobulin A deficiency. Ann Clin Biochem 2007;44(Pt 2):131–9.

82. Morell A, Muehlheim E, Schaad U, et al. Suscepti-bility to infections in children with selective IgA- and IgA-IgG subclass deficiency. Eur J Pediatr 1986;145(3):199–203.

83. Janzi M, Kull I, Sjoberg R, et al. Selective IgA defi-ciency in early life: association to infections and allergic diseases during childhood. Clin Immunol 2009;133(1):78–85.

84. Cassidy JT, Burt A, Petty R, et al. Selective IgA defi-ciency in connective tissue diseases. N Engl J Med 1969;280(5):275.

85. Bluestone R, Goldberg LS, Katz RM, et al. Juvenile rheumatoid arthritis–a serologic survey of 200 consecutive patients. J Pediatr 1970;77(1):98–102.

86. Meini A, Pillan NM, Villanacci V, et al. Prevalence and diagnosis of celiac disease in IgA-deficient children. Ann Allergy Asthma Immunol 1996;77(4):333–6.

87. Espanol T, Catala M, Hernandez M, et al. Develop-ment of a common variable immunodeficiency in IgA-deficient patients. Clin Immunol Immunopathol 1996;80(3 Pt 1):333–5.

88. Aghamohammadi A, Mohammadi J, Parvaneh N, et al. Progression of selective IgA deficiency to common variable immunodeficiency. Int Arch Al-lergy Immunol 2008;147(2):87–92.

89. Aghamohammadi A, Farhoudi A, Moin M, et al. Clinical and immunological features of 65 Iranian patients with common variable immunodeficiency. Clin Diagn Lab Immunol 2005;12(7):825–32.

90. Daniels JA, Lederman HM, Maitra A, et al. Gastro-intestinal tract pathology in patients with common variable immunodeficiency (CVID): a clinicopatho-logic study and review. Am J Surg Pathol 2007;31(12):1800–12.

91. Teahon K, Webster AD, Price AB, et al. Studies on the enteropathy associated with primary hypogam-maglobulinaemia. Gut 1994;35(9):1244–9.

92. Zullo A, Romiti A, Rinaldi V, et al. Gastric pathology in patients with common variable immunodefi-ciency. Gut 1999;45(1):77–81.

93. Rubio-Tapia A, Hernandez-Calleros J, Trinidad-Hernandez S, et al. Clinical characteristics of a group of adults with nodular lymphoid hyperplasia: a single center experience. World J Gastroenterol 2006;12(12):1945–8.

94. Pytrus T, Iwanczak B, Iwanczak F. Nodular lymphoid hyperplasia—underestimated problem of gastrointestinal tract pathology in children. Pol Merkur Lekarski 2008;24(143):449–52 [in Polish].

95. Heyman MB, Kirschner BS, Gold BD, et al. Children with early-onset inflammatory bowel disease (IBD): analysis of a pediatric IBD consortium registry. J Pediatr 2005;146(1):35–40.

96. Griffiths AM. Specificities of inflammatory bowel disease in childhood. Best Pract Res Clin Gastroenterol 2004;18(3):509–23.

97. Langholz E, Munkholm P, Krasilnikoff PA, et al. Inflammatory bowel diseases with onset in childhood. Clinical features, morbidity, and mortality in a regional cohort. Scand J Gastroenterol 1997; 32(2):139–47.

98. Dignass A, Eliakim R, Magro F, et al. Second European evidence-based consensus on the diagnosis and management of ulcerative colitis part 1: definitions and diagnosis. J Crohns Colitis 2012;6(10): 965–90.

99. Glickman JN, Bousvaros A, Farraye FA, et al. Pediatric patients with untreated ulcerative colitis may present initially with unusual morphologic findings. Am J Surg Pathol 2004;28(2):190–7.

100. Washington K, Greenson JK, Montgomery E, et al. Histopathology of ulcerative colitis in initial rectal biopsy in children. Am J Surg Pathol 2002;26(11): 1441–9.

101. Robert ME, Tang L, Hao LM, et al. Patterns of inflammation in mucosal biopsies of ulcerative colitis: perceived differences in pediatric populations are limited to children younger than 10 years. Am J Surg Pathol 2004;28(2):183–9.

102. Van Assche G, Dignass A, Panes J, et al. The second European evidence-based Consensus on the diagnosis and management of Crohn's disease: definitions and diagnosis. J Crohns Colitis 2010; 4(1):7–27.

103. Ruuska T, Vaajalahti P, Arajarvi P, et al. Prospective evaluation of upper gastrointestinal mucosal lesions in children with ulcerative colitis and Crohn's disease. J Pediatr Gastroenterol Nutr 1994;19(2): 181–6.

104. Abdullah BA, Gupta SK, Croffie JM, et al. The role of esophagogastroduodenoscopy in the initial evaluation of childhood inflammatory bowel disease: a 7-year study. J Pediatr Gastroenterol Nutr 2002; 35(5):636–40.

105. Markowitz J, Kahn E, Daum F. Prognostic significance of epithelioid granulomas found in rectosigmoid biopsies at the initial presentation of pediatric Crohn's disease. J Pediatr Gastroenterol Nutr 1989; 9(2):182–6.

106. Rubio CA, Orrego A, Nesi G, et al. Frequency of epithelioid granulomas in colonoscopic biopsy specimens from paediatric and adult patients with Crohn's colitis. J Clin Pathol 2007;60(11):1268–72.

107. Schmitz-Moormann P, Schag M. Histology of the lower intestinal tract in Crohn's disease of children and adolescents. Multicentric Paediatric Crohn's Disease Study. Pathol Res Pract 1990;186(4): 479–84.

108. Hummel TZ, ten Kate FJ, Reitsma JB, et al. Additional value of upper GI tract endoscopy in the diagnostic assessment of childhood IBD. J Pediatr Gastroenterol Nutr 2012;54(6):753–7.

109. De Matos V, Russo PA, Cohen AB, et al. Frequency and clinical correlations of granulomas in children with Crohn disease. J Pediatr Gastroenterol Nutr 2008;46(4):392–8.

110. Lemberg DA, Clarkson CM, Bohane TD, et al. Role of esophagogastroduodenoscopy in the initial assessment of children with inflammatory bowel disease. J Gastroenterol Hepatol 2005;20(11): 1696–700.

Polyposis Syndromes
Role of the Pathologist

Scott R. Owens, MD, Joel K. Greenson, MD*

KEYWORDS

- Gastrointestinal • Polyposis • Cancer • Syndrome

ABSTRACT

This article reviews the major gastrointestinal polyposis syndromes, with an emphasis on the molecular, clinical, and histopathological features of each. Salient features helpful in making or suggesting the diagnosis of these syndromes are discussed, as is the use of ancillary techniques, such as immunohistochemistry and molecular diagnostic studies in diagnosis confirmation and family screening.

Abbreviations: Polyposis	
APC	Adenomatous polyposis coli
CCS	Cronkhite-Canada syndrome
CHRPE	Congenital hypertrophy of the retinal pigment epithelium
CIMP	CpG island methylator phenotype
FAP	Familial adenomatous polyposis
GI	Gastrointestinal
HNPCC	"Hereditary non-polyposis colorectal cancer syndrome"
JPS	Juvenile polyposis syndrome
LS	Lynch syndrome
MLPA	Multiplex ligation-dependent probe amplification
MSI-H	High-level microsatellite instability
MutYH formerly MYH	"MutY homologue"
PHS	PTEN-hamartoma syndrome/ Cowden/Bannayan-Riley-Ruvalcaba
PJS	Peutz-Jeghers syndrome
SCTAT	Sex cord tumor with annular tubules

OVERVIEW

Gastrointestinal (GI) polyposis syndromes are a challenging group of diagnoses for both surgical pathologists and patients. The distribution of the polyps in these syndromes can vary throughout the GI tract, and different entities (or even different manifestations of the same syndrome) may have a handful of polyps or hundreds to thousands of polyps affecting 1 or more organs. In addition, some syndromes have extra-GI manifestations, many have polyps with overlapping histologic features, and not all are associated with an increased risk of GI cancer. Furthermore, important clinical and hereditary information that could provide a clue to diagnosis may not accompany biopsies sent to a surgical pathologist. Thus, a high index of suspicion for a microscopic appearance and any clinical clues to the possibility of a polyposis syndrome must be maintained to make (or even suggest) an accurate diagnosis.

Recent advances in molecular diagnostic techniques and in understanding the genetic basis of these syndromes provide an opportunity for ancillary studies that aid both patient care teams and, potentially, the families of affected patients. An understanding of the molecular genetic pathology underlying such syndromes can aid pathologists in seeking the appropriate histologic features to suggest the diagnosis and in providing advice to clinical colleagues for further studies and family counseling, an opportunity to provide personalized

Funding Sources: Nil.
Conflict of Interest: Nil.
Department of Pathology, University of Michigan Hospital and Health Systems, 1301 Catherine, Ann Arbor, MI 48109, USA
* Corresponding author.
E-mail address: facjkgmd@med.umich.edu

Surgical Pathology 6 (2013) 545–565
http://dx.doi.org/10.1016/j.path.2013.05.005

medicine. This review addresses the clinical, histologic, and molecular aspects of the major GI polyposis syndromes, with an emphasis on the role of surgical pathologists in tissue diagnosis and in understanding and guiding the appropriate use of ancillary modalities, such as molecular diagnostic pathology.

FAMILIAL ADENOMATOUS POLYPOSIS

Inherited in an autosomal dominant and highly penetrant fashion, familial adenomatous polyposis (FAP) usually results from an inherited germline mutation in the *adenomatous polyposis coli* (*APC*) gene on chromosome 5 (5q21-q22).[1-4] *APC* is a tumor suppressor gene that functions in the *Wnt* signaling pathway by down-regulating β-catenin, and loss of its function allows the accumulation of mutations in additional, important genetic loci, such as *TP53*, *RAS*, and others.[1,5] Although FAP is the most common genetic polyposis syndrome, its incidence is much less than 1% of the population.

CLINICAL AND GROSS FEATURES

Most patients with the classic syndrome present by age 20 with hundreds or thousands of adenomatous colonic polyps (more than 100 polyps, by definition) that carpet the mucosa (**Fig. 1**), although there is an attenuated version in which patients tend to present later and have fewer polyps (fewer than 100 by definition but most often fewer than 30) that tend to concentrate in the right colon. The attenuated phenotype results from mutations at either end of the *APC* gene.[2,5] In addition to its manifestations in the colon, FAP has other characteristic features. First, adenomas can occur elsewhere in the GI tract, especially the duodenum. In the stomach, true adenomas can occur, as can fundic gland polyps, with or without epithelial dysplasia (**Fig. 2**). Extra-GI manifestations include osteomas of the mandible, desmoid fibromatosis (**Fig. 3**), and other soft tissue tumors, including leiomyomas and lipomas, as well as CHRPE. The constellation of adenomatous polyposis with prominent extracolonic manifestations, such as these (especially desmoid fibromatosis) is termed, *Gardner syndrome*. In addition, some FAP patients may have brain tumors (especially medulloblastomas in children), a combination termed, *Turcot syndrome*. A variety of other tumors have been associated with FAP, including hepatocellular carcinoma, hepatoblastoma, papillary thyroid carcinoma, adrenal cortical neoplasms, and nasopharyngeal angiofibromas.[2,6]

MICROSCOPIC FEATURES

The adenomas and tumors occurring in the setting of FAP are histologically indistinguishable from their sporadic counterparts, with crowded, pseudostratified, elongated, and hyperchromatic epithelial nuclei (**Fig. 4**). The histologic hallmark of FAP patients is the so-called unicryptal adenoma (**Fig. 5**), which can be seen on routine biopsy sections but is most easily identified by submission of en face mucosal (Bussey) sections (**Fig. 6**).[5]

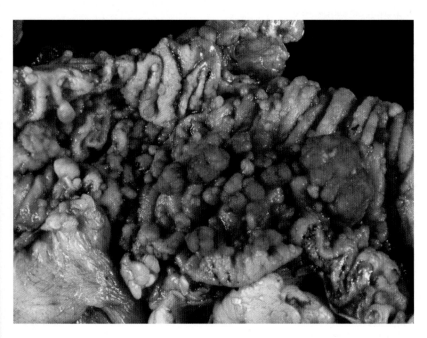

Fig. 1. Colectomy specimen from patient with FAP, with innumerable polyps of variable size and morphology carpeting the mucosal surface.

Fig. 2. Photomicrograph of a gastric fundic gland polyp from a patient with FAP, showing superimposed low-grade dysplasia characterized by crowded and hyperchromatic nuclei, involving the superficial epithelium (H&E, ×20).

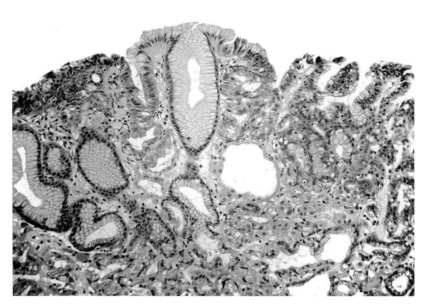

DIAGNOSIS AND DIFFERENTIAL DIAGNOSIS

Because the adenomas in FAP are identical to sporadic adenomas, it is incumbent on surgical pathologists to recognize unique histologic appearances and, especially, unusual combinations of histopathological findings, to be able to raise the possibility of the diagnosis and suggest ancillary studies and, potentially, genetic counseling. Examples include numerous adenomas found and biopsied at endoscopic examination, soft tissue tumors in patients with numerous adenomas, combined duodenal and colonic adenomas, and gastric fundic gland polyps with dysplasia. There is almost no differential diagnosis for the fully developed syndrome, but the attenuated version can mimic MutYH-associated polyposis (MAP) (described later).[2,3] In addition to the clinicopathologic clues (described previously), molecular assays for *APC* mutations are available, using peripheral blood. These can be used in a stepwise manner to confirm the diagnosis and

Fig. 3. Desmoid tumor from a patient with FAP/Gardner syndrome. This benign but locally aggressive tumor consists of dense collagen with admixed myofibroblasts (H&E, ×20).

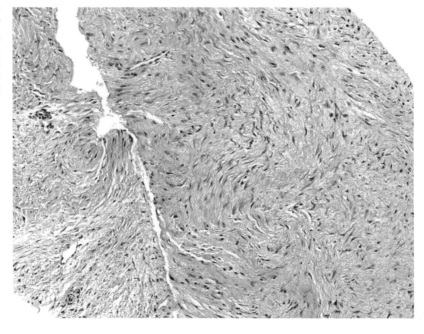

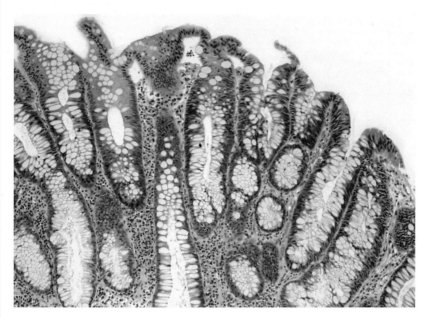

Fig. 4. Photomicrograph of an adenoma from a patient with FAP. The crowded crypts are lined by dysplastic epithelium with elongated and hyperchromatic nuclei. Despite a syndromic manifestation, this adenoma is indistinguishable from a sporadic example (H&E, ×20).

test family members and include protein truncation assay for abnormalities in exon 15, polymerase chain reaction assay for mutations in exons 1–14, and multiplex ligation-dependent probe amplification aimed at finding large deletions/duplications.[7] The diagnosis can be definitively made clinically when a patient is found to have more than 100 colorectal adenomas, a germline *APC* mutation, and/or a family history of FAP with at least 1 of the extraintestinal manifestations of desmoid fibromatosis, an osteoma, or an epidermoid cyst.[5]

PROGNOSIS

Patients diagnosed with FAP typically undergo early prophylactic total colectomy, because the risk of colonic adenocarcinoma is essentially 100% by age 40 in untreated individuals.[3,4] Once a patient receives the diagnosis, family genetic counseling and mutation testing are crucial to identifying additional cases. Although most cases of FAP are inherited, it is thought that 25% to 33% of cases result from sporadic *APC* mutations.[3–5]

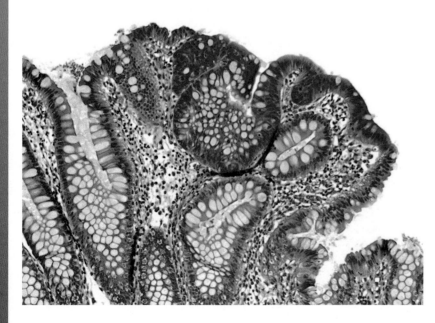

Fig. 5. Unicryptal adenoma from a patient with FAP. This type of tiny adenoma is a hallmark of the syndrome (H&E, ×20).

> ### *Key Features*
> #### FAMILIAL ADENOMATOUS POLYPOSIS
>
> 1. *APC* gene mutations
> 2. Autosomal dominant inheritance
> 3. 100s of polyps throughout GI tract
>   - Adenomas
>   - Fundic gland polyps in stomach
> 4. Other tumors: desmoid fibromatosis, brain tumors, many others
> 5. 100% GI cancer risk if untreated by colectomy

> ### *Key Features*
> #### ATTENUATED FAMILIAL ADENOMATOUS POLYPOSIS
>
> 1. *APC* gene mutations (near ends of the gene)
> 2. Autosomal dominant inheritance
> 3. <100 Colon adenomas (often <30; may favor right colon)
> 4. Other tumors less common than in true FAP
> 5. 80%–100% GI cancer risk

MUTYH-ASSOCIATED POLYPOSIS

CLINICAL AND GROSS FEATURES

This autosomal recessive disorder clinically mimics attenuated FAP, with patients typically having 20 to 100 adenomas and presenting in the middle of the 5th decade.[2,3] It results from biallelic mutation of the MutY homolog (*MutYH*, formerly *MYH*) gene on chromosome 1p, which encodes a base excision DNA repair enzyme that mends oxidative damage to guanine residues. Oxidized guanine binds to adenine rather than cytosine, resulting in G:C to T:A transversion mutations, which can be found using molecular techniques in the resulting adenomas.[2] In addition, the loss of DNA repair function can allow mutations to other crucial genes, such as *APC* and *RAS*. MAP patients may have duodenal adenomas but do not suffer the extraintestinal manifestations characteristic of FAP.

MICROSCOPIC FEATURES, DIAGNOSIS, AND PROGNOSIS

As with FAP, the adenomas in MAP syndrome are histologically indistinguishable from their sporadic counterparts, so vigilant surgical pathologists are essential. Some evidence suggests that MAP patients are at increased risk of extraintestinal malignancies; however, the lifetime risk of colorectal cancer for these patients is as high as 100% without treatment.[3,8] Given the recessive inheritance, the risk to family members is smaller than in FAP, although the risk of colorectal cancer to heterozygote carriers of *MutYH* mutations is being investigated.

> ### *Key Features*
> #### MUTYH-ASSOCIATED POLYPOSIS
>
> 1. *MutYH* gene mutations
> 2. Autosomal recessive inheritance
> 3. Few polyps to >100; occur throughout GI tract
>   - Adenomas
> 4. 80%–100% GI cancer risk
> 5. Questionable risk of non-GI malignancies

PEUTZ-JEGHERS SYNDROME

In contrast to FAP and MAP, Peutz-Jeghers syndrome (PJS) is one of several GI polyposis syndromes that present not with adenomas but with so-called hamartomatous polyps.[2,3,9] Its incidence is estimated at 1/25,000 to 1/300,000, and it is an autosomal dominant syndrome resulting from germline mutations in the *STK11* (also known as *LKB1*) gene on chromosome 19p13.3, which encodes a serine-threonine kinase (hence, *STK*) involved in chromatin remodeling, cell cycle activities, and *Wnt* signaling.[10,11] Functionally, this product is thought to behave as a tumor suppressor, regulating the mTOR (mammalian target of rapamycin) pathway, and loss of its function results in mTOR dysregulation.

CLINICAL AND GROSS FEATURES

Patients with PJS have a variety of manifestations, including characteristic polyps throughout the GI tract, and mucocutaneous pigmentation (melanotic macules, especially on the lips and buccal mucosa, but found in other sites, including

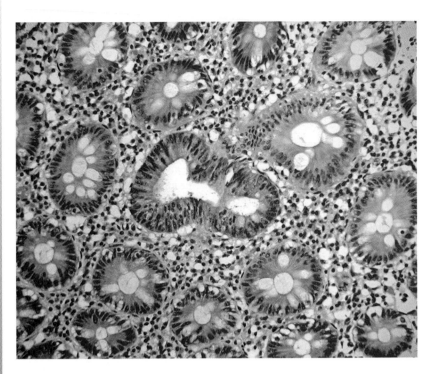

Fig. 6. Unicryptal adenoma cut en face, in a so-called Bussey section (H&E, ×20).

facial skin and extremities). In addition, polyps sometimes are found in the nasobronchial tree, the urinary bladder, and the renal pelvis, and some patients have skeletal abnormalities, such as scoliosis or clubfoot.[2,3,6,12] Depending on their size and number, the GI polyps can lead to bleeding, obstruction, or intussusception, and rectal polyps may suffer the ravages of prolapse.

MICROSCOPIC FEATURES

The polyps of PJS have a characteristic morphology, particularly those occurring in the small intestine. They do not typically carpet the mucosa as in FAP but often occur in clusters. At low magnification, PJS polyps have arborizing smooth muscle bundles that separate nondysplastic epithelial elements into disorganized lobules, imparting a cauliflower-like appearance (**Fig. 7**). The admixture of smooth muscle and epithelial elements (**Fig. 8**) can mimic invasive carcinoma, so care must be taken to avoid overcalling malignancy. At higher magnification, the epithelial elements, which are the normal constituents of the mucosa of the organ in which the polyp arises, may have reactive atypia. The epithelium is not dysplastic by definition, but dysplasia has been occasionally reported to occur.[11,13] The disorganized mixture of tissue types has led to the classification of PJS polyps as hamartomas, although there has been some recent debate as to whether the smooth muscle proliferation is the result of mucosal prolapse rather than a hamartomatous process, based on evidence that suggests an expanded epithelial stem cell compartment predisposing to both benign polyps and epithelial neoplasms.[14] In any case, a hamartoma-dysplasia-carcinoma sequence is not necessarily thought to occur in a stepwise fashion. PJS polyps most often occur in the small intestine, and it is here they achieve their best morphologic expression. The classic arborizing smooth muscle that is so characteristic may not be as apparent in colonic or gastric polyps, meaning that polyps outside the small intestine may not be as easily recognized on morphologic grounds alone.[12] In these locations, they may mimic juvenile-type polyps (discussed later) or hyperplastic polyps.

DIAGNOSIS AND DIFFERENTIAL DIAGNOSIS

Surgical pathologists must be able to recognize the classic PJS polyp morphology and must take care not to overinterpret the mixture of smooth muscle and epithelial elements as invasive carcinoma (**Fig. 9**). Similarly, they must not overdiagnose prolapse-type changes in benign distal colon polyps, which can have striking smooth muscle bundles extending up into the overlying mucosa, as absolutely indicative of PJS. In addition to recognizing the possibility of PJS based on polyp morphology, pathologists can aid in

Fig. 7. Low-magnification photomicrograph of a Peutz-Jeghers polyp, with admixed mucosal elements and bands of smooth muscle that divide the polyp into lobules, imparting a cauliflower-like appearance (H&E, ×2).

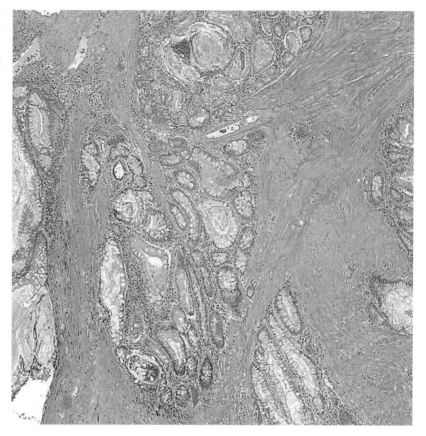

making the diagnosis by recognizing other characteristic tumors that occur in these patients. These include sex cord tumor with annular tubules (SCTATs) occurring in the ovaries of PJS patients (**Fig. 10**), testicular Sertoli cell tumors, and minimal deviation adenocarcinoma (adenoma malignum) of the uterine cervix.[3,4,11] A clinical diagnosis of PJS, usually made in the 2nd to 3rd decade of life, requires either the presence of at least 5 classic PJS polyps, any number of PJS polyps in a patient with characteristic mucocutaneous pigmentation, or a family history of PJS along with either a PJS polyp or mucocutaneous pigmentation. In addition to these clinical criteria, molecular assays for *STK11* gene abnormalities are available for diagnostic confirmation and testing of family members.

PROGNOSIS

As suggested previously, patients with PJS have a markedly increased risk of several types of malignancy. In addition to the genitourinary tumors (described previously), PJS patients may develop

Key Features
PEUTZ-JEGHERS SYNDROME

1. *STK11/LKB1* gene mutations

2. Autosomal dominant inheritance

3. Typically <25 hamartomatous polyps throughout GI tract

4. Polyps have characteristic arborizing smooth muscle and lobulated appearance

5. Patients have perioral pigmentation, characteristic gonadal tumors

   • SCTATs in ovary

   • Sertoli cell tumors in testes

   • Minimal deviation adenocarcinoma of uterine cervix

6. Up to 50% GI cancer risk

cancers throughout the luminal GI tract, pancreas, and breast.[4,11,15] The risk of malignancy is not as high as in patients with FAP, but relative risk of all tumors is approximately 15 in those with PJS.[11] The occurrence of sporadic PJS-type polyps is somewhat controversial, with a recent report suggesting that even patients with only a single PSJ-type polyp had a cancer risk similar to those with full-blown PJS, suggesting that even 1 characteristic polyp may imply the full syndromic risk.[16] Screening and therapy center on endoscopic removal of the GI polyps, resection of any malignancies, and identification of at-risk first-degree relatives with clinical and genetic studies.

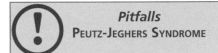

Pitfalls
PEUTZ-JEGHERS SYNDROME

! Peutz-Jeghers polyps outside the small intestine may not have characteristic morphology with arborizing smooth muscle and may more closely resemble juvenile polyps

! Admixture of smooth muscle bundles with epithelial elements in Peutz-Jeghers polyps may mimic invasive adenocarcinoma

! Prolapse-type changes in distal colon polyps may mimic Peutz-Jeghers polyp morphology

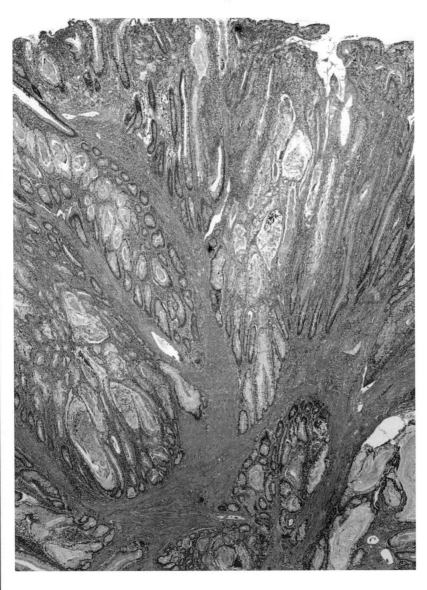

Fig. 8. Medium-magnification view of a Peutz-Jeghers polyp, highlighting the prominent, arborizing smooth muscle component (H&E, ×4).

Fig. 9. High-magnification view of a Peutz-Jeghers polyp, with an island of mucosa that is almost completely surrounded by muscle and which has reactive epithelial atypia. Such foci can be mistaken for invasive carcinoma (H&E, ×10).

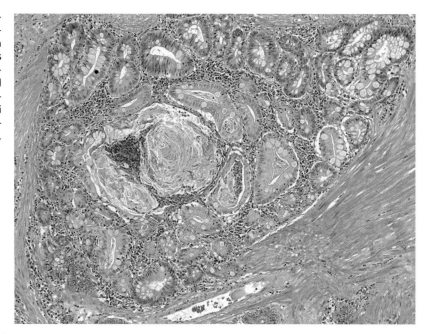

JUVENILE POLYPOSIS SYNDROME

Similar to PJS, juvenile polyposis syndrome (JPS) is a syndrome of autosomal dominant inheritance that manifests with hamartomatous polyps and increased cancer risk, which usually presents in the first or second decade of life.[2,3] JPS seems to be the result of mutations in one of several genes. Between 50% and 60% of JPS patients have a germline mutation in either *SMAD4* (also known as *DPC4*) or *BMPR1A*, both of which are involved in the transforming growth factor β/bone morphogenic protein signaling pathway.[17–19] A third gene, *ENG*, has more recently been implicated

Fig. 10. SCTATs from the ovary of a patient with PJS (H&E, ×40).

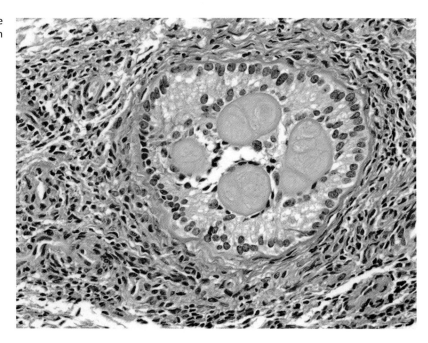

and is also involved in the transforming growth factor β signaling pathway.[20] There are some patients, allegedly with JPS, who harbor germline *PTEN* mutations, but recent evidence points to these patients having *PTEN* hamartoma syndrome (PHS) (discussed later) rather than true JPS.

CLINICAL AND GROSS FEATURES

Patients with JPS present with numerous polyps that can occur throughout the GI tract, although most occur in the colon and rectum. JPS patients with *SMAD4* mutations are thought more likely to harbor gastric and small intestinal (in addition to colonic) polyps than those without mutations in this gene.[3,21] These polyps may number up to the hundreds and can lead to melenic bleeding or hematochezia, depending on their location. Despite their syndromic association, however, sporadic juvenile-type polyps can occur in patients of any age and are the most common type of polyp in children, occurring in 1% to 2%.

MICROSCOPIC FEATURES

Histologically, juvenile polyps are characteristic of, but not specific to, JPS. They tend to be pedunculated and have a round contour when viewed endoscopically.[22] They are composed of a disorganized mixture of variably dilated, irregular crypts or glands, lined by epithelium appropriate to the anatomic site (**Fig. 11**). These may be mucin-filled, can have a serrated profile reminiscent of that seen in colonic hyperplastic polyps, and are embedded in a prominently inflamed stroma containing lymphocytes, plasma cells, eosinophils, and occasional lymphoid follicles. The polyps often have surface erosions with subjacent dilated capillaries that have a granulation tissue-like appearance. Smooth muscle bundles are conspicuously sparse or even absent. Despite these characteristics, the polyps are essentially indistinguishable from inflammatory-type polyps that can be seen sporadically or in the setting of inflammatory bowel disease. Furthermore, juvenile polyps may masquerade as hyperplastic polyps in either the colon or the stomach. This nonspecific appearance means that JPS is impossible to diagnose (or even suggest) based on the histologic appearance of 1 polyp in isolation. In contrast to PJS, cytologic dysplasia (and even invasive carcinoma) is more commonly found in the polyps of JPS patients (**Fig. 12**), although it is morphologically identical to that seen in sporadic adenomas (**Fig. 13**).[22] Reactive atypia can accompany the frequent surface erosions in juvenile polyps, so pathologists must be wary of overdiagnosing dysplasia in this setting. One study indicated that juvenile polyps with *SMAD4* mutations have a higher crypt-to-stroma ratio that those with *BMPR1A* mutations.[21] Recent evidence has also connected other genotype-phenotype relationships, such as prominent gastric manifestations and clinical features of Osler-Weber-Rendu disease (hereditary hemorrhagic telangiectasia) in patients with *SMAD4* mutation.[3,19]

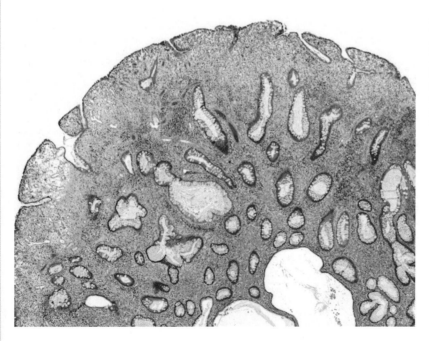

Fig. 11. Low-magnification view of a juvenile polyp from the colon. The irregular crypts are surrounded by a prominent stroma with mixed inflammation, and several are dilated and mucin-filled (H&E, ×4).

Fig. 12. Cytologic dysplasia arising in a juvenile polyp from a patient with JPS. The dysplastic crypts are at the upper left (H&E, ×4).

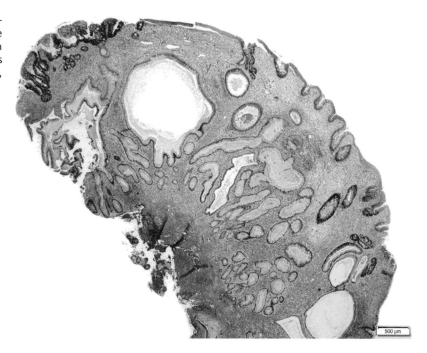

DIAGNOSIS AND DIFFERENTIAL DIAGNOSIS

Surgical pathologists should recognize the salient histologic features of juvenile polyps, although their lack of diagnostic specificity when seen in isolation must be admitted. Thus, it may be prudent to use a diagnostic phrase, such as juvenile/inflammatory-type polyp, when these features are encountered in a single polyp biopsy. When seen in multiple polyps, either from the same endoscopic examination or over the course of multiple examinations, however, such features should prompt the suggestion of JPS. Unfortunately, even this is not specific, because the polyps in other polyposis syndromes, such as PHS and Cronkhite-Canada syndrome (CCS), can have an appearance identical to those

Fig. 13. Medium-magnification view of dysplasia arising in a juvenile polyp. Apart from the background in which it occurs, the dysplasia is essentially identical to that seen in a sporadic adenoma (H&E, ×10).

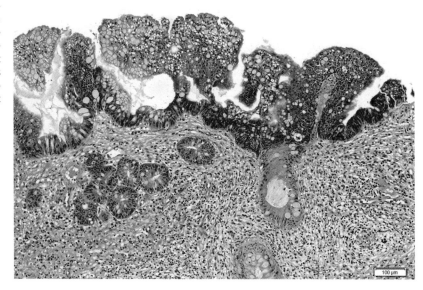

seen in JPS.[23,24] The latter is a noninherited polyposis syndrome with a controversial cancer association that is commonly associated with protein-losing enteropathy and several ectodermal abnormalities, such as hyperpigmentation, onychodystrophy, vitiligo, and alopecia. The key histologic difference between CCS and JPS is that the intervening mucosa between the polyps in CCS has an identical appearance to the polyps whereas that in JPS is normal. The diagnosis of JPS can be made definitively when there are more than 3 to 5 juvenile polyps in the colon, when there are juvenile polyps throughout the GI tract, or when any number of juvenile polyps is found in a patient with a positive family history for the disorder. The absolute number of colonic polyps needed for the diagnosis is somewhat labile, with 3, 5, and 10 all suggested.

PROGNOSIS

JPS patients have a relative risk of colorectal carcinoma of approximately 34 and an overall risk of 40% to 70%.[23] Although not as well studied, there is likely an increased risk of other GI cancers, such as gastric, small intestinal, and pancreatic. The rate of dysplasia development seems similar regardless of whether there is a mutation in SMAD4 or BMPR1A.[2] Surgical resection may be performed if a patient's polyp burden is heavy and/or for the development of dysplasia or neoplasia. If polyps are few in number, endoscopic removal is appropriate. JPS patients should be endoscopically screened at least every 3 years, and molecular genetic tests for SMAD4 and BMPR1A mutations are available for diagnostic confirmation and family testing.[22]

Key Features
JUVENILE POLYPOSIS SYNDROME

1. SMAD4, BMPR1A gene mutations

2. Autosomal dominant inheritance

3. Few hamartomatous polyps to >100; occur throughout GI tract

4. Juvenile polyp has abundant inflamed lamina propria with mixed inflammatory cells, round contour, surface erosions

5. SMAD4-mutated patients may have hereditary telangiectasia, gastric tumors

6. 40%–70% GI cancer risk

Pitfalls
JUVENILE POLYPOSIS SYNDROME

! Morphology of juvenile polyps is not specific to the syndrome

! Inflammation and surface erosions may induce epithelial atypia that can mimic dysplasia in juvenile polyps

! Juvenile polyps are identical to polyps seen in CCS, but intervening mucosa between polyps is also abnormal in CCS

PTEN HAMARTOMA/COWDEN/BANNAYAN-RILEY-RUVALCABA

Mutations in the PTEN gene on chromosome 10q23 underlie a family of syndromes that are inherited in an autosomal dominant fashion.[2,3,25,26] PTEN is a tumor suppressor gene whose product is a phosphatase involved in the cell cycle and that is mutated in a variety of human cancers. PHS is an umbrella term for these rare disorders, 2 of which (Cowden syndrome and Bannayan-Riley-Ruvalcaba syndrome, essentially allelic variants of one another) involve hamartomatous polyposis of the GI tract.

CLINICAL AND GROSS FEATURES

PHS patients may have a variety of polyps involving the GI tract. Other syndromic manifestations, however, are more prominent than GI polyps in PHS patients and include soft tissue tumors, cutaneous abnormalities, and tumors of the breast, endometrium, and thyroid.

MICROSCOPIC FEATURES AND DIAGNOSIS

The GI polyps of PHS can be subtle and are often essentially indistinguishable from juvenile or inflammatory polyps (Fig. 14). Thus, surgical pathologists should not expect to make the diagnosis in isolation but must recognize and correlate the other tumor types and clinical manifestations to suggest the possibility of PHS. Other GI polyps may include examples identical to hyperplastic polyps as well as ganglioneuromas, submucosal lipomas, and hemangiomas.[3] In addition to these GI entities, patients may have similar soft tissue tumors outside the GI tract as well as pigmented macules on the glans penis (in Bannayan-Riley-Ruvalcaba), facial trichilemmomas, and acral keratoses.

Fig. 14. Low-magnification photomicrograph of a colon polyp from a patient with Cowden syndrome (PHS). It is basically indistinguishable from a juvenile-type polyp (H&E, ×2).

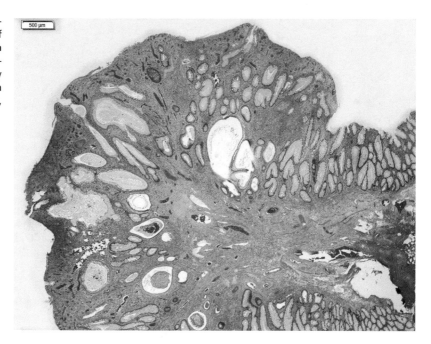

Prognosis

The GI polyps of PHS are a minor feature of the disorder, tend to present late in the course of disease, and may lead to a significantly increased risk of GI and other cancers.[3,25,27] There is an increased risk of extra-GI malignancies, including breast carcinoma, endometrial carcinoma, and follicular carcinoma of the thyroid.

Key Features
PTEN HAMARTOMATOUS POLYPOSIS

1. *PTEN* gene mutations

2. Autosomal dominant inheritance

3. Polyps often a minor feature but may have multiple polyps throughout GI tract
   - Juvenile-like
   - Hyperplastic polyp–like
   - Ganglioneuromatous
   - Other polyp types

4. Cutaneous, breast, endometrial, other tumors

5. Increased GI cancer risk (approximately 28% in a recent study)

HYPERPLASTIC POLYPOSIS SYNDROME

CLINICAL AND GROSS FEATURES

The term, *hyperplastic polyposis syndrome (HPS)*, originally referred to a polyposis thought to be a rare, benign disorder that could endoscopically mimic FAP and which presented with numerous colonic polyps with serrated crypt profiles (**Fig. 15**).[28,29] With the advent of the concept of a so-called serrated pathway to colorectal neoplasia, however, the idea of HPS has been turned on its head. Although sporadic hyperplastic polyps are a common (and benign, as currently understood) finding in the colon, at least a subset of patients with HPS is now thought at increased risk for colorectal cancer.[30–32] The evolution of understanding of what morphologic features constitute a serrated adenoma or sessile serrated adenoma/polyp (**Fig. 16**) and the morphologic overlap among these entities with both benign polyps and other adenomas has led to much confusion in the definition of HPS and the grasp of its genetic underpinnings and clinical implications. Other putative or ill-defined syndromes, including hereditary mixed polyposis and serrated polyposis, have been described and have considerable overlap with HPS, augmenting the confusion, and many of the polyps (discussed previously), such as those in JPS, can mimic hyperplastic polyps under the

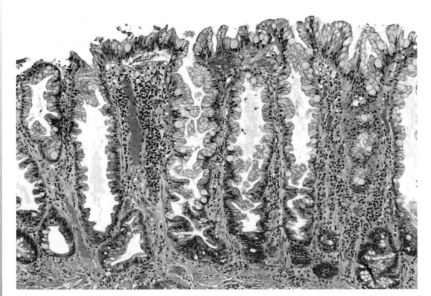

Fig. 15. Medium-magnification view of a polyp with serrated crypt profiles from a patient with hyperplastic polyposis. The patient had dozens of similar-appearing polyps of variable size (H&E, ×10).

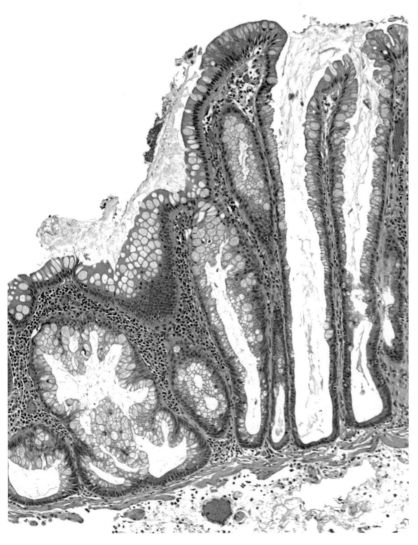

Fig. 16. Medium-magnification view of a sessile serrated adenoma/polyp, characterized by dilated and branched basal crypts that spread along the muscularis mucosae (H&E, ×20).

microscope. Finally, several different genes (*PTEN*, *EBPH2*, *MutYH*, *BMPR1A*, and others) have been implicated in these syndromes, and both autosomal dominant and recessive inheritance patterns have been described.[2]

MICROSCOPIC FEATURES AND DIAGNOSIS

Clinically, HPS is currently defined as having

1. At least 5 histologically diagnosed serrated polyps proximal to the sigmoid colon, of which 2 are more than 10 mm in diameter, or
2. More than 20 serrated polyps in a pancolonic distribution, or
3. Any number of serrated polyps proximal to the sigmoid colon in a patient with a first-degree relative diagnosed with HPS

Colectomy specimens from HPS patients often have multiple traditional adenomas, serrated polyps, and, sometimes, polyps with a mixture of serrated, nondysplastic crypts and those with true adenomatous dysplasia. There is considerable overlap with a syndrome described as "hereditary mixed polyposis" in which patients have a mixture of serrated polyps, adenomas, and juvenile polyps. *BMPR1A* mutations as well as abnormalities in another gene, called *CRAC1*, have been described in hereditary mixed polyposis.[2,33]

PROGNOSIS

With all of the confusion surrounding HPS, the tangle of potential entities encompassed by the term has been difficult to study. Nonetheless, it seems safe to suppose that many, if not all, patients presenting with a polyposis syndrome in which the polyps have a serrated architecture reminiscent of hyperplastic polyps should be closely followed for the risk of colorectal carcinoma, potentially via the serrated neoplasia pathway (**Fig. 17**). Thus, surgical

---

Key Features
HYPERPLASTIC POLYPOSIS

1. Unknown mutations (many possible genes identified)
2. Unknown inheritance pattern and cancer risk
3. Variable number of colonic polyps
   - Serrated crypt profiles

Pitfalls
HYPERPLASTIC POLYPOSIS

! HPS is currently a poorly understood and confusing entity

! Because of recent upheaval regarding the diagnosis of serrated polyps (including sessile serrated adenoma/polyp), many pathologists are confused about the clinical significance of colon polyps with serrated architecture

! Because of the innocuous history of the hyperplastic polyp in colonic biopsy diagnosis, it may be difficult to recognize the possibility of HPS when multiple hyperplastic polyps are encountered in a patient's colon

---

pathologists should be aware of this entity (or entities) and recognize the potential implications of multiple serrated colon polyps. A variety of molecular abnormalities, including *BRAF* mutations, DNA mismatch repair (MMR) protein mutations, and the so-called CpG island methylator phenotype, have been implicated in the serrated neoplasia pathway and may be operative in HPS as well.

LYNCH SYNDROME

Lynch syndrome (LS) is an old term, later supplanted by hereditary nonpolyposis colorectal cancer (HNPCC), but which made a resurgence when it became clear that many LS patients have GI polyps and that the syndrome resulted in a risk of several other non-GI cancers. First described by Aldred Scott Warthin in 1913, the syndrome is now known to be the result of mutations or deletion in 1 of 4 major DNA MMR genes—*MLH1*, *PMS2*, *MSH2*, or *MSH6*.[2,3,34,35] The protein products of these genes function in the repair of DNA synthesis errors and double-stranded DNA breaks, among other tasks and, as such, function as tumor suppressors. A fifth gene, *MSH3*, may also be involved in a few cases.[36] LS is an autosomal dominant disorder that is thought the most common inherited cause of cancer and is responsible for 3% to 5% of all colon cancers.[4] Although inheritance of 1 abnormal (mutated or deleted) copy of an MMR gene that functions as a tumor suppressor might be presumed to lead to an autosomal recessive inheritance pattern, in reality, it is fairly easy to undergo loss of heterozygosity in the other allele in any given epithelial cell leading to the development of cancer, and the syndrome, therefore, follows an autosomal

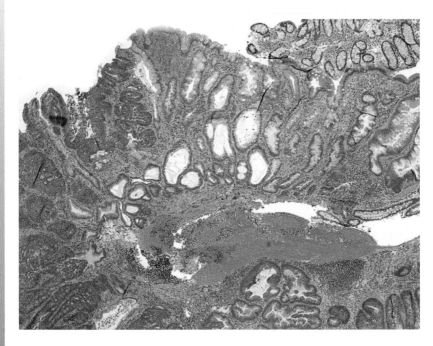

Fig. 17. High-grade dysplasia (*left*) arising in a serrated polyp from a patient with hyperplastic polyposis. This particular polyp had morphologic features of a sessile serrated adenoma/polyp, seen on the right (H&E, ×4).

dominant pattern. Some rare cases of biallelic MMR mutation/deletion, however, have been reported in children who present in early childhood with hematolymphoid neoplasms, café au lait spots, and GI malignancies.[37]

CLINICAL AND GROSS FEATURES

The former term, HNPCC, implies that LS patients do not present with colonic polyps, but this is variable, with patients harboring anywhere from 0 to fewer than 30 colonic adenomas, depending on the specific case.[3] Other tumors, including small intestinal, gastric, endometrial, ovarian, pancreaticobiliary, and urothelial (involving the renal pelvis and ureters), have also been reported, and there is some genotype-phenotype association, such as increased endometrial cancer risk and later colon cancer onset in LS patients with *MSH6* mutations.[38] LS patients with brain tumors are put into the eponymous category of Turcot syndrome, sharing this designation with similar FAP patients and those who also have sebaceous tumors of the skin receive the designation, Muir-Torre syndrome.

MICROSCOPIC FEATURES AND DIAGNOSIS

Because the adenomas and carcinomas arising in LS patients are morphologically similar to those seen in patients without the syndrome, it can be difficult for surgical pathologists to recognize the possibility of LS based on histologic evidence

alone. Clinical history can serve as a guide, and clinical criteria suggestive of the diagnosis have been published. The revised Amsterdam criteria are a useful screen to search for LS patients.[4] Each of the following criteria must be fulfilled:

1. Three or more relatives must have an LS-associated cancer (colorectal, endometrial, gastric, ovarian, small intestinal, ureteric/renal pelvic, and others).
2. Two or more successive generations must be affected.
3. One or more relatives must be diagnosed before age 50.
4. One relative (in line 1) should be a first-degree relative of the other 2.
5. FAP should be excluded in colorectal cancer cases.
6. Tumors should be histologically verified, if possible.

Patients fulfilling these criteria can be tested for MMR gene abnormalities using molecular techniques. Specifically, tumors arising in the setting of LS tend to have high-level microsatellite instability (MSI-H), and 90% to 95% of colon cancers arising in this setting manifest this abnormality. Microsatellites are short tandem repeats of 2 to 6 base pair DNA sequences, and MSI is a change in length of 1 or more of these sequences by insertion or deletion of the repeating units. By testing several important microsatellite loci in both tumor and normal tissue from the same patient, the presence and degree of MSI in the tumor can be determined. This assay can be performed on formalin-fixed, paraffin-embedded tissue and is correlated with immunohistochemical staining for the 4 major MMR gene products (hMLH1, hPMS2, hMSH2, and hMSH6) to provide a degree of likelihood that a patient has LS. The normal state for the immunohistochemical stains is positive nuclear expression and, thus, the stain results require a negative-is-positive interpretation (ie, loss of nuclear expression is the abnormal result) (**Fig. 18**).

Although these testing modalities provide a reliable way to confirm the suspicion of LS, they are not perfect. First, the MMR protein immunostains have a not insignificant false-negative rate.[39] Second, and most importantly, a substantial number of sporadic colorectal cancers have high-level MSI. Approximately 15% of all colon cancers are MSI-H and the vast majority of these are not related to LS. Current evidence indicates that the majority of sporadic MSI-H colon cancers result from methylation of the promoter of the *MLH1* gene, which is accompanied by an activating mutation (the V600E mutation) in the *BRAF* gene, whose product is a serine-threonine kinase involved in transduction of growth signals through the RAS-RAF-MAP kinase pathway. Thus, *BRAF* mutation analysis is typically ordered in conjunction with MSI and MMR protein testing to determine whether a given tumor is likely LS related (negative for the *BRAF* V600E mutation) or sporadic (majority positive for the mutation).[40] **Table 1** provides the interpretations for combined molecular MSI testing, MMR protein immunohistochemistry, and *BRAF* mutation analysis.

There are subtle histologic clues to the presence of MSI in colorectal adenomas and carcinomas (**Fig. 19**). MSI-H cancers tend to have a prominent infiltrate of intraepithelial lymphocytes (2 or more per high-power microscopic field, infiltrating the tumor epithelium), a nodular (Crohn-like) peritumoral lymphoid infiltrate, a pushing border, and mucinous or signet-ring morphology (at least in areas). They also tend to be at the extremes of differentiation (either poorly or well differentiated).[41,42] Similarly, the adenomas in LS tend to have adenoma-infiltrating lymphocytes (greater than 5/high-power field in the epithelium) and fewer apoptotic bodies than sporadic adenomas.[43] These histologic clues can be used to guide pathologists in ordering (or recommending) ancillary testing for LS in a given tumor, as can the revised Bethesda criteria[4]:

1. Colorectal cancer in a patient less than age 50 years.
2. Presence of synchronous or metachronous colorectal or other LS-associated tumor in a patient of any age

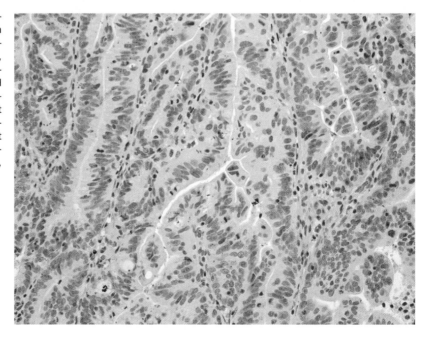

Fig. 18. High-magnification photomicrograph of an immunohistochemical stain for hMLH1, illustrating loss of nuclear expression in MSI-H carcinoma. A positive internal control is present in the admixed inflammatory cell nuclei that have brown staining (hematoxylin counterstain, ×40).

Table 1
Interpretation of molecular and immunohistochemical results for microsatellite instability testing in colorectal carcinomas

hMLH1	hPMS2	hMSH2	hMSH6	Molecular MSI	BRAF V600E	Interpretation
+	+	+	+	Stable	ND	Microsatellite stable; unlikely to be LS
+	+	+	+	MSI-H	WT	Likely LS; specific mutation unknown
−	−	+	+	MSI-H	WT	Likely LS with germline MLH1 mutation
−	−	+	+	MSI-H	Mutated	Likely sporadic MSI-H tumor (methylation-related)
+	−	+	+	MSI-H	WT	Likely LS with germline PMS2 mutation
+	+	+	−	MSI-H	WT	Likely LS with germline MSH6 mutation
+	+	−	−	MSI-H	WT	Likely LS with germline MSH2 mutation

Abbreviations: ND, not done; WT, wild type.

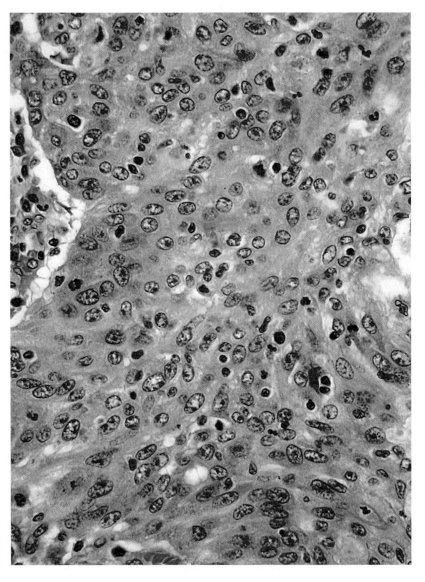

Fig. 19. Poorly differentiated adenocarcinoma with numerous tumor-infiltrating lymphocytes (small, dark nuclei with surrounding haloes that infiltrate the neoplastic epithelium). These morphologic features are among those suggestive of MSI in colon cancers (H&E, ×50).

3. Colorectal cancer with MSI-H histology in a patient less than age 60 years
4. Colorectal or other LS-associated tumor diagnosed in at least 1 first-degree relative <50 years of age
5. Colorectal or other LS-associated tumor diagnosed at any age in 2 first-degree or second-degree relatives

Following these guidelines, however, still results in missing some proportion of LS patients, and the cost-effectiveness of LS screening has been studied several times. In reality, many clinicians and pathologists are now advocating a priori testing of all colorectal cancers, regardless of the clinical scenario or histologic findings. The exact method of testing remains somewhat unsettled, however, with advocates for MMR protein immunohistochemistry alone, molecular MSI testing alone, or the full combination coupled with reflexive BRAF mutation analysis for tumors found MSI-H.

PROGNOSIS

Patients diagnosed with LS have a high risk of neoplasm development, both within and outside the GI tract. In addition to colorectal cancer, LS patients are at high risk for endometrial carcinomas, and these 2 cancers together are the most common malignancies in those with the syndrome.[4]

Key Features
LYNCH SYNDROME

1. DNA MMR gene mutations (*MLH1, PMS2, MSH2, MSH6*)

2. Autosomal dominant inheritance

3. Variable number of colonic polyps (zero–dozens)

   • Adenomas, when present

4. Many other tumors possible (endometrial, ovarian, gastric, and so forth)

5. High GI and endometrial cancer risk

   • Accounts for 3%–5% of all colorectal cancers

6. Thought the most common inherited cause of cancer

Pitfalls
LYNCH SYNDROME

! LS cases with dozens of adenomas can be confused with FAP based on clinicopathologic findings alone

! Strict adherence to the revised Bethesda criteria for determining which patients to test for LS results in missing some diagnoses

---

SUMMARY

The GI polyposis syndromes can be a challenge for surgical pathologists to diagnose, because most have at least some increased risk of cancer, and many have overlapping histologic features and/or polyps that mimic benign processes. Furthermore, certain types of polyposis may be a common manifestation of more than 1 syndrome or disease. Thus, pathologists encountering endoscopic biopsies of GI polyps must use a basic understanding of these syndromes and their features to be able to correlate the variety of both GI and extraintestinal findings and to even entertain the possibility of a syndromic condition. Once such connections are made, ancillary tests using immunohistochemistry and molecular techniques are available to confirm the diagnosis and screen family members for heritable syndromes.

REFERENCES

1. Fearon ER. Molecular genetics of colorectal cancer. Annu Rev Pathol 2011;6:479–507.
2. Jass JR. Colorectal polyposis: from phenotype to diagnosis. Pathol Res Pract 2008;204:431–47.
3. Aretz S. The differential diagnosis and surveillance of hereditary gastrointestinal polyposis syndromes. Dtsch Arztebl Int 2010;107:163–73.
4. Shah NB, Lindor NM. Lower gastrointestinal tract cancer predisposition syndromes. Hematol Oncol Clin North Am 2010;24:1229–52.
5. Owens SR. Familial adenomatous polyposis. In: Putnam AR, Wallentine JC, Polydorides AD, et al, editors. Diagnostic pathology: pediatric neoplasms. Salt Lake City, Utah: Amirsys, Inc; 2012. p. 12-12–12-15.
6. Anaya DA, Chang GJ, Rodriquez-Bigas MA. Extracolonic manifestations of hereditary colorectal cancer syndromes. Clin Colon Rectal Surg 2008;21:263–72.
7. Meuller J, Kanter-Smoler G, Nygren AO, et al. Identification of genomic deletions of the APC gene in familial adenomatous polyposis by two independent quantitative techniques. Genet Test 2004;8:248–56.

8. Vogt S, Jones N, Christian D, et al. Expanded extracolonic tumor spectrum in MUTYH-associated polyposis. Gastroenterology 2009;137:1976–85.

9. McGarrity TJ, Amos C. Peutz-Jeghers syndrome: clinicopathology and molecular alterations. Cell Mol Life Sci 2006;63:2135–44.

10. Jansen M, Langeveld D, De Leng WW, et al. LKB1 as the ghostwriter of crypt history. Fam Cancer 2011;10:437–46.

11. Owens SR. Peutz-Jeghers polyps. In: Putnam AR, Wallentine JC, Polydorides AD, et al, editors. Diagnostic pathology: pediatric neoplasms. Salt Lake City, Utah: Amirsys, Inc; 2012. p. 12-16–12-19.

12. Lam-Himlin D, Park JY, Cornish TC, et al. Morphologic characterization of syndromic gastric polyps. Am J Surg Pathol 2010;34:1656–62.

13. Entius MM, Westerman AM, Giardeilla FM, et al. Peutz-Jeghers polyps, dysplasia, and K-ras codon 12 mutations. Gut 1997;41:320–2.

14. De Leng WW, Jansen M, Keller JJ, et al. Peutz-Jeghers syndrome polyps are polyclonal with expanded progenitor cell compartment. Gut 2007;56:1475–6.

15. Geggs AD, Latchford AR, Vasen HF, et al. Peutz-Jeghers syndrome: a systematic review and recommendations for management. Gut 2010;59:975–86.

16. Burkart AL, Sheridan T, Lewin M, et al. Do sporadic Peutz-Jeghers polyps exist? Experience of a large teaching hospital. Am J Surg Pathol 2007;31:1209–14.

17. Chen HM, Fang JY. Genetics of the hamartomatous polyposis syndromes: a molecular review. Int J Colorectal Dis 2009;24:865–74.

18. Zbuk MM, Eng C. Hamartomatous polyposis syndromes. Nat Clin Pract Gastroenterol Hepatol 2007;4:492–502.

19. Van Hattem WA, Brosens LA, de Leng WW, et al. Large genomic deledtions of SMAD4, BMPR1A and PTEN in juvenile polyposis. Gut 2008;57:623–7.

20. Lee ST, Kim JA, Jang SY, et al. Clinical features and mutations in the ENG, ACVRL1, and SMAD4 genes in Korean patients with hereditary hemorrhagic telangiectasia. J Korean Med Sci 2009;24:69–76.

21. Van Hattem WA, Langeveld D, de Leng WW, et al. Histologic variations in juvenile polyp phenotype correlate with genetic defect underlying juvenile polyposis. Am J Surg Pathol 2011;35:530–6.

22. Owens SR. Juvenile polyps. In: Putnam AR, Wallentine JC, Polydorides AD, et al, editors. Diagnostic pathology: pediatric neoplasms. Salt Lake City, Utah: Amirsys, Inc; 2012. p. 12-10–12-11.

23. Owens SR. Cronkhite-Canada syndrome. In: Putnam AR, Wallentine JC, Polydorides AD, et al, editors. Diagnostic pathology: pediatric neoplasms. Salt Lake City, Utah: Amirsys, Inc; 2012. p. 12-24–12-25.

24. Burke AP, Sobin LH. The pathology of Cronkhite-Canada polyps. A comparison to juvenile polyposis. Am J Surg Pathol 1989;13:940–6.

25. Heald B, Mester J, Rybicki L, et al. Frequent gastrointestinal polyps and colorectal adenocarcinomas in a prospective series of PTEN mutation carriers. Gastroenterology 2010;139:1927–33.

26. Stanich PP, Owens VL, Sweetser S, et al. Colonic polyposis and neoplasia in Cowden syndrome. Mayo Clin Proc 2011;86:489–92.

27. Tan MH, Mester JL, Ngeow J, et al. Lifetime cancer risks in individuals with germline PTEN mutations. Clin Cancer Res 2012;18:400–7.

28. Williams GT, Arthur JF, Bussey HJ, et al. Metaplastic polyps and polyposis of the colorectum. Histopathology 1980;4:155–70.

29. Jeevaratnam P, Cottier DS, Browett PF, et al. Familial giant hyperplastic polyposis predisposing to colorectal cancer: a new hereditary bowel cancer syndrome. J Pathol 1996;179:20–5.

30. Boparai KS, Dekker E, Polak MM, et al. A serrated colorectal cancer pathway predominates over the class WNT pathway in patients with hyperplastic polyposis syndrome. Am J Pathol 2011;178:2700–7.

31. Kalady MF, Jarrar A, Leach B, et al. Defining phenotypes and cancer risk in hyperplastic polyposis syndrome. Dis Colon Rectum 2011;54:164–70.

32. Boparai KS, Reitsma JB, Lemmens V, et al. Increased colorectal cancer risk during follow-up in patients with hyperplastic polyposis syndrome: a multicentre cohort study. Gut 2010;59:1094–100.

33. O'Riordan JM, O'Donoghue D, Green A, et al. Hereditary mixed polyposis syndrome due to a BMPR1A mutation. Colorectal Dis 2009;12:570–3.

34. Warthin AS. Heredity with reference to carcinoma as shown by the study of the cases examined in the pathological laboratory of the University of Michigan, 1895-1913. Arch Intern Med 1913;12:546–55.

35. Lynch HT, Lynch PM, Lanspa SJ, et al. Review of the Lynch syndrome: history, molecular genetics, screening differential diagnosis, and medicolegal ramifications. Clin Genet 2009;76:1–18.

36. Duraturo F, Liccardo R, Cavallo A, et al. Association of low-risk MSH3 and MSH2 variant alleles with Lynch syndrome: probability of synergistic effects. Int J Cancer 2011;129:1643–50.

37. Durno CA, Holter S, Sherman PM, et al. The gastrointestinal phenotype of germline biallelic mismatch repair gene mutations. Am J Gastroenterol 2010;105:2449–56.

38. Pollock J, Welsh JS. Clinical cancer genetics. Part I: gastrointestinal. Am J Clin Oncol 2011;34:332–6.

39. De La Chapelle A. Microsatellite instability phenotype of tumors: genotyping or immunohistochemistry? The jury is still out. J Clin Oncol 2002;20:897–9.

40. Snover DC. Update on the serrated pathway to colo-rectal carcinoma. Hum Pathol 2011;42:1–10.

41. Greenson JK, Bonner JD, Ben-Yzhak O, et al. Phenotype of microsatellite unstable colorectal car-cinomas: well-differentiated and focally mucinous tumors and the absence of dirty necrosis correlate with microsatellite instability. Am J Surg Pathol 2003;27:563–70.

42. Greenson JK, Huang SC, Heron C, et al. Patho-logic predictors of microsatellite instability in colorectal cancer. Am J Surg Pathol 2009;33:126–33.

43. Polydorides AD, Mukherjee B, Gruber SB, et al. Adenoma-infiltrating lymphocytes are a potential marker of HNPCC. Am J Surg Pathol 2008;32:1661–6.

Immunohistochemistry in Gastroenterohepatopancreatobiliary Epithelial Neoplasia
Practical Applications, Pitfalls, and Emerging Markers

Andrew M. Bellizzi, MD

KEYWORDS

- Immunohistochemistry • Differential diagnosis • Tumor classification • Site of origin
- Predictive markers • DNA mismatch repair • p53 • HER2

ABSTRACT

Immunohistochemistry (IHC) has broad applications in neoplastic gastrointestinal surgical pathology. Although classically used as a diagnostic tool, IHC increasingly provides prognostic and predictive information. This review highlights 11 key uses of IHC (Box 1). Emphasis is placed on specific clinical applications and qualitative aspects of interpretation. Common pitfalls are specifically highlighted. The potential application of emerging markers is discussed in relation to several of the 11 topics. In many instances, an immunostain serves as a surrogate for specific molecular genetic events. Survey of relevant articles forms the evidence basis for this review.

DIAGNOSIS AND RISK STRATIFICATION OF DYSPLASIA IN BARRETT'S ESOPHAGUS

CLINICAL OVERVIEW

Barrett's esophagus (BE) represents the replacement of some length of the squamous lining of the distal esophagus by intestinalized columnar mucosa. It is common in the West, seen in up to 2% of the general population and 10% of those with chronic gastroesophageal reflux disease. Adenocarcinoma of the esophagus arises in BE through

---

Box 1
Selected applications of immunohistochemistry in neoplastic gastrointestinal pathology

1. Diagnosis and risk stratification of dysplasia in BE

2. Determination of tumor type in poorly differentiated esophageal carcinomas

3. Distinguishing primary from metastatic poorly cohesive carcinomas in the stomach

4. Prediction of response to anti-HER2 therapy in gastroesophageal adenocarcinomas

5. Diagnosis of serrated colon polyps

6. Assessment of MMR function in CRCs

7. Diagnosis of well-differentiated hepatocellular lesions

8. Determination of tumor type in poorly differentiated liver tumors

9. Diagnosis of cellular epithelioid neoplasms of the pancreas

10. Determining site of origin of neuroendocrine tumors of unknown primary

11. Determining site of origin of adenocarcinomas

Department of Pathology, University of Iowa Hospitals and Clinics, University of Iowa Carver College of Medicine, 200 Hawkins Drive, Iowa City, IA 52242, USA
E-mail address: andrew-bellizzi@uiowa.edu

Surgical Pathology 6 (2013) 567–609
http://dx.doi.org/10.1016/j.path.2013.06.003

Abbreviations: Immunohistochemistry in Gastroenterohepatopancreatobiliary Epithelial Neoplasia	
ACC	Acinar cell carcinoma
AMACR	Alpha-methylacyl-CoA racemase
Arg-1	Arginase-1
BCAT	β-catenin
BE	Barrett's esophagus
CRC	Colorectal cancer
dMMR	Mismatch repair deficiency
EpCAM	Epithelial cell adhesion molecule
ER	Estrogen receptor
FNH	Focal nodular hyperplasia
GEJ	Gastroesophageal junction
GI	Gastrointestinal
GPC3	Glypican-3
GS	Glutamine synthetase
HA	Hepatocellular adenoma
HCC	Hepatocellular carcinoma
Hep Par 1	Hepatocyte paraffin 1
HER2	Human epidermal growth factor receptor 2
H&E	hematoxylin-and-eosin
HP	Hyperplastic polyp
HSP70	Heat shock protein-70
ICC	Intrahepatic cholangiocarcinoma
IHC	Immunohistochemistry
LAMN	Low-grade appendiceal mucinous neoplasm
LBC	Lobular breast carcinoma
LS	Lynch syndrome
MMR	Mismatch repair
MoAb	Monoclonal antibody
MSI-H	High-level microsatellite unstable
MSI	Microsatellite instability
NEC	Neuroendocrine carcinoma
NET	Neuroendocrine tumor
OITMBT	Ovarian intestinal-type mucinous borderline tumor
PB	Pancreatoblastoma
pCEA	Polyclonal CEA
PDA	Pancreatic ductal adenocarcinoma
PNET	Pancreatic neuroendocrine tumor
RCC	Renal cell carcinoma
SATB2	Special AT-rich sequence-binding protein 2
SCC	Squamous cell carcinoma
SPN	Solid-pseudopapillary neoplasm
SSA/P	Sessile serrated adenoma/polyp
ToGA	Trastuzumab for Gastric Cancer
TTF-1	Thyroid transcription factor-1

an inflammation → metaplasia → dysplasia → carcinoma sequence. The risk of progression to adenocarcinoma was historically estimated at 0.5% per year (relative risk 30–60), the evidence base for the standard practice of placing BE patients into endoscopic surveillance. More recent population-based cohort studies suggest that this figure is a 2- to 4-fold overestimate.[1,2] Given this finding and current health care financial constraints, there is invigorated interest in improving selection of those patients most likely to benefit from the allocation of scarce medical resources (eg, endoscopic surveillance and endoscopic ablative techniques).

Histologic dysplasia assessment represents the gold standard for BE risk stratification. Unfortunately, there is significant interobserver variability, especially in fine distinctions at extreme ends of the morphologic spectrum. For example, interobserver agreement for the diagnoses of low-grade dysplasia and indefinite for dysplasia are fair and slight, respectively.[3] A host of biomarkers aiming to supplement hematoxylin-and-eosin (H&E) diagnosis have been studied. p53 immunohistochemistry (IHC) is among the most promising and has the additional advantage of widespread availability. p53 IHC has been shown to improve the reproducibility of dysplasia assessment,[4] and several studies have shown it prognostically significant, especially in low-grade dysplasia.[4–7]

P53 IMMUNOHISTOCHEMISTRY

p53 is a transcription factor that mediates cell cycle arrest or apoptosis in the setting of cellular stresses, including DNA damage. TP53 inactivation is among the most frequent molecular genetic events in neoplasia, most commonly by missense mutation involving its DNA binding core domain coupled with loss of the wild-type allele.[8] Most missense mutations result in a conformational change that prolongs the half-life of the protein, leading to increased expression,[9] whereas occasional large deletions or truncating mutations may result in complete absence of expression.[10,11] Wild-type p53 is stabilized in response to cellular stresses.

I occasionally use p53 IHC in the assessment of atypical BE foci, particularly when I am considering a differential of indefinite for dysplasia versus low-grade dysplasia, including cases in which atypia is confined to the crypt compartment. In evaluating the p53 immunostain, I am seeking to colocalize a histologically atypical focus with patterns of expression in keeping with TP53 inactivation. Diffuse, strong staining, obscuring nuclear detail, suggests a missense mutation (**Fig. 1A, B**), whereas complete absence of staining (null pattern) in a background of wild-type pattern staining may represent a large deletion or truncating mutation (see **Fig. 1**C, D). Given an inflammatory milieu, increased expression of wild-type p53 in nondysplastic BE is not surprising. This takes the form of diffuse expression of weak intensity, often punctuated by scattered more darkly staining nuclei. I use the mouse monoclonal antibody (MoAb), DO-7, which, among several commercially available p53 antibodies, has been shown to correlate well with *TP53* mutation status.[10] The finding of a pattern of p53 expression characteristic of *TP53* inactivation supports a diagnosis of low-grade dysplasia over indefinite for dysplasia. Given variability in histologic dysplasia assessment and lack of standardized p53 IHC scoring criteria, the reported frequency of p53 positivity in low-grade dysplasia has varied from 9% to 89%, making it impossible to confidently comment on the negative predictive value of wild-type pattern staining. Abnormal p53 staining is typical of high-grade dysplasia and carcinoma, and, thus, I do not consider the result useful for dysplasia grading.

PITFALLS

Errors in interpretation are rooted in failure to use p53 IHC as a surrogate for *TP53* mutation status. The wild-type pattern is often misinterpreted as a positive result, whereas the less familiar null pattern may be misinterpreted as a negative result.

Pitfalls
Pitfalls INTERPRETATION OF P53 IMMUNOHISTOCHEMISTRY
! Wild-type pattern staining should not be considered a positive result.
! Null pattern staining is abnormal, suggesting *TP53* deletion or truncating mutation.

DETERMINATION OF TUMOR TYPE IN POORLY DIFFERENTIATED ESOPHAGEAL CARCINOMAS

CLINICAL OVERVIEW

In the West, most esophageal carcinomas are BE-associated adenocarcinomas. Not uncommonly, solid, poorly differentiated examples are

---

⚠⚠ Differential Diagnosis
IMMUNOPHENOTYPE OF ESOPHAGEAL ADENOCARCINOMA VERSUS SQUAMOUS CELL CARCINOMA

	Adenocarcinoma, % (n)	Squamous Cell Carcinoma, % (n)
p63	8 (7/92)	99 (66/67)
CK5/6	21 (19/92)	97 (65/67)
CDX2	63 (58/92)	19 (13/67)
CK7	91 (62/68)	34 (14/41)
MUC5AC	64 (44/69)	2 (1/41)
SOX2	29 (27/92)	84 (56/57)

Data from Long KB, Hornick JL. SOX2 is highly expressed in squamous cell carcinomas of the gastrointestinal tract. Hum Pathol 2009;40(12):1768–73; and DiMaio MA, Kwok S, Montgomery KD, et al. Immunohistochemical panel for distinguishing esophageal adenocarcinoma from squamous cell carcinoma: a combination of p63, cytokeratin 5/6, MUC5AC, and anterior gradient homolog 2 allows optimal subtyping. Hum Pathol 2012;43(11):1799–807.

difficult to definitively distinguish from squamous cell carcinoma (SCC) on H&E. In addition, primary poorly differentiated neuroendocrine carcinomas (NECs), fairly evenly split between those representing divergent differentiation in an adenocarcinoma or SCC and pure tumors, are rare although not extraordinary (3.8% of 1105 in a recent series).[12] Somewhat surprisingly, until recently, the distinction of esophageal adenocarcinoma from SCC has had no therapeutic relevance. This has changed with the uptake of anti–human epidermal growth factor receptor 2 (anti-HER2) therapy in esophageal and gastric adenocarcinomas, and accurate histologic typing is important going forward (eg, for clinical trial eligibility). Although many NEC patients with locoregional disease undergo neoadjuvant therapy followed by resection,

Diagnostic Algorithm: Immunohistochemistry in Poorly Differentiated Esophageal Carcinoma

- Primary panel to include
  - p63 (SCC marker)
  - MUC5AC (adenocarcinoma marker)
  - Chromogranin and synaptophysin (as needed)

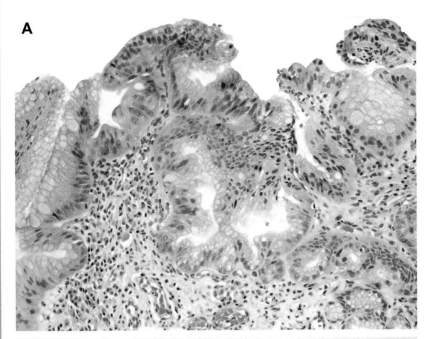

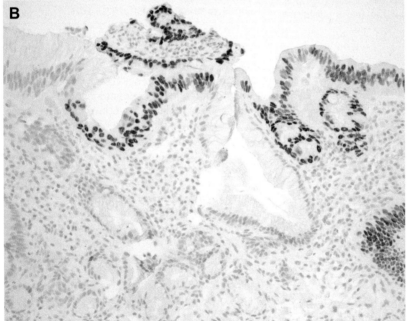

Fig. 1. p53 IHC in BE. (*A*) BE with focus (*center*) characterized by slight nuclear enlargement and stratification, originally considered indefinite for dysplasia (H&E, ×200). (*B*) Clonal-appearing areas of diffuse, strong staining in keeping with a *TP53* missense mutation adjacent to areas of weak, patchy, wild-type pattern staining (×200).

in patients with systemic disease, recognition of the neuroendocrine phenotype directs the initiation of appropriate platinum-based small cell chemotherapy.

IMMUNOHISTOCHEMICAL FEATURES

Commonly used markers for the distinction of esophageal adenocarcinoma from SCC include

Fig. 1. (*C*) BE with atypia largely confined to the crypt region, referred for consideration of "indefinite for dysplasia versus low-grade dysplasia" (H&E, ×200). (*D*) Columnar epithelium with complete absence of staining in keeping with a large deletion or truncating mutation (right two-thirds) abruptly transitioning to wild-type pattern staining (left one-third) (×200). The results in both cases favor a diagnosis of dysplasia.

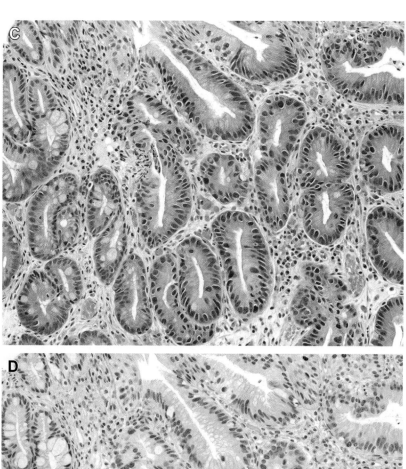

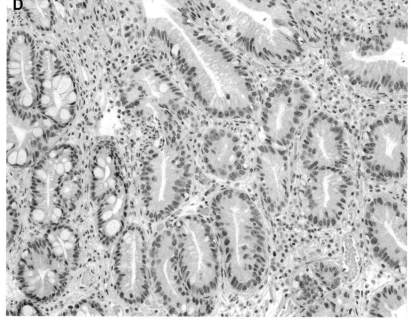

p63, CK5/6, and CDX2. The general neuroendocrine markers, chromogranin and synaptophysin, can be added if a NEC component is in question. In especially poorly differentiated tumors, immunostains for broad-spectrum keratins (eg, AE1/AE3 and CAM5.2) are appropriate. Histochemical stains for mucin (eg, PAS-D and mucicarmine) may also be applied, but in poorly differentiated tumors, mucin, if present at all, is typically quite focal. Although p63 and CK5/6 are both incredibly sensitive for the diagnosis of SCC (vs adenocarcinoma), specificity, especially for CK5/6, is less than perfect.[13,14] CDX2 is only reasonably sensitive for the diagnosis of adenocarcinoma (quoted by the editor of this issue as "40% in biopsies, 60% in resections"), and I was surprised to learn in reading for this review that it is expressed in up to 20% of esophageal SCCs and that staining can be intense.[13–15] Based on the results of a recent study, I would consider substituting MUC5AC (the gastric foveolar mucin core protein) for CDX2 as the positive adenocarcinoma marker in this differential (expressed in 64% of 69 adenocarcinomas vs 2% of 41 SCCs).[14]

PITFALLS

I have encountered 3 main pitfalls in this setting:

1. Assuming the specificity of the commonly used markers
2. Confusion regarding the immunophenotype of extrapulmonary visceral NECs
3. Incorrect interpretation of the results of so-called adenocarcinoma markers, in particular MOC-31

The first of these pitfalls has been adequately addressed. I have seen pathologists unfamiliar with the diagnosis of primary esophageal NEC assume the lesion is metastatic from lung and apply thyroid transcription factor-1 (TTF-1) IHC to support their impression. Although TTF-1 is expressed by the vast majority of small cell lung carcinomas (approximately 80%–90%), it is also frequently expressed by extrapulmonary examples (approximately 35%), especially esophageal tumors (60%–70%).[12,16]

MOC-31, one of several MoAbs to the transmembrane glycoprotein epithelial cell adhesion molecule (EpCAM), has, based on its performance in the selected differential diagnoses of (1) mesothelioma versus adenocarcinoma and (2) hepatocellular carcinoma (HCC) versus

---

> ## Pitfalls
> ### IMMUNOHISTOCHEMISTRY IN POORLY DIFFERENTIATED ESOPHAGEAL CARCINOMA
>
> ! p63 and especially CK5/6 are occasionally expressed by esophageal adenocarcinomas.
>
> ! CDX2 positivity is seen in up to 20% of esophageal SCCs.
>
> ! TTF-1 positivity is often seen in extrapulmonary visceral poorly differentiated NECs and does not imply a lung origin.
>
> ! MOC-31 expression is not confined to adenocarcinomas; it is frequently seen in SCCs and poorly differentiated NECs.

---

adenocarcinoma (discussed later), gained an undue reputation as an adenocarcinoma marker. I frequently see MOC-31 applied to the adenocarcinoma versus SCC differential (at diverse anatomic sites). Ironically, MOC-31 was initially raised against a small cell lung carcinoma cell line,[17] and, although data are somewhat limited, expression is not uncommon in SCC. For example, Pai and West[18] reported MOC-31 expression in 5 of 5 pulmonary and 3 of 4 esophageal SCCs.

DISTINGUISHING PRIMARY FROM METASTATIC POORLY COHESIVE CARCINOMAS IN THE STOMACH

CLINICAL OVERVIEW

Primary gastric adenocarcinomas present as 2 main histologic types, a dyshesive one (diffuse-type in the Laurén classification and poorly cohesive in the World Health Organization 2010 classification) and a gland-forming one (intestinal-type in the Laurén classification and tubular, papillary, or mucinous in the World Health Organization 2010 classification).[19] Similarly, breast cancer occurs as dyshesive (lobular) and gland-forming (ductal) types. Although stage and grade

---

> ### Differential Diagnosis
> #### IMMUNOPHENOTYPE OF POORLY COHESIVE GASTRIC CANCER VERSUS METASTATIC LOBULAR BREAST CANCER
>
> | | Poorly Cohesive Gastric Cancer, % (n) | Metastatic Lobular Breast Cancer, % (n) |
> |---|---|---|
> | CDX2 | 78 (42/54) | 0 (0/51) |
> | Estrogen receptor (ER) | 0 (0/58) | 76 (42/55) |
> | Hepatocyte paraffin 1 (Hep Par 1) | 83 (25/30) | 0 (0/21) |
> | GCDFP-15 | 0 (0/28) | 76 (26/34) |
> | MUC1 | 20 (10/51) | 100 (27/27) |
> | MUC2 | 51 (40/79) | 13 (8/60) |
> | MUC5AC | 54 (43/79) | 5 (3/60) |
> | MUC6 | 35 (17/49) | 10 (4/39) |
> | CK7 | 66 (38/58) | 100 (21/21) |
> | CK20 | 53 (31/58) | 5 (1/20) |
> | E-cadherin (intact) | 57 (17/30) | 29 (6/21) |
>
> Data from Refs.[20–22]

Diagnostic Algorithm: Poorly Cohesive Gastric Cancer Versus Metastatic Lobular Breast Cancer

- Primary panel to include
  - CDX2 (gastric cancer marker)
  - ER (breast cancer marker)
- Additional useful markers, if the primary panel markers are negative
  - Hep Par 1, MUC5AC, and CK20 (gastric cancer markers)
  - GCDFP-15, mammaglobin, and GATA3 (breast cancer markers)
- Generally not useful in this setting
  - E-cadherin

are more important than tumor type in determining patient prognosis and therapy, dyshesive and gland-forming lesions have unique biologies. While gland-forming tumors tend to metastasize hematogenously (eg, to liver and lung), dyshesive ones have a propensity to spread transperitoneally to involve the gastrointestinal (GI) tract, peritoneal surfaces, and ovaries. Thus, secondary gastric involvement by invasive lobular breast carcinoma (LBC) is not an especially uncommon occurrence, and I encounter at least a couple examples in my practice each year. Diffuse-type/poorly cohesive gastric cancer and metastatic LBC are not readily separable on the H&E, and failure to recognize a tumor as metastatic can have serious clinical consequences (a patient undergoes a gastrectomy instead of receiving appropriate medical [antiestrogenic] therapy). Before levying a diagnosis of diffuse-type/poorly cohesive gastric cancer, especially in women, I always consider the possibility of a metastasis and seek out a histologic context in keeping with gastric cancer (eg, gastritis, *Helicobacter* infection). I have a low threshold for ordering immunostains in this setting, which are well suited to the distinction of these 2 tumor types.

IMMUNOHISTOCHEMICAL FEATURES

My primary immunopanel in this diagnostic context consists of antibodies to CDX2 and ER. The former is positive in up to 80% of gastric cancers, although staining is typically weaker and less extensive than in colon cancer, and it is negative in LBC.[20,21] ER immunostains are positive in approximately three-quarters of LBCs and are nearly always negative in gastric cancers (**Fig. 2**) (discussed

later). If both markers are negative, additional useful immunostains include Hep Par 1, MUC5AC, and CK20 (each expressed in half to three-quarters of dyshesive gastric cancers and rarely, if ever, in LBC) as well as GCDFP-15, mammaglobin, and GATA3 (positive breast cancer markers).[20–22] Although absent E-cadherin expression is seen in most LBCs, it is also common in dyshesive gastric cancers (seen in just under half), such that it is not an especially useful marker in this context.[20]

PITFALLS

The biggest pitfall in this setting is failing to recognize a metastasis. Beyond this, I have encountered a misconception about the specificity of ER immunostains that may potentially interfere with diagnosis—namely that ER is expressed by 15% of gastric cancers. As is often the case in diagnostic IHC, the specificity lies in the clone. In studies published in the late 1980s and throughout the 1990s, including more than 400 gastric and esophageal adenocarcinomas, the frequency of ER positivity with the rat MoAb H222 was closer to 30%, whereas rates in more contemporary series using the mouse MoAbs 1D5 and 6F11 (tested in a similar number of tumors) are less than 1%.[23] Rabbit MoAbs are increasingly used, and some concern has been raised as to their specificity.[24] To this end, I recently tested 160 gastric cancers with the anti-ER rabbit MoAb SP1, none (0%) of which were reactive.

Pitfalls
POORLY COHESIVE GASTRIC CANCER VERSUS METASTATIC LOBULAR BREAST CANCER

! Metastatic lobular breast cancer can perfectly simulate primary poorly cohesive gastric cancer.

! There is no significant ER expression by gastric cancers using the ID5, 6F11, and SP1 clones.

PREDICTION OF RESPONSE TO ANTI-HER2 THERAPY IN GASTROESOPHAGEAL ADENOCARCINOMAS

CLINICAL OVERVIEW

HER2, although most familiar in the context of breast cancer, was known to be overexpressed at a similar frequency in gastric cancer.[25]

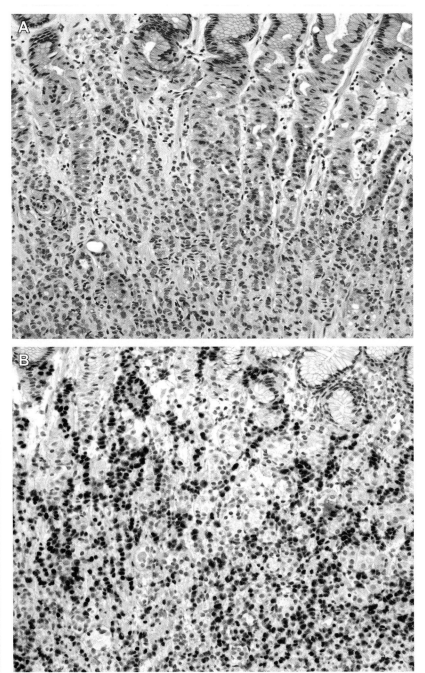

Fig. 2. Poorly cohesive carcinoma in the stomach—primary versus metastatic. (*A*) Cellular infiltrate disposed as single cells surrounding and merging with the gastric glands (H&E, ×200). (*B*) Tumor cells express ER (and not CDX2—not depicted), supporting a diagnosis of metastatic breast cancer (×200). The patient had undergone a mastectomy and received chemotherapy for breast cancer 15 years prior.

Furthermore, trastuzumab (Herceptin) had shown efficacy in preclinical models of gastric cancer. These findings, combined with the only modest efficacy of existing medical therapies, were the impetus behind the conduct of an international, phase 3, open-label, randomized controlled trial comparing trastuzumab plus standard chemotherapy (fluoropyrimidine + cisplatin) versus chemotherapy alone in advanced (ie, locally advanced, metastatic, or recurrent) gastric and gastroesophageal junction (GEJ) adenocarcinomas (Trastuzumab for Gastric Cancer [ToGA] trial).[26] For the purpose of the trial, tumors were tested by both HER2 IHC and fluorescence in situ hybridization (FISH), and patients with an IHC score of 3+ (positive) or who were HER2 FISH positive (defined here as HER2:centromeric probe 17 ratio ≥2) were randomized. Among 3807 tumors screened for enrollment, HER2 positivity was found in 20.9% of gastric and 33.2% of GEJ tumors. The addition of trastuzumab in HER2-positive patients improved median survival by 2.7 months (13.8 months vs 11.1 months). Based on this positive study, HER2 testing has become standard of care in patients with advanced gastric and GEJ adenocarcinomas who are candidates for trastuzumab. The National Comprehensive Cancer Network has further extended this recommendation to patients with esophageal adenocarcinomas.[27]

HER2 IMMUNOHISTOCHEMISTRY

In the ToGA trial, the survival benefit from trastuzumab was even greater in patients with IHC 3+ or IHC 2+/FISH-positive tumors (4.2 months), whereas patients with HER2 amplification in the absence of protein overexpression (IHC 0/1+) derived no survival benefit. These results served to establish HER2 IHC as the first-line test, with FISH primarily reserved for IHC 2+ (equivocal) cases.

There are 3 key differences between HER2 IHC testing in gastroesophageal and breast cancer. These are based, in part, on observations made in the context of a validation study performed in anticipation of the ToGA trial.[28] The group observed more frequent HER2 heterogeneity (areas of positive and negative staining) in gastroesophageal tumors than had been seen in breast tumors (**Fig. 3**). They also noted several cases of basolateral (U-shaped) or lateral membrane staining, some of which were HER2 amplified. Because of heterogeneity, there are different scoring criteria for biopsies and resections (key difference 1); in a biopsy specimen, any amount of 2+ staining warrants FISH, whereas any 3+ staining is considered positive (one group has suggested the need of at least 5 cells staining to improve reproducibility). Because of cases with biologically significant (ie, HER2-amplified) basolateral and lateral membrane staining, the strict requirement of complete membrane staining, as seen with breast cancer, is relaxed (key difference 2). For resections, the threshold for significant reactivity is 10% or greater (ie, staining of any intensity in less than 10% of tumor cells is considered 0/negative), whereas in the 2007 American Society of Clinical Oncology/College of American Pathologists HER2 breast guideline, the threshold is 30% or greater (key difference 3) (see review on this topic by Davison and Pai elsewhere in this issue).[29]

PITFALLS

Errors in interpretation are mainly due to failure to apply the gastroesophageal-specific HER2 IHC

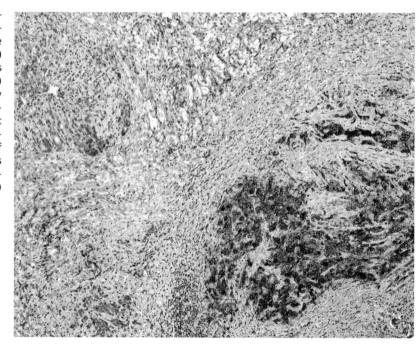

Fig. 3. HER2 IHC in gastroesophageal adenocarcinoma. Strong, complete membrane staining (3+) (*right side*) alternates with faint staining (1+) (*left side*). Heterogeneity is seen more often in gastroesophageal than breast tumors. Given strong reactivity in 10% or more of tumor cells, tumor in this resection is given an overall score of 3+ (positive) (×100).

Diagnostic Algorithm: HER2 Immunohistochemistry Scoring Criteria in Gastroesophageal Adenocarcinoma

Biopsy	Resection	Score	Interpretation
No reactivity	No reactivity or reactivity in <10% of tumor cells	0	Negative
Tumor cell cluster with faint/barely perceptible reactivity (ie, only discernible at 40×)	Faint/barely perceptible reactivity in ≥10% of tumor cells	1+	Negative
Tumor cell cluster with weak to moderate reactivity (ie, discernible at 10×–20×)	Weak to moderate reactivity in ≥10% of tumor cells	2+	Equivocal (reflex to FISH testing)
Tumor cell cluster with strong reactivity (ie, visible with the naked eye or discernible at 2.5×–5×)	Strong reactivity in ≥10% of tumor cells	3+	Positive

Note: significant reactivity includes complete, lateral, or basolateral membrane staining; in one study, a tumor cell cluster was defined as ≥5 cells.

criteria. Rüschoff and colleagues[29] have also emphasized staining in foci of intestinal metaplasia, false staining due to edge artifact, and nonspecific nuclear and cytoplasmic staining as potential sources of a false-positive result. The College of American Pathologists now offers proficiency testing for gastroesophageal HER2 IHC.

Pitfalls
INTERPRETATION OF HER2 IMMUNOHISTOCHEMISTRY IN GASTROESOPHAGEAL ADENOCARCINOMA

! HER2 immunohistochemistry scoring criteria are different in gastroesophageal and breast cancers.

! In gastroesophageal adenocarcinoma, there are different scoring criteria for biopsies and resections.

! The threshold for significant reactivity in gastroesophageal resections (≥10%) is lower than in breast specimens (≥30%).

! In gastroesophageal adenocarcinomas, in addition to complete membrane staining, basolateral and lateral membrane staining should be considered.

DIAGNOSIS OF SERRATED COLON POLYPS

CLINICAL OVERVIEW

For the first 2 decades of endoscopic mucosal biopsy diagnosis there existed 2 main classes of colon polyps: adenomas, the main precursor lesion of colorectal cancer (CRC); and hyperplastic polyps (HPs), trivial, benign lesions of the distal colon. Throughout the 1970s and 1980s, however, rare cases of dysplasia and carcinoma arising in association with HPs were reported, and in 1990, an additional polyp type, the serrated adenoma, was born.[30] The subsequent 2-plus decades have seen the unraveling of the serrated pathway of colorectal neoplasia. Today, the sessile serrated adenoma/polyp (SSA/P) is the recognized precursor of sporadic high-level microsatellite unstable (MSI-H) CRC (discussed later). Lu and colleagues[31] recently reported a longitudinal outcome study of SSA/P, in which the risk of subsequent colon cancer in the subset of patients originally diagnosed with HPs (between 1980 and 2001) in whom polyps were reclassified as SSA/P was nearly 7 times higher than in control groups with either hyperplastic or adenomatous polyps. A National Institutes of Health–sponsored expert panel has issued surveillance guidelines for patients with serrated polyps.[32] The SSA/P is considered an adenoma equivalent, with the diagnosis triggering a 5-year surveillance interval, whereas the presence of 3 or more polyps or any

Pathologic Key Features: Sessile Serrated Adenoma/Polyp Versus Hyperplastic Polyp

Sessile Serrated Adenoma/Polyp	Hyperplastic Polyp
Typically right sided	Typically rectosigmoid colon
Often >5 mm	Usually <5 mm
Serration/crypt dilatation involving full thickness of lesion	Serration/crypt dilatation confined to upper half of lesion
Transverse-lying and anchor-shaped crypts	Crypts oriented perpendicular to muscularis mucosae
Mucous cells in crypt bases	Progressive mucus accumulation toward the surface
Mitotic figures in upper crypt region	Mitotic figures confined to crypt bases
BRAF V600E mutation	*BRAF* V600E mutation (in microvesicular subtype)
Frequent CpG island methylation	Infrequent CpG island methylation

polyp 1 cm or larger in size prompts a 3-year interval. In the face of 2 or more SSA/Ps 1 cm or larger, an interval of 1 to 3 years is recommended. Thus, the recognition of SSA/P has significant prognostic and management implications. Unfortunately, the reproducibility of the diagnosis of SSA/P is only fair to moderate, even among GI pathologists, which is not surprising given that the lesion exists in a morphologic continuum with HP.[33]

MUC6 IMMUNOHISTOCHEMISTRY

In 2008, Owens and colleagues[34] published a stunning result—expression of the gastric pyloric gland mucin core protein MUC6 perfectly distinguished SSA/P (33 of 33 positive) from HP (0 of 48 positive) and traditional serrated adenoma (0 of 13 positive). Although other groups have consistently shown the preferential expression of MUC6 in SSA/P relative to HP, the findings have been less dramatic. Collectively, MUC6 expression has been noted in 71% of 237 SSA/Ps (including 44 cases with cytologic dysplasia), 23% of 277 HPs, and 9% of 124 traditional serrated adenomas.[34–38] Expression is confined to the crypt bases, and the percentage of crypts staining may vary widely from case to case (**Fig. 4**). I occasionally request a MUC6 immunostain when evaluating challenging serrated polyps, particularly in the left colon, where the diagnosis of SSA/P is uncommon and where superimposed mucosal prolapse complicates assessment of

Differential Diagnosis
MUC6 EXPRESSION IN SERRATED COLON POLYPS

Study	Sessile Serrated Adenoma/Polyp, % (n)	Sessile Serrated Adenoma/Polyp with Cytologic Dysplasia, % (n)	Hyperplastic Polyp, %, (n)	Traditional Serrated Adenoma, % (n)	Conventional Adenoma, % (n)
Mochizuka et al,[35] 2007	76 (22/29)	NE	27 (4/15)	0 (0/12)	6 (1/16)
Owens et al,[34] 2008	100 (26/26)	100 (7/7)	0 (0/48)	0 (0/13)	NE
Bartley et al,[36] 2010	53 (23/43)	NE	17 (16/92)	18 (2/11)	NE
Fujita et al,[37] 2010	39 (20/51)	NE	17 (11/65)	4 (3/72)	NE
Gibson et al,[38] 2011	91 (40/44)	84 (31/37)	60 (34/57)	38 (6/16)	43 (15/35)
Totals	68 (131/193)	86 (38/44)	23 (65/277)	9 (11/124)	31 (16/51)

Note: all 5 studies used the anti-MUC6 MoAb CLH5.
Abbreviation: NE, not evaluated.

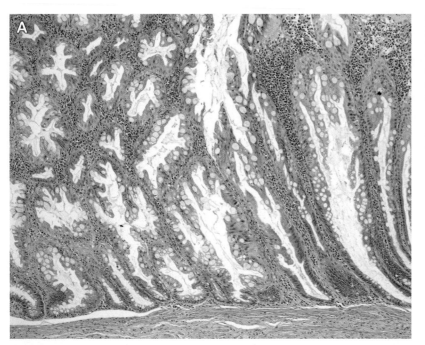

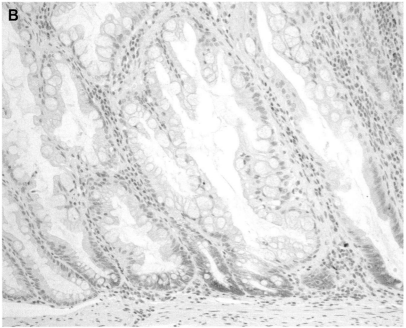

Fig. 4. MUC6 in serrated polyps. (*A*) Serrated polyp with serration/crypt dilatation involving full thickness of the lesion and with goblet cells noted in crypt bases (H&E, ×100). (*B*) MUC6 is expressed by cells in the crypt bases, seen more often with SSA/P than with HP (×200).

the architectural features critical to the distinction of SSA/P from HP.[39]

ASSESSMENT OF MISMATCH REPAIR FUNCTION IN COLORECTAL CANCERS

CLINICAL OVERVIEW

Genomic instability is a hallmark of cancer. CRCs are broadly divided into those that demonstrate chromosomal instability (85%) and those that demonstrate microsatellite instability (MSI) (15%). The latter of these groups is the focus of this section. MSI is a phenotypic consequence of deficient DNA mismatch repair (MMR) function (one of several DNA repair mechanisms). The MMR apparatus recognizes mispaired bases and insertion-deletion loops and directs their repair. Failure of this mechanism leads to accumulation of innumerable point and frameshift mutations, fertile soil for neoplastic progression. MMR deficiency (dMMR) occurs as sporadic and hereditary forms. In sporadic MSI tumors (approximately 15% of all CRCs) dMMR is due to transcriptional silencing of *MLH1* via promoter hypermethylation. Lynch syndrome (LS),

> ### Pathologic Key Features: Colon Cancers with Deficient Mismatch Repair Function
>
> Right sided
>
> Well or poorly differentiated
>
> Mucinous, signet ring cell, or medullary histology
>
> Heterogeneous histologic patterns
>
> Prominent tumor-infiltrating lymphocytes
>
> Prominent Crohn-like reaction
>
> Pushing border

accounting for 2% to 4% of all CRCs, is an autosomal dominant hereditary cancer syndrome in which dMMR is due to germline mutations in the MMR genes *MLH1*, *PMS2*, *MSH2*, or *MSH6* (and rarely due to *EPCAM* deletions and exceptionally due to *MLH1* or *MSH2* epimutations).[40] Characteristics of the LS phenotype include early cancer onset, tumor multiplicity (synchronous and

Diagnostic Algorithm: Mismatch Repair Function Testing in Colorectal Cancers

Immunohistochemistry Result	Frequency	Interpretation	Action(s)
All 4 proteins intact	80%–85%	Normal MMR function Unlikely LS	Consider follow-up MSI testing to confirm normal result Refer to Cancer Genetics if clinically appropriate
MLH1/PMS2 lost MSH2/MSH6 intact	15%	Abnormal MMR function Likely sporadic dMMR due to *MLH1* promoter methylation Less likely LS due to *MLH1* (usually) or *PMS2* (rarely) mutation	*BRAF* V600E and/or *MLH1* promoter methylation testing If above are normal: Refer to Cancer Genetics *MLH1* mutation testing (followed by *PMS2* if needed)
MSH2/MSH6 lost MLH1/PMS2 intact	1%–2%	Abnormal MMR function Likely LS due to *MSH2* (usually) or *EPCAM* deletion or *MSH6* mutation (rarely)	Refer to Cancer Genetics *MSH2* mutation testing (followed by *EPCAM* and *MSH6* if needed)
MSH6 lost MLH1/PMS2/MSH2 intact	Up to 0.5%	Abnormal MMR function Likely LS due to *MSH6* (usually) or *MSH2* (rarely) mutation	Refer to Cancer Genetics *MSH6* mutation testing (followed by *MSH2* if needed)
PMS2 lost MLH1/MSH2/MSH6 intact	Up to 0.5%	Abnormal MMR function Likely LS due to *PMS2* (usually) or *MLH1* (rarely) mutation	Refer to Cancer Genetics *PMS2* mutation testing (followed by *MLH1* if needed)

metachronous tumors), and occurrence of extracolonic tumors at defined anatomic sites (including endometrium, stomach, ovary, hepatobiliary tree, upper urinary tract, small intestine, skin [sebaceous neoplasms], and brain [gliomas]).

Identification of patients with LS is desirable because it may have an impact on cancer management (eg, patients with CRC due to LS are advised to undergo subtotal colectomy), directs appropriate surveillance (eg, intensive colonoscopy and endometrial sampling), and, perhaps most importantly, facilitates the detection of affected family members. Identification of all dMMR CRCs (including the much larger group of sporadic tumors) has also become desirable because dMMR is associated with superior stage-for-stage survival (hazard ratio 0.65) relative to MMR-proficient tumors as well as a lack of benefit from 5-fluorouracil–based chemotherapy (reviewed by Bellizzi[25]). Medical oncologists are increasingly incorporating the results of MMR testing into their decision making regarding recommending adjuvant chemotherapy in patients with high-risk stage II (lymph node negative) CRC.

Tumors with dMMR are identified using MMR IHC or MSI testing (a molecular diagnostic test). The 2 tests may be used singly or in combination, and their performance characteristics regarding identifying LS are similar (greater than 90% sensitive).[25,40] Concerning which tumors to test, a variety of strategies exist. Until recently, the principal goal was to identify LS. This is the basis of clinical criteria (eg, revised Bethesda guidelines) and use of an age-based cutoff (eg, less than 50 years old). Given prognostic and especially therapeutic relevance, the thrust of testing is shifting toward identifying all dMMR tumors. Histology-based prediction models (taking advantage of the characteristic histologic features shared by sporadic and hereditary dMMR tumors) perform well in this setting. Examples include the MsPath,[41] MSI Probability,[42] and PREDICT models.[43] Universal testing (ie, testing all new CRCs) is gaining traction. This strategy has been officially endorsed by the Evaluation of Genomic Applications in Practice and Prevention Working Group[44] and the Association for Molecular Pathology,[45] the former of which has also published a favorable cost-effectiveness analysis. At the University of Iowa Hospitals and Clinics, my colleagues and I have adopted an MMR-IHC–based universal testing strategy.

MISMATCH REPAIR PROTEIN IMMUNOHISTOCHEMISTRY

The MMR proteins function as heterodimers, with MSH2-MSH6 recognizing the replication error

and MLH1-PMS2 directing the repair. Each heterodimer is composed of a dominant (expressed regardless of the status of its partner) and dependent (not expressed in the absence of its partner) protein. MLH1 and MSH2 are dominant, whereas PMS2 and MSH6 are dependent. This results in 5 main patterns of MMR IHC (nuclear) staining:

1. All 4 proteins expressed
2. Loss of MLH1/PMS2; intact MSH2/MSH6
3. Loss of MSH2/MSH6; intact MLH1/PMS2
4. Loss of MSH6; intact MLH1/PMS2/MSH2
5. Loss of PMS2; intact MLH1/MSH2/MSH6

Pattern 2 is seen with sporadic *MLH1* promoter hypermethylation (usually) or LS due to an *MLH1* mutation (occasionally). Molecular testing that takes advantage of phenotypic characteristics of sporadic MSI-H tumors, including *BRAF* mutation analysis and *MLH1* promoter methylation testing, are useful in this distinction. Patterns 3 through 5 are nearly always LS, due to *MSH2*, *MSH6*, and *PMS2* mutations, respectively (**Fig. 5**). This can be confirmed with mutation analysis. Although the majority of LS mutations (approximately 95%) destabilize the protein, leading to absent expression, in up to 5% nonfunctional protein is still detected (pattern 1). Thus, given a strong clinical suspicion despite a normal IHC result, follow-up MSI testing should be considered.

Absent protein expression in LS requires silencing of the wild-type allele and, in sporadic neoplasms, meeting some critical threshold of *MLH1* promoter methylation. Both of these may occur before invasion. Absent MMR protein expression is seen in approximately two-thirds of adenomas in LS patients.[40] Although it tends to correlate with polyp size and the presence of high-grade dysplasia, it may be seen in polyps as small as a few millimeters. In SSA/P, neoplastic progression manifests morphologically as superimposed cytologic dysplasia (**Fig. 6**A). I order an MLH1 immunostain in lesions I am otherwise certain are SSA/Ps in 2 diagnostic contexts:

1. To evaluate a focus indeterminate for reactive change versus superimposed cytologic dysplasia
2. In fragmented specimens in which it is unclear whether an adenomatous focus in the same tissue block as an SSA/P represents a separate adenoma versus superimposed cytologic dysplasia

Although I am unaware of the frequency of MLH1 loss in SSA/P with superimposed low-grade cytologic dysplasia (and I suspect it may be infrequent) (see **Fig. 6**B), it is not uncommon

Fig. 5. MMR IHC—LS. (*A*) Low-grade adenocarcinoma with frequent tumor-infiltrating lymphocytes arising in the cecum of a 73-year-old man (H&E, ×200). (*B*) PMS2 is not expressed by tumor cells, with normal expression in lymphocytes and stromal cells (×200). (*C*) Intact expression of MLH1 (depicted), MSH2, and MSH6 (×200). The results support a diagnosis of LS due to *PMS2* mutation.

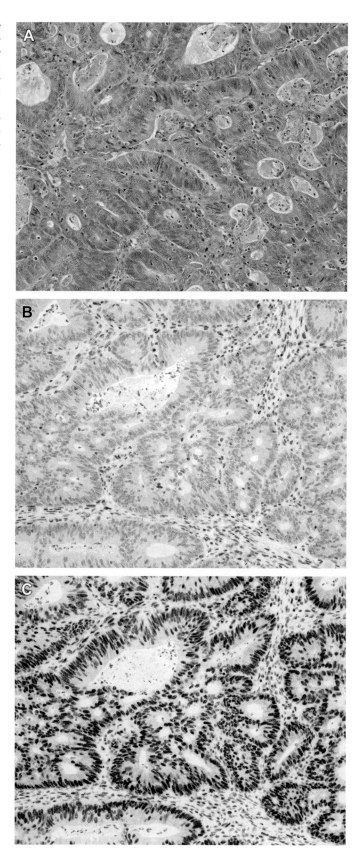

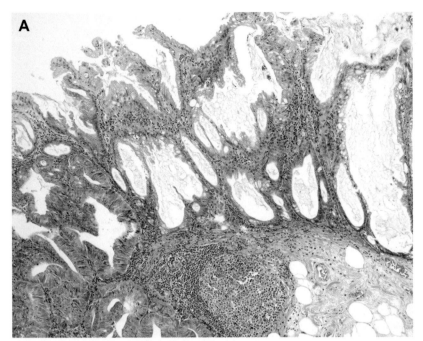

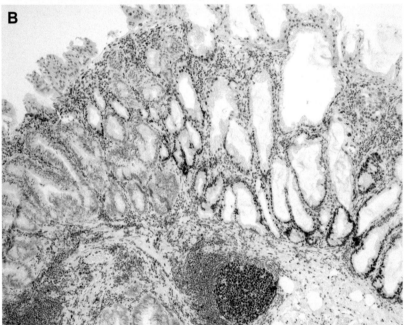

Fig. 6. MLH1 in SSA/P. (*A*) SSA/P (*right side*) abruptly transitions to adenomatous-appearing area (*left side*) (H&E, ×100). (*B*) MLH1 expression is intact in the background SSA/P but lost in the superimposed cytologic dysplasia due to transcriptional silencing of the gene by promoter hypermethylation (×100). This polyp type is the precursor of sporadic, MSI-H colon cancers.

with superimposed high-grade dysplasia and early invasive carcinoma. Regardless, it is certainly specific, and it has helped me on a few occasions. Owens and colleagues[34] reported absent MLH1 expression in 5 of 7 SSA/Ps with cytologic dysplasia, which was confined to areas of high-grade dysplasia or carcinoma. Sheridan and colleagues[46] reported absent MLH1 expression in 7 of 11 SSA/Ps with superimposed cytologic dysplasia or early invasive carcinoma, including 1 (of 1) case of SSA/P with low-grade cytologic dysplasia.

PITFALLS

MMR proteins should generally be interpreted as intact (expressed) or lost (not expressed). In most instances, I interpret any definite nuclear staining as probably normal. In tissue sections, especially from resections, staining is occasionally weak and/or heterogeneous. This is probably attributable to variability in fixation, because expression in biopsy specimens has been shown to be more strongly uniform.[47] Several groups have observed diminution in staining intensity for all 4 markers and, especially for MSH6, in rectal cancers status post–neoadjuvant chemoradiotherapy (**Fig. 7**A, B). Furthermore, in this setting, MSH6 expression may be concentrated in the nucleolus (see **Fig. 7**C).

Pitfalls
INTERPRETATION OF MISMATCH
REPAIR PROTEIN
IMMUNOHISTOCHEMISTRY

! Staining is occasionally weak/heterogeneous, especially in resection specimens; any definite nuclear staining should be interpreted as intact (normal).

! There is reduced expression of all 4 markers, especially MSH6, in rectal cancers status post–neoadjuvant chemoradiotherapy.

EMERGING MARKER—*BRAF* V600E-SPECIFIC IMMUNOHISTOCHEMISTRY

A mouse MoAb specific for the *BRAF* V600E mutant protein has recently become commercially available (VE1; Spring Bioscience, Pleasanton, California). A few groups have published near-perfect to perfect sensitivity and specificity in a couple hundred CRCs.[48–50] All 3 of these successes made use of a Ventana autostainer (Tucson, Arizona). By comparison, a group using manual staining (which was favored over the weak staining seen with a Dako autostainer [Carpinteria, California]) reported a sensitivity and specificity of only 71% and 74%, respectively, in 52 tumors and observed weak staining in 17% of *KRAS*-mutant and 35% of wild-type cases.[51] Another group, having published in abstract form, achieved perfect sensitivity/specificity in 76 tumors but noted that the antibody had a "narrow range for optimal conditions" and that "repeat attempts to optimize the staining by manual processing did not generate reproducible results."[52] Like the first 3 groups, their success came on a Ventana autostainer. Similar positive studies have been published in papillary thyroid carcinoma and melanoma.[53,54] In laboratories that are able to successfully implement *BRAF* V600E-specific IHC, advantages include faster turnaround time and possibly superior analytical sensitivity. As alluded to previously, its key application in neoplastic GI pathology is in the distinction of sporadic from LS-associated MLH1-deficient CRCs.

DIAGNOSIS OF WELL-DIFFERENTIATED HEPATOCELLULAR LESIONS

CLINICAL OVERVIEW

Well-differentiated hepatocellular lesions include regenerative nodule, focal nodular hyperplasia (FNH), hepatocellular adenoma (HA), dysplastic

Pathologic Key Features/Differential Diagnosis: Focal Nodular Hyperplasia Versus Hepatocellular Adenoma Versus Well-Differentiated Hepatocellular Carcinoma

Focal Nodular Hyperplasia	Hepatocellular Adenoma	Well-Differentiated Hepatocellular Carcinoma
Central scar	Isolated arterioles	May have adenoma-like vascular pattern
Fibrous bands containing malformed vessels and with peripheral bile ductular proliferation	Inflamed portal-like areas, peliosis (inflammatory/telangiectatic subtype) Prominent steatosis (HNF1α-inactivated subtype) Cytologic atypia, pseudoglands (BCAT-activated subtype)	Small cell change (ie, increased nucleus:cytoplasm ratio) Mitotic activity
Absent portal areas	Absent portal areas	Absent portal areas
1–2 cell–thick cell plates (reticulin stain)	2–3 cell–thick cell plates (reticulin stain)	Thickened cell plates (reticulin stain)

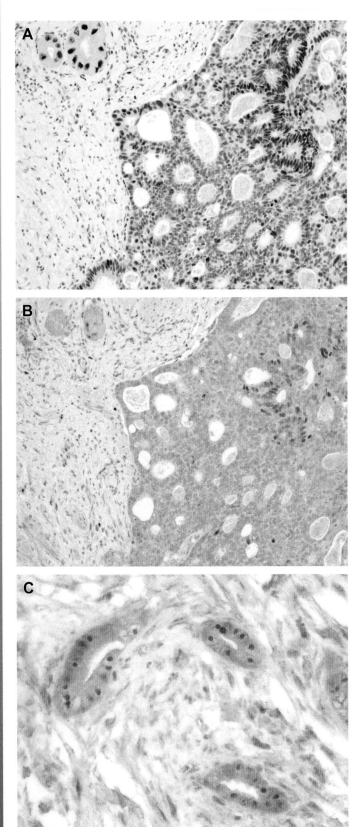

Fig. 7. MMR IHC after neoadjuvant chemoradiation. (*A*) Uniform, strong PMS2 expression in a treated rectal cancer (×200). (*B*) MSH6 expression, detected in only a few tumor nuclei, should be interpreted as intact (×200). (*C*) In some cases, MSH6 expression is dot-like/nucleolar (×600), which should also be interpreted as intact. MSH6 IHC in pretreatment biopsies from these patients showed uniform, strong staining (not depicted).

Diagnostic Algorithm: Well-Differential Hepatocellular Lesions

Differential Diagnosis	Stain	Result → Interpretation
Benign vs malignant	Reticulin	Intact → Benign
		Diminished → Malignant
	GPC3	Negative → Benign
		Positive → Malignant
If benign, proceed to		
Regenerative nodule vs FNH vs HA	CD34	Areas of diffuse staining → favors FNH or HA
	GS	Map-like pattern → FNH
If hepatocellular adenoma, consider subtyping		
Inflammatory/telangiectatic vs HNF1α-inactivated vs BCAT-activated vs unclassified	GS	Diffuse staining → BCAT-activated
	If GS-positive:	
	SAA and/or CRP	Positive → combined BCAT-activated–inflammatory/telangiectatic
		Negative → pure BCAT-activated
	If GS-negative:	
	SAA and/or CRP	Positive → inflammatory/telangiectatic
	L-FABP	Lost → HNF1α-inactivated
		Both sets of markers normal → unclassified

Abbreviations: CRP, C-reactive protein; GPC3, glypican-3; GS, glutamine synthetase; L-FABP, liver fatty acid–binding protein; SAA, serum amyloid A.

nodule, and well-differentiated HCC. While HA is a benign neoplasm associated with a significant risk of hemorrhage and some risk of progression to HCC, warranting extirpation, FNH, an exaggerated hyperplastic response to localized increased arterial flow, is not associated with these risks. FNH need not be excised, and, given a confident diagnosis, no long-term follow-up is necessary. It was classically taught that the distinction of these lesions on core biopsy was treacherous and that, in particular, the distinction of FNH from HA nearly impossible. Improved ability to positively identify FNH on small biopsies would spare patients a surgery from which they would not derive benefit. Prompt diagnosis of HA and well-differentiated HCC triages patients to appropriate therapy.

A multi-institutional French group has unified and extended several previous observations, resulting in a new molecular-based classification of HAs.[55] HA subtypes include HNF1α-inactivated, inflammatory/telangiectatic, β-catenin (BCAT)-activated, and unclassified tumors. BCAT-activated tumors are associated with an increased risk of concurrent or subsequent HCC. Some HNF1α-inactivated tumors arise in the setting of a germline mutation, which was known to cause maturity-onset diabetes

of the young type 3. Inflammatory/telangiectatic HAs were previously considered variants of FNH and are now recognized as neoplastic.

IMMUNOHISTOCHEMICAL FEATURES—BENIGN VERSUS MALIGNANT

In the noncirrhotic liver, HCC must be distinguished from background liver, FNH, and HA, whereas in the cirrhotic liver, the main distinctions are from dysplastic and regenerative nodules. Histologic features of HCC include increased nucleus:cytoplasm ratio (ie, small cell change) and mitotic activity. Reticulin staining may reveal thickened cell plates. Traditional diagnosis can be supplemented with IHC for CD34, GPC3, GS, and heat shock protein-70 (HSP70).

CD34 is normally expressed by the endothelium lining hepatic artery and portal vein branches and central veins and is restricted to sinusoidal endothelium extending along the first few hepatocytes emanating from the limiting plate (so-called inflow pattern) (**Fig. 8**A). HCC is characterized by a phenotypic alteration of its sinusoidal endothelium (capillarization of the sinusoids), resulting in (re) expression of CD34. Although areas of diffuse

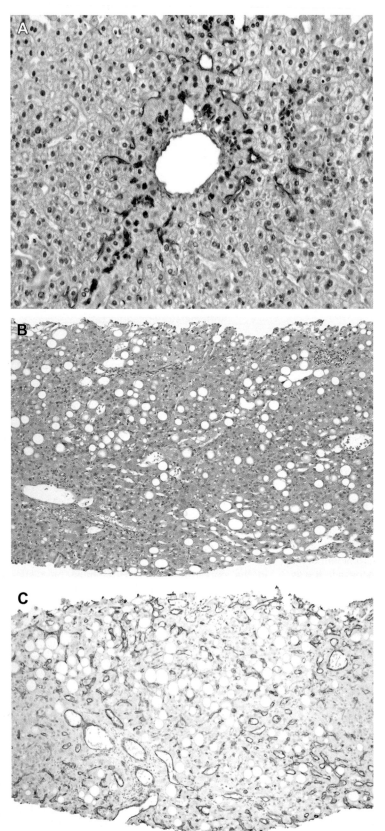

Fig. 8. CD34 in well-differentiated hepatocellular lesions. (*A*) In the liver, CD34 is normally expressed by endothelium lining portal vein and hepatic artery branches and central veins; expression by sinusoidal endothelium abruptly ceases at a distance of a few hepatocytes from the limiting plate (×200). (*B*) This core biopsy of a clinical mass lesion was referred questioning whether the lesion had been sampled and asking for comment on probable fatty liver disease (H&E, ×100). (*C*) Diffuse sinusoidal CD34 staining in this case confirms sampling of a mass lesion, which was favored for an HNF1α-inactivated HA (×100).

staining are common in HA and even FNH, limiting its application in the benign versus malignant differential, in my experience, it is useful in separating lesional from nonlesional liver, especially in limited samples (see **Fig. 8**B, C).[56]

GPC3 is a glycosyl phosphatidylinositol–linked cell surface heparan sulfate proteoglycan that is highly expressed in embryonic liver and re-expressed in many HCCs (ie, it is an oncofetal protein). Staining is detected in approximately 60% of well-differentiated HCCs, variably in dysplastic nodules, rarely in regenerative nodules, and not at all in FNH and HA.[57–60] Expression is cytoplasmic with membranous or canalicular pattern accentuation.

GS and HSP70 were both identified as HCC markers through gene expression profiling. GS catalyzes the formation of glutamine from glutamate and ammonia. In normal liver, GS expression (cytoplasmic) is limited to hepatocytes immediately adjacent to the central vein (**Fig. 9**A). HSP70 participates in protein folding and, as with p53, increased expression is induced by cellular stresses. It is strongly anti-apoptotic. Nuclear and cytoplasmic staining is normally seen in bile duct epithelium and oval cells. In hepatocytes, areas of diffuse GS expression and any HSP70 expression are considered abnormal. A recent prospective study of these markers in 60 cirrhotics with solitary liver nodules less than 2 cm demonstrated the following test characteristics for a diagnosis of HCC: GS 50% sensitive and 90% specific; HSP70 57.5% sensitive and 85% specific.[61]

IMMUNOHISTOCHEMICAL FEATURES—FOCAL NODULAR HYPERPLASIA

Areas of map-like, anastomosing GS expression are characteristic of FNH (see **Fig. 9**B, C), reliably demonstrated even in core biopsies.[62] This is believed to occur secondary to BCAT activation unrelated to *CTNNB1* (the gene encoding BCAT) mutation.[63] This pattern of GS staining must be distinguished from normal staining of pericentrivenular hepatocytes and diffuse staining seen in BCAT-activated HAs (discussed later) and some HCCs.

IMMUNOHISTOCHEMICAL FEATURES—HEPATOCELLULAR ADENOMA SUBTYPING

HNF1α-inactivated HAs are characterized by absent L-FABP expression (an HNF1α downstream target), with intact expression in background liver. Inflammatory/telangiectatic HAs overexpress SAA and CRP, with lack of significant expression in non-tumor liver (**Fig. 10**). GS is a downstream target of BCAT, and overexpression is seen in the setting of *CTNNB1*-activating mutations. Diffuse

GS expression has been shown to be a more reliable marker of BCAT-activated HAs than BCAT IHC itself.[62] HAs with intact L-FABP staining and lack of SAA, CRP, or GS overexpression are unclassified. Occasional HAs share a combined inflammatory/telangiectatic and BCAT-activated phenotype.

PITFALLS

Abdul-Al and colleagues[64] reported GPC3 expression in 25 of 30 (83%) cases of chronic hepatitis C with high-grade inflammatory activity and 0 of 30 (0%) low-grade cases. GS and HSP70 overexpression are not limited to hepatocellular tumors, and, thus, unlike GPC3, they are not applicable to determining the site of origin of a carcinoma. GS and HSP70 expression were recently reported in most intrahepatic cholangiocarcinomas (ICCs) (76% and 88%, respectively) and tumors metastatic to the liver (71% and 88%, respectively).[65]

> ## Pitfalls
> ### INTERPRETATION OF GLYPICAN-3, GLUTAMINE SYNTHETASE, AND HEAT SHOCK PROTEIN-70 IMMUNOHISTOCHEMISTRY
>
> ! GPC3 expression may be seen in severely active hepatitis.
>
> ! GS and HSP70 expression are frequently seen in non-hepatocellular carcinomas.

EMERGING MARKERS—GLUTAMINE SYNTHETASE, HSP70, L-FABP, SAA, AND CRP

Aside from CD34 and possibly GPC3, all of the markers discussed in the previous section can be considered emerging markers. GPC3 is also an excellent marker of hepatoblastomas and non-seminomatous germ cell tumors, in particular yolk sac tumors. Of the remaining immunostains, GS is arguably the most important given its usefulness in distinguishing HCC from benign, establishing a confident diagnosis of FNH, and subtyping HAs.

DETERMINATION OF TUMOR TYPE IN POORLY DIFFERENTIATED LIVER TUMORS

CLINICAL OVERVIEW

At the opposite end of the differentiation spectrum, HCC must be reliably distinguished from ICC and metastatic adenocarcinoma. Patients with chronic liver disease and early-stage HCC may be candidates for liver transplantation, while this therapy is not pursued in ICC outside of

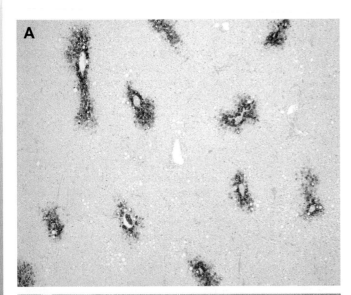

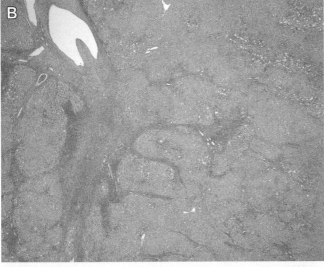

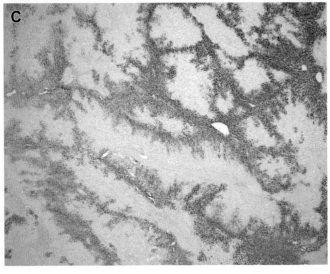

Fig. 9. GS in well-differentiated hepatocellular lesions. (*A*) GS expression in normal liver is restricted to pericentrivenular hepatocytes (×40). (*B*) Well-differentiated hepatocellular lesion with a central scar containing malformed vessels dissecting surrounding liver (H&E, ×20). (*C*) Map-like, anastomosing GS expression supports the diagnosis of FNH (×20).

Fig. 10. SAA in inflamma-
tory/telangiectatic   HA.
(*A*)   Well-differentiated
hepatocellular   lesion
with prominent sinusoi-
dal dilatation, congestion,
parenchymal hemorrhage
and   easily   identified
isolated   arterioles (H&E,
×100). (*B*) SAA is overexpressed in the adenoma
(*top*) relative to adjacent
normal   liver   (*bottom*)
(×40).

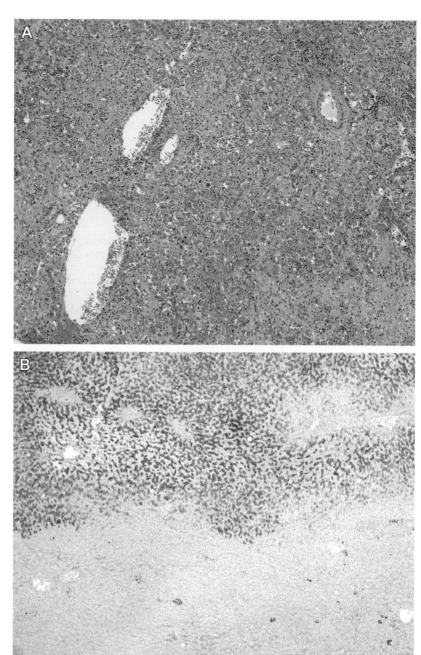

Differential Diagnosis
Immunophenotype of Hepatocellular Carcinoma Versus Adenocarcinoma

	Hepatocellular Carcinoma	Adenocarcinoma
Hep Par 1	>80%	Occasional
Polyclonal carcinoembryonic antigen (pCEA) (canalicular pattern)	60%–90%	−
CD10 (canalicular pattern)	50%	−
AFP	30%–50%	Rare
GPC3	60%–90%	Occasional
MOC-31	Occasional	80%–100%

− indicates negative.

Data from Kakar S, Gown AM, Goodman ZD, et al. Best practices in diagnostic immunohistochemistry: hepatocellular carcinoma versus metastatic neoplasms. Arch Pathol Lab Med 2007;131(11):1648–54.

Diagnostic Algorithm: Hepatocellular Carcinoma Versus Adenocarcinoma

- Primary panel to include
  - Hep Par 1 (HCC marker)
  - MOC-31 (non-HCC marker)
- Consider substituting arginase 1 (Arg-1) for Hep Par 1 in this primary panel
- Additional useful markers in this differential include
  - GPC3, canalicular pCEA or CD10 (HCC markers)
  - Claudin-4 (non-HCC marker)
- Additional IHC to distinguish tumor type/site of origin indicated if MOC-31 (claudin-4) positive/Hep Par 1 (Arg-1) negative

antigen, the urea cycle enzyme, carbamoyl phosphate synthetase I, is a mitochondrial protein, explaining the granular, cytoplasmic staining with this immunostain.[69] TTF-1 cross-reactivity with this same antigen is the basis of cytoplasmic staining in some HCCs. GPC3 is also relevant to this differential. One potential advantage of this marker is its possibly increased sensitivity in poorly differentiated HCCs (89% in one series) relative to Hep Par 1 (63%).[59] This immunopanel is complemented by markers expressed in adenocarcinoma and generally not in HCC, including MOC-31 and claudin-4 (1 of 24 members of the claudin family, which represent key components of tight junctions) (see later discussion of the immunophenotype of metastatic adenocarcinoma).

PITFALLS

Pathologists occasionally lose sight of the fact that canalicular staining for pCEA and CD10 and Hep

clinical trials. Treatment of metastatic tumors is determined by site of origin.

IMMUNOHISTOCHEMICAL FEATURES

Traditional HCC markers include AFP, pCEA, and CD10.[66] AFP is limited by poor sensitivity, and weak, patchy cytoplasmic staining may be difficult to interpret.[67] pCEA stains HCCs in a canalicular pattern, attributable to cross-reactivity with biliary glycoprotein.[68] CD10 demonstrates a similar staining pattern. Although pCEA is generally favored over CD10 due to its superior sensitivity, CD10 staining is often cleaner. Hep Par 1 was first described 20-years ago and over the past decade has become a mainstream HCC marker. Its target

Pitfalls
Interpretation of Immunohistochemistry in Poorly Differentiated Liver Tumors

! Only canalicular pCEA/CD10 staining is specific for hepatocellular differentiation.

! Hep Par 1 is occasionally expressed by non-hepatocellular tumors, especially gastric and small intestinal adenocarcinomas and adrenal cortical tumors.

! GPC3 staining is often seen in SCCs and melanomas (30%) and may occasionally be seen in adenocarcinomas.

ΔΔ
Differential Diagnosis
IMMUNOPHENOTYPE OF CELLULAR EPITHELIOID NEOPLASMS OF THE PANCREAS

	Pancreatic Neuroendocrine Tumor	Solid-Pseudopapillary Neoplasm	Acinar Cell Carcinoma	Pancreatoblastoma
Broad-spectrum keratins	+	70%	+	+
Synaptophysin	95%	20%–70%	30% (scattered cells)	80%
Chromogranin	90%	Rare +	30% (scattered cells)	80%
Trypsin	Scattered cells	Rare +	95%	95%
BCAT (nuclear)	<5%	>95%	10%	>90%

+ indicates positive.

Par 1 expression only suggest the presence of hepatocellular differentiation; they do not distinguish benign from malignant. For pCEA and CD10, attention to the pattern of staining is critical, because most adenocarcinomas demonstrate cytoplasmic and/or membranous positivity for pCEA, whereas non-canalicular staining for CD10 is seen in several other tumor types, including lymphomas, carcinomas (especially renal cell carcinoma [RCC]), and sarcomas. Hep Par 1 expression is occasionally detected in non-hepatocellular tumors, notably adenocarcinomas of the stomach (discussed previously) and small intestine (the antibody also highlights non-neoplastic small intestinal epithelium) and adrenal cortical tumors, among others.[20,70,71] GPC3 positivity is described in approximately 30% of SCCs and melanomas, and I have seen this result in diagnostic errors. Expression in non-seminomatous germ cell tumors was discussed previously. Similar to Hep Par 1, staining is occasionally detected in adenocarcinomas.[72,73] The lack of perfect specificity for Hep Par 1 and GPC3 serves to highlight the importance of using a panel of immunostains in evaluating the HCC versus adenocarcinoma differential, which should include both positive and negative markers.

EMERGING MARKER—ARGINASE 1

Arg-1, another urea cycle enzyme, is the most recent addition to the HCC versus adenocarcinoma immunopanel. In 5 studies to date, its sensitivity for the diagnosis of HCC has ranged from 81% to 96% and, in these studies, Arg-1 incrementally but systematically

outperformed Hep Par 1 as an HCC maker by a factor of approximately 1.15.[74] As with Hep Par 1 and GPC3, Arg-1 is occasionally expressed by adenocarcinomas, although perhaps somewhat less frequently.

DIAGNOSIS OF CELLULAR EPITHELIOID NEOPLASMS OF THE PANCREAS

CLINICAL OVERVIEW

Cellular epithelioid neoplasms of the pancreas are characterized grossly by solid or solid and cystic

Diagnostic Algorithm: Diagnosis of Cellular Epithelioid Neoplasms of the Pancreas

- Primary panel to include

  ○ Broad-spectrum keratin (highly expressed in PNET, ACC, and PB; focally expressed in SPN)

  ○ Synaptophysin (highly expressed in PNET and PB; may be focally expressed in SPN and ACC)

  ○ Chromogranin (highly expressed in PNET and PB; focally expressed in ACC)

  ○ Trypsin (highly expressed in ACC and PB)

  ○ BCAT (cytoplasmic/nuclear expression is nearly universal in SPN and PB)

- E-cadherin may substitute for BCAT in this panel if the latter is unavailable growth and cytomorphologically by monomorphism and relative dyscohesion. This group of tumors includes pancreatic neuroendocrine tumor (PNET), solid-pseudopapillary neoplasm (SPN), acinar cell carcinoma (ACC), and pancreatoblastoma (PB). Of these, PNET is the most familiar (and the most common), and the other cellular epithelioid neoplasms are frequently misdiagnosed as PNET. Accurate tumor classification is prognostically and therapeutically important, with tumors in this class ranging from rarely metastasizing (SPN) to frankly malignant (ACC). A directed panel of immunohistochemical stains successfully classifies nearly all cases.

IMMUNOHISTOCHEMICAL FEATURES

When faced with a cellular epithelioid neoplasm of the pancreas, my immunopanel includes a broad-spectrum keratin, synaptophysin, chromogranin, trypsin, and BCAT, although I may not apply each of these in every case. PNETs are characterized by expression, typically strong, of broad-spectrum keratins and general neuroendocrine markers. SPNs variably stain with different keratin antibodies, and expression may be weak and patchy. Weak/patchy synaptophysin staining may also be observed, although chromogranin expression has only rarely been reported. The immunophenotypic hallmark of SPN is cytoplasmic and nuclear staining for BCAT, seen in greater than 95% of tumors (**Fig. 11**A, B). In non-neoplastic tissues, BCAT IHC demonstrates membranous staining, reflecting the protein's function in cell-cell adhesion. As with the BCAT-activated HAs (discussed previously), cytoplasmic and nuclear staining is a consequence of *CTNNB1*-activating mutations, which impede normal BCAT degradation.[75] BCAT accumulates in the cytoplasm and translocates to the nucleus, where it interacts with T-cell factor/lymphoid enhancer factor family transcription factors to activate target genes. Cytoplasmic and nuclear staining for BCAT has only been reported in a rare PNET, is seen in approximately 10% of ACCs, and is also characteristic of PB (greater than 90%). Expression of pancreatic exocrine enzymes typifies ACC; trypsin IHC is most commonly used.[76] One-third of tumors demonstrate scattered neuroendocrine cells. Rare biphasic tumors composed of greater than 30% neuroendocrine cells are classified as mixed acinar-neuroendocrine carcinomas. PB is a primitive, polyphenotypic tumor typically occurring in children (**Fig. 12**A). The diagnosis is suggested by the presence of squamoid nests. *CTNNB1* mutations have been described in approximately half

of cases, and even tumors without detectable mutations usually demonstrate cytoplasmic and nuclear BCAT staining, which tends to concentrate in the morular areas (see **Fig. 12**B).[77] Expression of broad-spectrum keratins, general neuroendocrine markers (see **Fig. 12**C), and pancreatic exocrine enzymes (see **Fig. 12**D) is also typical.

PITFALLS

As stated in the clinical overview, most errors in diagnosis relate to misclassifying SPN, ACC, or PB as PNET. For SPN, staining for synaptophysin is sometimes responsible. This favors the additional application of chromogranin, which is only rarely expressed in SPN. Perhaps the most useful protection against incorrect diagnosis is a low threshold for BCAT staining, with cytoplasmic and nuclear staining usually indicating SPN. The recognition of ACC and PB requires a high index of suspicion. ACC resembles PNET but with disappointing results on synaptophysin and chromogranin IHC, suggesting the possibility of an alternative diagnosis and prompting trypsin staining. PB also resembles PNET, with the incorrect morphologic impression corroborated by typically strong expression of the general neuroendocrine markers. As with SPN, cytoplasmic and nuclear expression of BCAT suggests the correct diagnosis, which can be further supported with a positive trypsin stain.

Pitfalls
CELLULAR EPITHELIOID
NEOPLASMS OF THE PANCREAS

! SPN, ACC, and PB are each not uncommonly misdiagnosed as PNETs.

! All of these tumor types may stain with general neuroendocrine markers, especially synaptophysin.

EMERGING MARKER—E-CADHERIN

E-cadherin is perhaps less of an emerging marker than it is an immunostain with an emerging application. Of all the dyscohesive pancreatic cellular epithelioid neoplasms, SPN is the most dyscohesive. Investigators had hypothesized that diminished E-cadherin function would contribute to this phenotype, and this proved correct. Antibodies that recognize E-cadherin's extracellular

Fig. 11. SPN. (*A*) Monomorphous epithelioid lesion with ependymoma-like relationship between tumor cells and small vessels (H&E, ×200). (*B*) Cytoplasmic and nuclear BCAT staining in keeping with a *CTNNB1*-activating mutation; normal membranous staining in background pancreas noted at left (×200). (*C*) Abnormal E-cadherin staining (absent with antibodies to the protein's extracellular domain) is also characteristic of this tumor type; again, background pancreas demonstrates intact membranous staining (×400).

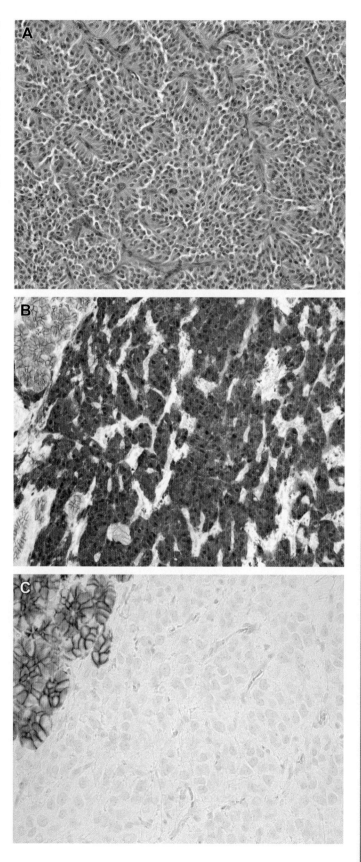

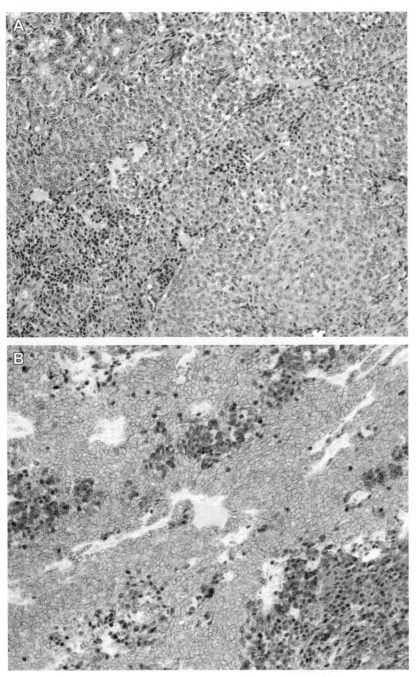

Fig. 12. PB. (*A*) Cellular epithelioid tumor, predominantly sheet-like but with foci of ductal (*upper left*) and morular (*upper center, lower right*) growth (H&E, ×200). (*B*) Areas of abnormal cytoplasmic/nuclear BCAT staining alternate with those with normal, membranous staining (×200).

domain show complete absence of staining in SPN (see **Fig. 11**C), whereas those that bind to its cytoplasmic domain demonstrate nuclear staining.[78] This aberrant E-cadherin staining is sensitive and specific for the diagnosis of SPN (among the cellular epitheloid neoplasms), which is especially applicable to those laboratories that do not have BCAT IHC on their test menu.

DETERMINING SITE OF ORIGIN OF NEUROENDOCRINE TUMORS OF UNKNOWN PRIMARY

CLINICAL OVERVIEW

Well-differentiated neuroendocrine epithelial neoplasms (ie, neuroendocrine tumors [NETs]) are

Fig. 12. (*C*) Chromogranin and (*D*) trypsin expression are also characteristic of this tumor type (each ×200). This case was originally diagnosed as a neuroendocrine tumor based on the extensive chromogranin staining.

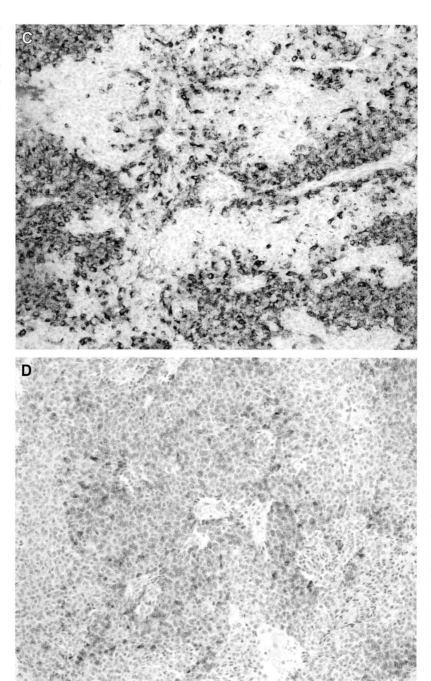

encountered at most anatomic sites, although gastroenteropancreatic and lung primaries predominate. Metastases of unknown primary are common, representing 10% to 20% of all NETs in contemporary series.[16,79] Determining the site of origin is therapeutically critical. For example, although medical treatment in patients with metastatic midgut (ie, jejunoileal and appendiceal) tumors is largely limited to the somatostatin analog, octreotide, patients with pancreatic tumors have been shown to additionally benefit from streptozocin (alkylating agent) and, more recently, temozolomide (alkylating agent), everolimus (mTOR inhibitor), and sunitinib (multiple

Differential Diagnosis
△△ IMMUNOPHENOTYPE OF WELL-DIFFERENTIATED NEUROENDOCRINE TUMORS BY SITE OF ORIGIN

	Lung (%)	Jejunoileum (%)	Pancreas (%)	Rectum (%)
TTF-1	30	<1	<1	<1
CDX2	<5	90	15	30
pPAX8	5	<1	60	60
Islet 1	10	<5	75	85
PDX1	5	<1	55	10
NESP55	5	<1	50	10

Abbreviation: pPAX8, polyclonal PAX8.
Data from Bellizzi AM. Assigning site of origin in metastatic neuroendocrine neoplasms: a clinically significant application of diagnostic immunohistochemistry. Adv Anat Pathol, in press.

tyrosine kinase inhibitor). For patients in whom conventional imaging modalities (eg, CT) fail to identify the primary, traditional somatostatin receptor imaging (ie, OctreoScan) performs surprisingly poorly (30%–40% sensitive).[80] Newer radionuclide tracers (eg, DOTA-NOC) coupled with improved scanning techniques hold promise for increased detection rates but are not widely available. A few off-the-shelf immunostains have been well vetted in this diagnostic context.

Diagnostic Algorithm: Assigning Site of Origin in Metastatic Well-Differentiated Neuroendocrine Tumors

- Primary panel to include
  - TTF-1 (lung origin)
  - CDX2 (midgut origin; may also be seen in pancreatoduodenal and rectal tumors)
  - Polyclonal PAX8 (pancreatoduodenal or rectal origin)
- Additional useful markers in this differential include
  - Islet 1 (pancreatoduodenal or rectal origin)
  - PDX1 (pancreatoduodenal origin)
  - NESP55 (pancreatoduodenal origin)

IMMUNOHISTOCHEMICAL FEATURES

When faced with a metastatic NET of unknown origin, my primary immunopanel includes TTF-1, CDX2, and polyclonal PAX8. TTF-1 positivity is incredibly specific (greater than 99%) although only modestly sensitive (30%) for assigning lung origin (**Fig. 13**).[16] These figures are based on staining with the widely used 8G7G3/1 clone. A few more recent studies have shown increased sensitivity with the SPT24 clone. Diffuse, strong CDX2 expression typifies midgut NETs (90% sensitive). CDX2 positivity is also seen in 15% of pancreatic and 30% of rectal tumors, which tends to be weaker and patchier. Polyclonal PAX8 IHC is positive in 60% of pancreatoduodenal and rectal tumors, whereas it is rarely and essentially never positive in lung and midgut tumors, respectively.

PITFALLS

I have seen pathologists extrapolate site-specific expression data for adenocarcinomas to NETs. Thus, many a CK7 and CK20 have been ordered in this setting despite limited utility, and comments that "CDX2 positivity in this tumor supports an intestinal primary" are often issued, when they should probably more specifically refer to the midgut. Regarding PAX8, choice of antibody is critical. Polyclonal PAX8 positivity in PNETs is likely due to cross-reactivity with PAX6 and possibly PAX4, and more recently developed PAX8 MoAbs are nonreactive.[81]

Pitfalls
IMMUNOHISTOCHEMISTRY TO ASSIGN SITE OF ORIGIN IN METASTATIC WELL-DIFFERENTIATED NEUROENDOCRINE TUMORS

- ! CK7 and CK20 are not especially useful in this diagnostic application.
- ! Diffuse, strong CDX2 positivity is typical of midgut tumors.
- ! Although polyclonal PAX8 is a good marker of pancreatoduodenal and rectal tumors, MoAbs are nonreactive.

EMERGING MARKERS—ISLET 1, PDX1, AND NESP55

Several other markers seem useful in this diagnostic context. Among the most promising are the transcription factors, Islet 1[82] and PDX1,[83]

Fig. 13. Well-differentiated neuroendocrine tumor—IHC to determine site of origin. (*A*) Biopsy of a hepatic metastasis of unknown origin demonstrates a tumor with amphophilic cytoplasm and fine chromatin growing in ribbon-like fashion (H&E, ×400). (*B*) TTF-1 expression in this neuroendocrine tumor suggests a lung origin; note also granular cytoplasmic staining in a few admixed hepatocytes (×400).

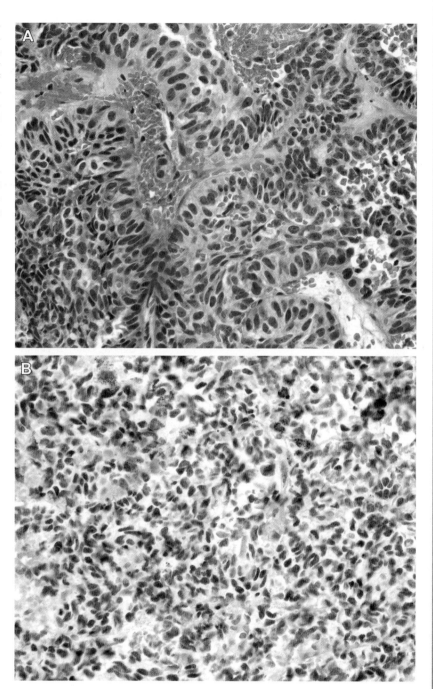

and the granin, NESP55.[84] Compared to polyclonal PAX8, Islet 1 boasts superior sensitivity for pancreatoduodenal or rectal origin (80%), although rare lung and midgut tumors are also positive. PDX1 and NESP55 perform similarly to polyclonal PAX8 regarding pancreatoduodenal tumors, with the distinct advantage that both are less often positive in rectal tumors (10%).

DETERMINING SITE OF ORIGIN OF ADENOCARCINOMAS

BROAD DIAGNOSTIC APPROACH

Use of IHC to determine tumor type and to suggest site of origin is a critical diagnostic application, with obvious impact on patient management. Before ordering IHC on any case, considerations include patient gender and age, the nature of tumor involvement (eg, anatomic site, solitary or multiple, small or large, and involving surface or tissue invasive), and, especially, the morphologic appearance of the tumor (eg, epithelial vs epithelioid vs spindled, monomorphous or polymorphous, and small or large cells). Main classes of tumors include

1. Carcinoma
2. Melanoma
3. Lymphoma
4. Sarcoma
5. Mesothelioma
6. Germ cell tumor
7. Non-epithelial neuroendocrine neoplasm

In particularly poorly differentiated neoplasms, the first 3 of these are often contemplated with a first-pass immunopanel including a broad-spectrum keratin, S-100, and leukocyte common antigen (the so-called big 3).

Carcinomas are grouped into

1. Squamotransitional (SCC and urothelial carcinoma)
2. Gland forming/mucin producing (adenocarcinoma)
3. Large polygonal cell (HCC, RCC, adrenal cortical carcinoma)
4. Neuroendocrine (NET and NEC)

The high sensitivity (and moderate specificity) of p63 and CK5/6 for SCC was discussed previously; urothelial carcinomas usually and often express these 2 markers, respectively (they also usually express the transcription factor GATA3 and often coexpress CK7 and CK20). Regarding the large polygonal cell tumors, in addition to the HCC markers reviewed previously, I often use PAX8 for RCC and some combination of melan-A (clone A103), inhibin, calretinin, and synaptophysin for adrenal cortical carcinoma. As discussed previously, TTF-1, CDX2, and polyclonal PAX8 are useful in assigning site of origin in NETs; IHC does not seem useful for this purpose in NECs (with the notable exception of the specificity of CK20 positivity for Merkel cell carcinoma).[16]

The site of origin of an adenocarcinoma must be distinguished in 2 main contexts—either presenting as metastatic carcinoma of unknown primary or at an anatomic site (eg, lung, bladder, uterine cervix, or ovary) where metastases, especially from the GI tract, exhibit significant morphologic overlap with a primary tumor type. In the first setting, carefully taking into account the clinicopathologic features as outlined previously, judicious application of a panel of immunostains with emphasis on those with greatest specificity for various tissue types is generally pursued. Many of these markers are transcription factors. Among my most widely used (ranked from most to least ordered) are the following:

- CDX2 (enteric differentiation)
- TTF-1 (lung or thyroid)
- ER and progesterone receptor (breast or Müllerian)
- PAX8 (kidney, Müllerian, or thyroid)
- p53 and WT-1 (serous carcinoma, with the latter also expressed by mesothelioma)

△△ *Differential Diagnosis*
CK7/CK20 COORDINATE EXPRESSION IN
GASTROENTEROPANCREATOBILIARY ADENOCARCINOMAS

	CK7−/CK20−	CK7+/CK20−	CK7+/CK20+	CK7−/CK20+
Esophagus	8% (7/85)	74% (63/85)	15% (13/85)	2% (2/85)
Stomach	14% (5/37)	19% (7/37)	32% (27/37)	35% (13/37)
Small intestine	0% (0/24)	33% (8/24)	67% (16/24)	0% (0/24)
Pancreas	3% (1/36)	28% (10/36)	64% (23/36)	6% (2/36)
Biliary tree	7% (1/14)	50% (7/14)	43% (6/14)	0% (0/14)
Colon	10% (6/60)	0% (0/60)	8% (5/60)	82% (49/60)

Data from Refs.[97–100]

- Napsin A (lung or papillary RCC)
- Prostate-specific antigen and prostatic acid phosphatase (prostate)

In the second setting, the resemblance of a potential metastasis to a primary tumor type often extends beyond morphology, as there may be substantial immunophenotypic overlap. Attention to the extent and intensity of immunoreactivity are important considerations in both these settings, but especially in the second. This review concludes with comment on the nature of CK7, CK20 (still the 2 most widely applied markers for assigning site of origin), and CDX2 expression in GI and pancreatobiliary tumors, especially as distinguished from expression of these same markers in tumors at potential metastatic sites.

CK7/CK20/CDX2 COORDINATE EXPRESSION

Colon

The classic CRC immunophenotype is CK7−/ CK20+/CDX2+ (seen in greater than 80%). CK20 and CDX2 expression are typically diffuse and strong. Up to 10% of CRCs are CK20−; many of these are poorly differentiated and/or MSI-H.[85,86] CDX2 expression is often intact in this subset, although staining may be focal. CK7+/CK20+ tumors similarly represent up to 10% of CRCs. This group is enriched in the rectum, where they comprise up to 25% of cases.[87] Second-line markers that have been used to suggest a colonic origin include BCAT (cytoplasmic and nuclear expression)[88,89] and α-methylacyl-CoA racemase (strong expression).[88,90]

Appendix

Non-neuroendocrine appendiceal epithelial neoplasms include invasive adenocarcinomas and low-grade appendiceal mucinous neoplasms (LAMNs) (**Fig. 14**A). Both tumor types characteristically demonstrate diffuse, strong CK20 (see **Fig. 14**B) and CDX2 staining. LAMNs tend to create the greatest diagnostic difficulty, because ruptured examples have a propensity to involve the ovaries, simulating OITMBTs. Reports of CK7 expression in LAMNs have varied from usually negative (see **Fig. 14**C)[91] to usually positive.[92] In cases where it is expressed, it can be strong. OITMBTs typically demonstrate diffuse, strong CK7 expression, whereas CK20 and CDX2 staining, if present at all, are characteristically weak and patchy. Key clinical features in the distinction of these 2 tumor types include tumor size and laterality. Bilateral ovarian involvement favors secondary spread, whereas large,

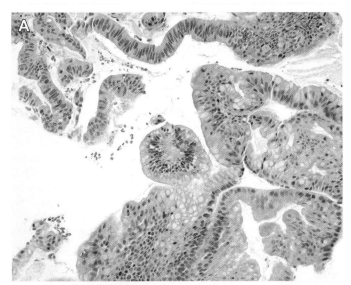

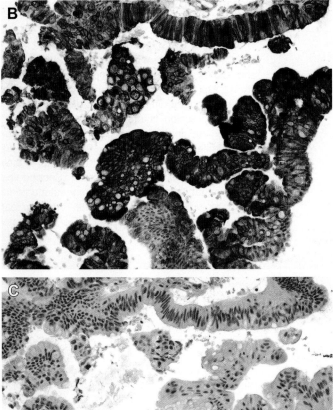

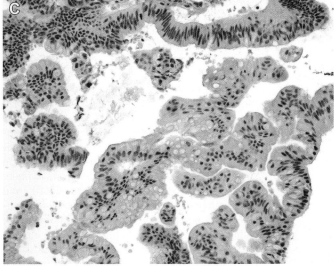

Fig. 14. CK7/CK20 coordinate expression—low-grade appendiceal mucinous neoplasm. (*A*) Strips of low-grade columnar epithelium with scattered goblet cells (H&E, ×200). (*B*) Extensive CK20 staining and (*C*) absent CK7 staining (each ×200). CDX2 expression (not performed) is expected to be diffuse and strong. This patient presented with a peritoneal recurrence 10-years after undergoing debulking for low-grade pseudomyxoma peritonei. At the time, the patient had been diagnosed with a mucinous borderline tumor, but the pattern of disease, morphology, and immunophenotype are most in keeping with an appendiceal origin. The patient had undergone remote appendectomy, the pathology of which was unavailable.

unilateral tumors (eg, greater than 13 cm) are typically primary.[93]

Pancreatobiliary Tree

Adenocarcinomas of the pancreatobiliary tree (ie, pancreatic ductal adenocarcinoma [PDA], extrahepatic cholangiocarcinoma, and ICC) usually demonstrate diffuse, strong CK7 expression. CK20 and CDX2 expression are variable, and when staining is present, it is often weak and patchy. Goldstein and Bassi[94] described CK20 positivity in 45% of pancreatobiliary tumors if any staining was considered positive, 30% of tumors at a threshold of greater than 25% cells staining, and 22% of tumors at a threshold of greater than 50%. Chu and colleagues[95] reported CDX2 positivity in 21% of ICCs and 22% of PDAs, with all positive cases demonstrating heterogeneous staining. For a strongly CK7+ adenocarcinoma presenting in the liver, a pancreatobiliary tumor is often a top consideration; the presence of weak, patchy CK20 or CDX2 staining lends further support. SMAD4 inactivation, reliably detected with SMAD4 IHC, is seen in half of PDAs and a smaller number of cholangiocarcinomas (and CRCs). Given a strong CK7+, weak CK20/CDX2+ tumor in the ovary, SMAD4 inactivation may favor a pancreatobiliary origin, because mucinous ovarian tumors are SMAD4 intact.[96]

Upper Gastrointestinal Tract

Although often conceived of as a CK7+/CK20+ group, the immunophenotype of adenocarcinomas of the upper GI tract is actually quite variable.[97,98] Distal gastric cancers are fairly evenly split among the 4 possible combinations of CK7/CK20 coordinate expression, with CK7−/CK20+ cases not uncommon. By comparison, in esophageal and GEJ tumors, the CK7+/CK20− group clearly predominates,[99] whereas small intestinal tumors are often CK7+/CK20+.[100] CDX2 is expressed in more than half of upper GI tract adenocarcinomas, although staining is generally neither as uniform nor as intense as in the colon or appendix.

Sites of Secondary Involvement

Sites of potential secondary involvement harboring primary tumor types with substantial morphologic overlap with GI and pancreatobiliary tumors include

1. Lung—mucinous adenocarcinoma in situ, invasive mucinous carcinoma, and enteric adenocarcinoma
2. Bladder and uterine cervix—each harboring intestinal-type adenocarcinomas

3. Ovary—mucinous carcinoma and OITMBT (**Fig. 15**A)

As a general rule, tumors at these sites demonstrate diffuse, strong CK7 staining (see **Fig. 15**B), distinguishing this group from most CRCs. CDX2, if it is expressed at all, is typically weak and patchy (see **Fig. 15**C, D), again in distinction to the homogenous, strong staining seen in most CRCs. The CK7/CK20/CDX2 immunophenotype of these tumors entirely overlaps with that seen in pancreatobiliary tree and upper GI tract tumors. Some of the primary lung tumors express TTF-1; in the uterine cervix p16 (driven by human papillomavirus) is often overexpressed, whereas in the ovary a minority may express PAX8.

PITFALLS

Errors in interpretation revolve around failure to recognize the diversity of CK7/CK20/CDX2 immunophenotypes seen in tubal gut and pancreatobiliary tumors. In addition, the well-documented infrequency of primary mucinous ovarian tumors relative to secondary involvement is still underappreciated in clinical practice.[93] One final tumor type is worthy of special note. Medullary carcinoma of the colon is an undifferentiated neoplasm nearly always showing MSI-H. It demonstrates circumscription at low power, is disposed as sheets of large cells with a syncytial quality (**Fig. 16**A), and contains large numbers of tumor-infiltrating lymphocytes. An intact precursor is rarely identified. Even more so than the typical MSI-H tumor, medullary carcinomas are especially

---

Pitfalls

CK7/CK20/CDX2 COORDINATE **E**XPRESSION IN **D**ETERMINING **S**ITE OF **O**RIGIN IN **A**DENOCARCINOMA

! Up to 10% of CRCs are CK20−, mainly poorly differentiated and MSI-H tumors.

! Up to 10% of CRCs are CK7+/CK20+, especially rectal tumors.

! Most cases of pseudomyxoma peritonei arise from ruptured low-grade appendiceal mucinous neoplasms.

! Metastasis should always be considered when evaluating a mucinous neoplasm in the ovary.

! Medullary carcinoma of the colon often deviates from the CK7−/CK20+/CDX2+ immunophenotype.

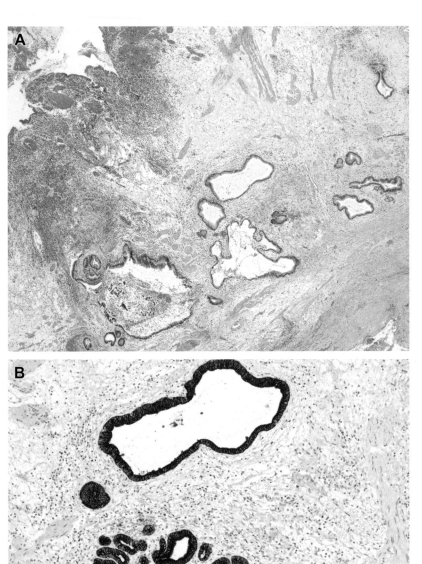

Fig. 15. CK7/CK20/CDX2 coordinate expression—mucinous ovarian neoplasm. (*A*) Metastatic adenocarcinoma involving the wall of the ureter; note inflamed urothelium at the upper left (H&E, ×40). (*B*) Diffuse, strong CK7 expression (×100).

prone to deviate from the CK7−/CK20+/CDX2+ immunophenotype (see **Fig. 16**B, C).[86] Given the odd histology, lack of identifiable precursor lesion, and atypical immunophenotype, examples are often incorrectly diagnosed as metastases. When the tumor type is considered, abnormal MMR IHC results support the diagnosis (see **Fig. 16**D).

Fig. 15. (*C*) Focal, weak CK20 expression; and (*D*) heterogeneous CDX2 expression (×100, ×200). This immunophenotype is in keeping with an ovarian, upper GI, or pancreatobiliary origin. In this case, the patient had undergone excision of a 15-cm, unilateral, ruptured mucinous ovarian tumor 6-years prior. Given an indolent biology and the distribution of disease at initial presentation, tumor in the current specimen is interpreted as spread from an ovarian origin.

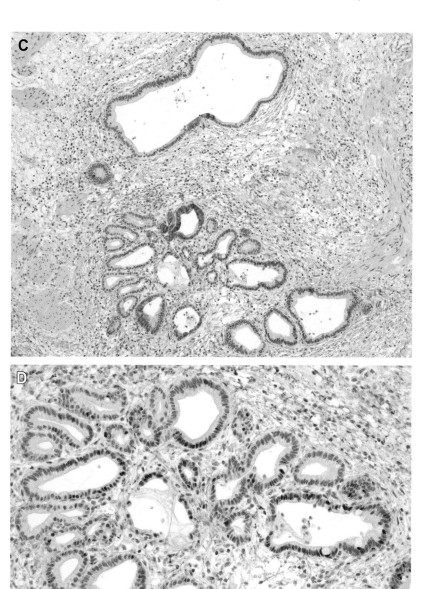

EMERGING MARKER—SATB2

Special AT-rich sequence-binding protein 2 (SATB2) is a homeodomain-containing transcription factor that forms part of the nuclear matrix and participates in epigenetic regulation through chromatin remodeling. In epithelial neoplasms, it has been proposed as a specific marker of colorectal origin.

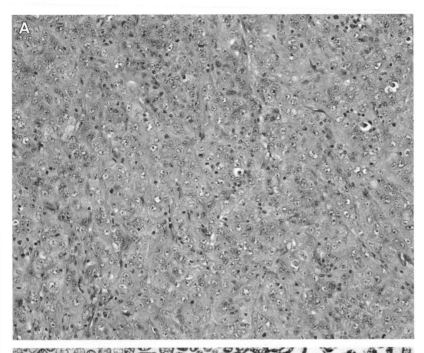

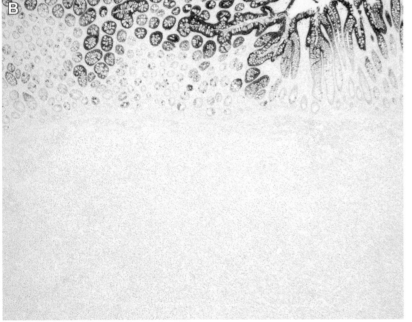

Fig. 16. Medullary carcinoma of the colon. (*A*) Undifferentiated carcinoma composed of sheets of large cells with vesicular chromatin (H&E, ×200). (*B*) The tumor fails to express CK20, with normal expression in overlying intestinal epithelium (×40).

Magnusson and colleagues[101] detected SATB2 expression in 86% of 1558 primary CRCs and 81% of 252 metastases. Gastric and pancreatic adenocarcinomas (25 of each) were uniformly negative (0%), as were 122 prostate cancers. A few breast (4%), ovarian (3%), lung (6%), and biliary tract (7%) carcinomas were positive. Interestingly, 5 of 9 (56%) sinonasal carcinomas expressed SATB2. Although additional studies are needed, SATB2 holds promise as a true lower GI tract marker.

Fig. 16. (*C*) CDX2 is focally, weakly expressed, which may not have been detected on a biopsy (×400). (*D*) MLH1 is not expressed by tumor nuclei, with intact expression by tumor-infiltrating lymphocytes and endothelium. This tumor type is often diagnosed as a metastasis by the unfamiliar.

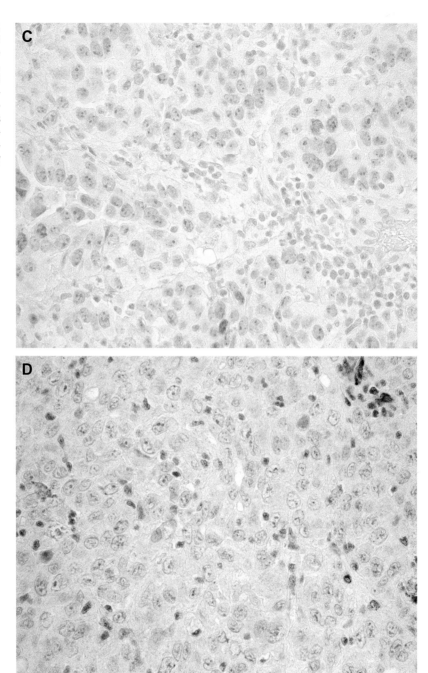

REFERENCES

1. Bhat S, Coleman HG, Yousef F, et al. Risk of malignant progression in Barrett's esophagus patients: results from a large population-based study. J Natl Cancer Inst 2011;103(13):1049–57.

2. Hvid-Jensen F, Pedersen L, Drewes AM, et al. Incidence of adenocarcinoma among patients with Barrett's esophagus. N Engl J Med 2011;365(15): 1375–83.

3. Montgomery E, Bronner MP, Goldblum JR, et al. Reproducibility of the diagnosis of dysplasia in

Barrett esophagus: a reaffirmation. Hum Pathol 2001;32(4):368–78.

4. Kaye PV, Haider SA, Ilyas M, et al. Barrett's dysplasia and the Vienna classification: reproducibility, prediction of progression and impact of consensus reporting and p53 immunohistochemistry. Histopathology 2009;54(6):699–712.

5. Weston AP, Banerjee SK, Sharma P, et al. p53 protein overexpression in low grade dysplasia (LGD) in Barrett's esophagus: immunohistochemical marker predictive of progression. Am J Gastroenterol 2001;96(5):1355–62.

6. Skacel M, Petras RE, Rybicki LA, et al. p53 expression in low grade dysplasia in Barrett's esophagus: correlation with interobserver agreement and disease progression. Am J Gastroenterol 2002; 97(10):2508–13.

7. Kastelein F, Biermann K, Steyerberg EW, et al. Aberrant p53 protein expression is associated with an increased risk of neoplastic progression in patients with Barrett's oesophagus. Gut 2012. [Epub ahead of print].

8. Nigro JM, Baker SJ, Preisinger AC, et al. Mutations in the p53 gene occur in diverse human tumour types. Nature 1989;342(6250):705–8.

9. Finlay CA, Hinds PW, Tan TH, et al. Activating mutations for transformation by p53 produce a gene product that forms an hsc70-p53 complex with an altered half-life. Mol Cell Biol 1988;8(2): 531–9.

10. Baas IO, Mulder JW, Offerhaus GJ, et al. An evaluation of six antibodies for immunohistochemistry of mutant p53 gene product in archival colorectal neoplasms. J Pathol 1994;172(1):5–12.

11. Kaye PV, Haider SA, James PD, et al. Novel staining pattern of p53 in Barrett's dysplasia–the absent pattern. Histopathology 2010;57(6):933–5.

12. Huang Q, Wu H, Nie L, et al. Primary high-grade neuroendocrine carcinoma of the esophagus: a clinicopathologic and immunohistochemical study of 42 resection cases. Am J Surg Pathol 2013; 37(4):467–83.

13. Long KB, Hornick JL. SOX2 is highly expressed in squamous cell carcinomas of the gastrointestinal tract. Hum Pathol 2009;40(12):1768–73.

14. DiMaio MA, Kwok S, Montgomery KD, et al. Immunohistochemical panel for distinguishing esophageal adenocarcinoma from squamous cell carcinoma: a combination of p63, cytokeratin 5/6, MUC5AC, and anterior gradient homolog 2 allows optimal subtyping. Hum Pathol 2012;43(11): 1799–807.

15. Borrisholt M, Nielsen S, Vyberg M. Demonstration of CDX2 is highly antibody dependant. Appl Immunohistochem Mol Morphol 2013;21(1):64–72.

16. Bellizzi AM. Assigning site of origin in metastatic neuroendocrine neoplasms: a clinically significant application of diagnostic immunohistochemistry. Adv Anat Pathol 2013;20(5):285–314.

17. Myklebust AT, Beiske K, Pharo A, et al. Selection of anti-SCLC antibodies for diagnosis of bone marrow metastasis. Br J Cancer Suppl 1991;14: 49–53.

18. Pai RK, West RB. MOC-31 exhibits superior reactivity compared with Ber-EP4 in invasive lobular and ductal carcinoma of the breast: a tissue microarray study. Appl Immunohistochem Mol Morphol 2009;17(3):202–6.

19. Lauwers GY, Carneiro F, Graham DY, et al. Gastric carcinoma. In: Bosman FT, Carneiro F, Hruban RH, et al, editors. World Health Organization Classification of Tumours WHO Classification of Tumours of the Digestive System. 4th edition. Lyon: IARC; 2010. p. 48–58.

20. Chu PG, Weiss LM. Immunohistochemical characterization of signet-ring cell carcinomas of the stomach, breast, and colon. Am J Clin Pathol 2004;121(6):884–92.

21. O'Connell FP, Wang HH, Odze RD. Utility of immunohistochemistry in distinguishing primary adenocarcinomas from metastatic breast carcinomas in the gastrointestinal tract. Arch Pathol Lab Med 2005;129(3):338–47.

22. Nguyen MD, Plasil B, Wen P, et al. Mucin profiles in signet-ring cell carcinoma. Arch Pathol Lab Med 2006;130(6):799–804.

23. Wei S, Said-Al-Naief N, Hameed O. Estrogen and progesterone receptor expression is not always specific for mammary and gynecologic carcinomas: a tissue microarray and pooled literature review study. Appl Immunohistochem Mol Morphol 2009;17(5):393–402.

24. Gomez-Fernandez C, Mejias A, Walker G, et al. Immunohistochemical expression of estrogen receptor in adenocarcinomas of the lung: the antibody factor. Appl Immunohistochem Mol Morphol 2010;18(2):137–41.

25. Bellizzi AM. Contributions of molecular analysis to the diagnosis and treatment of gastrointestinal neoplasms. Semin Diagn Pathol, in press.

26. Bang YJ, Van Cutsem E, Feyereislova A, et al. Trastuzumab in combination with chemotherapy versus chemotherapy alone for treatment of HER2-positive advanced gastric or gastro-oesophageal junction cancer (ToGA): a phase 3, open-label, randomised controlled trial. Lancet 2010;376(9742):687–97.

27. NCCN clinical practice guidelines in oncology. Esophageal and esophagogastric junction cancers. 2012 [7/12/12]; Version 2.2012. Available at: http://www.nccn.org/professionals/physician_gls/pdf/esophageal.pdf. Accessed July 12, 2012.

28. Hofmann M, Stoss O, Shi D, et al. Assessment of a HER2 scoring system for gastric cancer: results

from a validation study. Histopathology 2008;52(7): 797–805.

29. Rüschoff J, Dietel M, Baretton G, et al. HER2 diagnostics in gastric cancer-guideline validation and development of standardized immunohistochemical testing. Virchows Arch 2010;457(3):299–307.

30. Longacre TA, Fenoglio-Preiser CM. Mixed hyperplastic adenomatous polyps/serrated adenomas. A distinct form of colorectal neoplasia. Am J Surg Pathol 1990;14(6):524–37.

31. Lu FI, van Niekerk de W, Owen D, et al. Longitudinal outcome study of sessile serrated adenomas of the colorectum: an increased risk for subsequent right-sided colorectal carcinoma. Am J Surg Pathol 2010;34(7):927–34.

32. Rex DK, Ahnen DJ, Baron JA, et al. Serrated lesions of the colorectum: review and recommendations from an expert panel. Am J Gastroenterol 2012;107(9):1315–29 [quiz: 4, 30].

33. Farris AB, Misdraji J, Srivastava A, et al. Sessile serrated adenoma: challenging discrimination from other serrated colonic polyps. Am J Surg Pathol 2008;32(1):30–5.

34. Owens SR, Chiosea SI, Kuan SF. Selective expression of gastric mucin MUC6 in colonic sessile serrated adenoma but not in hyperplastic polyp aids in morphological diagnosis of serrated polyps. Mod Pathol 2008;21(6):660–9.

35. Mochizuka A, Uehara T, Nakamura T, et al. Hyperplastic polyps and sessile serrated 'adenomas' of the colon and rectum display gastric pyloric differentiation. Histochem Cell Biol 2007;128(5): 445–55.

36. Bartley AN, Thompson PA, Buckmeier JA, et al. Expression of gastric pyloric mucin, MUC6, in colorectal serrated polyps. Mod Pathol 2010;23(2): 169–76.

37. Fujita K, Hirahashi M, Yamamoto H, et al. Mucin core protein expression in serrated polyps of the large intestine. Virchows Arch 2010;457(4):443–9.

38. Gibson JA, Hahn HP, Shahsafaei A, et al. MUC expression in hyperplastic and serrated colonic polyps: lack of specificity of MUC6. Am J Surg Pathol 2011;35(5):742–9.

39. Huang CC, Frankel WL, Doukides T, et al. Prolapse-related changes are a confounding factor in misdiagnosis of sessile serrated adenomas in the rectum. Hum Pathol 2013;44(4):480–6.

40. Bellizzi AM, Frankel WL. Colorectal cancer due to deficiency in DNA mismatch repair function: a review. Adv Anat Pathol 2009;16(6):405–17.

41. Jenkins MA, Hayashi S, O'Shea AM, et al. Pathology features in Bethesda guidelines predict colorectal cancer microsatellite instability: a population-based study. Gastroenterology 2007;133(1):48–56.

42. Greenson JK, Huang SC, Herron C, et al. Pathologic predictors of microsatellite instability in colorectal cancer. Am J Surg Pathol 2009;33(1): 126–33.

43. Hyde A, Fontaine D, Stuckless S, et al. A histology-based model for predicting microsatellite instability in colorectal cancers. Am J Surg Pathol 2010; 34(12):1820–9.

44. Evaluation of Genomic Applications in Practice and Prevention (EGAPP) Working Group. Recommendations from the EGAPP Working Group: genetic testing strategies in newly diagnosed individuals with colorectal cancer aimed at reducing morbidity and mortality from Lynch syndrome in relatives. Genet Med 2009;11(1):35–41.

45. Funkhouser WK Jr, Lubin IM, Monzon FA, et al. Relevance, pathogenesis, and testing algorithm for mismatch repair-defective colorectal carcinomas: a report of the association for molecular pathology. J Mol Diagn 2012;14(2):91–103.

46. Sheridan TB, Fenton H, Lewin MR, et al. Sessile serrated adenomas with low- and high-grade dysplasia and early carcinomas: an immunohistochemical study of serrated lesions "caught in the act". Am J Clin Pathol 2006;126(4):564–71.

47. Shia J, Stadler Z, Weiser MR, et al. Immunohistochemical staining for DNA mismatch repair proteins in intestinal tract carcinoma: how reliable are biopsy samples? Am J Surg Pathol 2011;35(3): 447–54.

48. Capper D, Voigt A, Bozukova G, et al. BRAF V600E-specific immunohistochemistry for the exclusion of Lynch syndrome in MSI-H colorectal cancer. Int J Cancer 2013;133(7):1624–30.

49. Affolter K, Samowitz W, Tripp S, et al. BRAF V600E mutation detection by immunohistochemistry in colorectal carcinoma. Genes Chromosomes Cancer 2013;52(8):748–52.

50. Sinicrope FA, Smyrk TC, Tougeron D, et al. Mutation-specific antibody detects mutant BRAF protein expression in human colon carcinomas. Cancer 2013;119(15):2765–70.

51. Adackapara CA, Sholl LM, Barletta JA, et al. Immunohistochemistry using a BRAF V600E mutation-specific monoclonal antibody is not a useful surrogate for genotyping in colorectal adenocarcinoma. Histopathology 2013;63(2):187–93.

52. Kuan SF, Pai RK, Navina S, et al. Assessment of BRAF V600E mutation-specific antibody (VE1) in colorectal cancers. Mod Pathol 2013;26(Suppl 2): 161A.

53. Koperek O, Kornauth C, Capper D, et al. Immunohistochemical detection of the BRAF V600E-mutated protein in papillary thyroid carcinoma. Am J Surg Pathol 2012;36(6):844–50.

54. Long GV, Wilmott JS, Capper D, et al. Immunohistochemistry is highly sensitive and specific for the detection of V600E BRAF mutation in melanoma. Am J Surg Pathol 2013;37(1):61–5.

55. Zucman-Rossi J, Jeannot E, Nhieu JT, et al. Geno-type-phenotype correlation in hepatocellular ade-noma: new classification and relationship with HCC. Hepatology 2006;43(3):515–24.

56. Kong CS, Appenzeller M, Ferrell LD. Utility of CD34 reactivity in evaluating focal nodular hepatocellular lesions sampled by fine needle aspiration biopsy. Acta Cytol 2000;44(2):218–22.

57. Yamauchi N, Watanabe A, Hishinuma M, et al. The glypican 3 oncofetal protein is a promising diag-nostic marker for hepatocellular carcinoma. Mod Pathol 2005;18(12):1591–8.

58. Wang XY, Degos F, Dubois S, et al. Glypican-3 expression in hepatocellular tumors: diagnostic value for preneoplastic lesions and hepatocellular carcinomas. Hum Pathol 2006;37(11):1435–41.

59. Shafizadeh N, Ferrell LD, Kakar S. Utility and lim-itations of glypican-3 expression for the diagnosis of hepatocellular carcinoma at both ends of the differentiation spectrum. Mod Pathol 2008;21(8):1011–8.

60. Wang HL, Anatelli F, Zhai QJ, et al. Glypican-3 as a useful diagnostic marker that distinguishes hepatocellular carcinoma from benign hepatocellular mass lesions. Arch Pathol Lab Med 2008;132(11):1723–8.

61. Tremosini S, Forner A, Boix L, et al. Prospective validation of an immunohistochemical panel (glypi-can 3, heat shock protein 70 and glutamine synthe-tase) in liver biopsies for diagnosis of very early hepatocellular carcinoma. Gut 2012;61(10):1481–7.

62. Bioulac-Sage P, Cubel G, Taouji S, et al. Immuno-histochemical markers on needle biopsies are helpful for the diagnosis of focal nodular hyperpla-sia and hepatocellular adenoma subtypes. Am J Surg Pathol 2012;36(11):1691–9.

63. Rebouissou S, Couchy G, Libbrecht L, et al. The beta-catenin pathway is activated in focal nodular hyperplasia but not in cirrhotic FNH-like nodules. J Hepatol 2008;49(1):61–71.

64. Abdul-Al HM, Makhlouf HR, Wang G, et al. Glypi-can-3 expression in benign liver tissue with active hepatitis C: implications for the diagnosis of hepatocellular carcinoma. Hum Pathol 2008;39(2):209–12.

65. Lagana SM, Moreira RK, Remotti HE, et al. Gluta-mine synthetase, heat shock protein-70, and glypican-3 in intrahepatic cholangiocarcinoma and tumors metastatic to liver. Appl Immunohisto-chem Mol Morphol 2013;21(3):254–7.

66. Kakar S, Gown AM, Goodman ZD, et al. Best practices in diagnostic immunohistochemistry: hepatocellular carcinoma versus metastatic neo-plasms. Arch Pathol Lab Med 2007;131(11):1648–54.

67. Lau SK, Prakash S, Geller SA, et al. Comparative immunohistochemical profile of hepatocellular carcinoma, cholangiocarcinoma, and metastatic adenocarcinoma. Hum Pathol 2002;33(12):1175–81.

68. Sheahan K, O'Brien MJ, Burke B, et al. Differential reactivities of carcinoembryonic antigen (CEA) and CEA-related monoclonal and polyclonal anti-bodies in common epithelial malignancies. Am J Clin Pathol 1990;94(2):157–64.

69. Butler SL, Dong H, Cardona D, et al. The antigen for Hep Par 1 antibody is the urea cycle enzyme carbamoyl phosphate synthetase 1. Lab Invest 2008;88(1):78–88.

70. Fan Z, van de Rijn M, Montgomery K, et al. Hep par 1 antibody stain for the differential diagnosis of hepatocellular carcinoma: 676 tumors tested using tissue microarrays and conventional tissue sec-tions. Mod Pathol 2003;16(2):137–44.

71. Lugli A, Tornillo L, Mirlacher M, et al. Hepatocyte paraffin 1 expression in human normal and neoplastic tissues: tissue microarray analysis on 3,940 tissue samples. Am J Clin Pathol 2004;122(5):721–7.

72. Baumhoer D, Tornillo L, Stadlmann S, et al. Glypi-can 3 expression in human nonneoplastic, preneo-plastic, and neoplastic tissues: a tissue microarray analysis of 4,387 tissue samples. Am J Clin Pathol 2008;129(6):899–906.

73. Mounajjed T, Zhang L, Wu TT. Glypican-3 expres-sion in gastrointestinal and pancreatic epithelial neoplasms. Hum Pathol 2013;44(4):542–50.

74. Yan BC, Gong C, Song J, et al. Arginase-1: a new immunohistochemical marker of hepatocytes and hepatocellular neoplasms. Am J Surg Pathol 2010;34(8):1147–54.

75. Abraham SC, Klimstra DS, Wilentz RE, et al. Solid-pseudopapillary tumors of the pancreas are genetically distinct from pancreatic ductal adenocarcinomas and almost always harbor beta-catenin mutations. Am J Pathol 2002;160(4):1361–9.

76. La Rosa S, Adsay V, Albarello L, et al. Clinicopath-ologic study of 62 acinar cell carcinomas of the pancreas: insights into the morphology and immu-nophenotype and search for prognostic markers. Am J Surg Pathol 2012;36(12):1782–95.

77. Tanaka Y, Kato K, Notohara K, et al. Significance of aberrant (cytoplasmic/nuclear) expression of beta-catenin in pancreatoblastoma. J Pathol 2003;199(2):185–90.

78. Chetty R, Serra S. Membrane loss and aberrant nu-clear localization of E-cadherin are consistent fea-tures of solid pseudopapillary tumour of the pancreas. An immunohistochemical study using two antibodies recognizing different domains of the E-cadherin molecule. Histopathology 2008;52(3):325–30.

79. Yao JC, Hassan M, Phan A, et al. One hundred years after "carcinoid": epidemiology of and

prognostic factors for neuroendocrine tumors in 35,825 cases in the United States. J Clin Oncol 2008;26(18):3063–72.

80. Savelli G, Lucignani G, Seregni E, et al. Feasibility of somatostatin receptor scintigraphy in the detection of occult primary gastro-entero-pancreatic (GEP) neuroendocrine tumours. Nucl Med Commun 2004;25(5):445–9.

81. Lorenzo PI, Jimenez Moreno CM, Delgado I, et al. Immunohistochemical assessment of Pax8 expression during pancreatic islet development and in human neuroendocrine tumors. Histochem Cell Biol 2011;136(5):595–607.

82. Graham RP, Shrestha B, Caron BL, et al. Islet-1 is a sensitive but not entirely specific marker for pancreatic neuroendocrine neoplasms and their metastases. Am J Surg Pathol 2013;37(3):399–405.

83. Chan ES, Alexander J, Swanson PE, et al. PDX-1, CDX-2, TTF-1, and CK7: a reliable immunohistochemical panel for pancreatic neuroendocrine neoplasms. Am J Surg Pathol 2012;36(5):737–43.

84. Srivastava A, Hornick JL. Immunohistochemical staining for CDX-2, PDX-1, NESP-55, and TTF-1 can help distinguish gastrointestinal carcinoid tumors from pancreatic endocrine and pulmonary carcinoid tumors. Am J Surg Pathol 2009;33(4):626–32.

85. Lugli A, Tzankov A, Zlobec I, et al. Differential diagnostic and functional role of the multi-marker phenotype CDX2/CK20/CK7 in colorectal cancer stratified by mismatch repair status. Mod Pathol 2008;21(11):1403–12.

86. Winn B, Tavares R, Fanion J, et al. Differentiating the undifferentiated: immunohistochemical profile of medullary carcinoma of the colon with an emphasis on intestinal differentiation. Hum Pathol 2009;40(3):398–404.

87. Saad RS, Silverman JF, Khalifa MA, et al. CDX2, cytokeratins 7 and 20 immunoreactivity in rectal adenocarcinoma. Appl Immunohistochem Mol Morphol 2009;17(3):196–201.

88. Logani S, Oliva E, Arnell PM, et al. Use of novel immunohistochemical markers expressed in colonic adenocarcinoma to distinguish primary ovarian tumors from metastatic colorectal carcinoma. Mod Pathol 2005;18(1):19–25.

89. Wang HL, Lu DW, Yerian LM, et al. Immunohistochemical distinction between primary adenocarcinoma of the bladder and secondary colorectal adenocarcinoma. Am J Surg Pathol 2001;25(11):1380–7.

90. Suh N, Yang XJ, Tretiakova MS, et al. Value of CDX2, villin, and alpha-methylacyl coenzyme A racemase immunostains in the distinction between primary adenocarcinoma of the bladder and secondary colorectal adenocarcinoma. Mod Pathol 2005;18(9):1217–22.

91. Vang R, Gown AM, Barry TS, et al. Cytokeratins 7 and 20 in primary and secondary mucinous tumors of the ovary: analysis of coordinate immunohistochemical expression profiles and staining distribution in 179 cases. Am J Surg Pathol 2006;30(9):1130–9.

92. Nonaka D, Kusamura S, Baratti D, et al. CDX-2 expression in pseudomyxoma peritonei: a clinicopathological study of 42 cases. Histopathology 2006;49(4):381–7.

93. Yemelyanova AV, Vang R, Judson K, et al. Distinction of primary and metastatic mucinous tumors involving the ovary: analysis of size and laterality data by primary site with reevaluation of an algorithm for tumor classification. Am J Surg Pathol 2008;32(1):128–38.

94. Goldstein NS, Bassi D. Cytokeratins 7, 17, and 20 reactivity in pancreatic and ampulla of vater adenocarcinomas. Percentage of positivity and distribution is affected by the cut-point threshold. Am J Clin Pathol 2001;115(5):695–702.

95. Chu PG, Schwarz RE, Lau SK, et al. Immunohistochemical staining in the diagnosis of pancreatobiliary and ampulla of Vater adenocarcinoma: application of CDX2, CK17, MUC1, and MUC2. Am J Surg Pathol 2005;29(3):359–67.

96. Ji H, Isacson C, Seidman JD, et al. Cytokeratins 7 and 20, Dpc4, and MUC5AC in the distinction of metastatic mucinous carcinomas in the ovary from primary ovarian mucinous tumors: Dpc4 assists in identifying metastatic pancreatic carcinomas. Int J Gynecol Pathol 2002;21(4):391–400.

97. Wang NP, Zee S, Zarbo RJ, et al. Coordinate expression of cytokeratins 7 and 20 defined unique subsets of carcinomas. Appl Immunohistochem 1995;3(2):99–107.

98. Chu P, Wu E, Weiss LM. Cytokeratin 7 and cytokeratin 20 expression in epithelial neoplasms: a survey of 435 cases. Mod Pathol 2000;13(9):962–72.

99. Taniere P, Borghi-Scoazec G, Saurin JC, et al. Cytokeratin expression in adenocarcinomas of the esophagogastric junction: a comparative study of adenocarcinomas of the distal esophagus and of the proximal stomach. Am J Surg Pathol 2002;26(9):1213–21.

100. Chen ZM, Wang HL. Alteration of cytokeratin 7 and cytokeratin 20 expression profile is uniquely associated with tumorigenesis of primary adenocarcinoma of the small intestine. Am J Surg Pathol 2004;28(10):1352–9.

101. Magnusson K, de Wit M, Brennan DJ, et al. SATB2 in combination with cytokeratin 20 identifies over 95% of all colorectal carcinomas. Am J Surg Pathol 2011;35(7):937–48.

Index

Note: Page numbers for article titles are in **boldface** type.

Surgical Pathology 6 (2013) 611–617
http://dx.doi.org/10.1016/S1875-9181(13)00077-9
1875-9181/13/$ – see front matter © 2013 Elsevier Inc. All rights reserved.

Moving?

Make sure your subscription moves with you!

To notify us of your new address, find your **Clinics Account Number** (located on your mailing label above your name), and contact customer service at:

Email: journalscustomerservice-usa@elsevier.com

800-654-2452 (subscribers in the U.S. & Canada)
314-447-8871 (subscribers outside of the U.S. & Canada)

Fax number: 314-447-8029

Elsevier Health Sciences Division
Subscription Customer Service
3251 Riverport Lane
Maryland Heights, MO 63043

*To ensure uninterrupted delivery of your subscription, please notify us at least 4 weeks in advance of move.